Veterinary Treatment of Llamas and Alpacas

2nd Edition

I would like to dedicate this book to all the veterinary surgeons who are mothers and have to juggle looking after their families with practicing veterinary surgery in all its many forms.

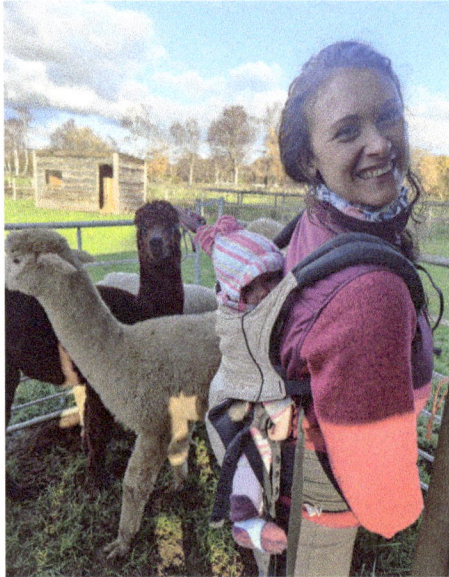

'Taking your daughter to work'.
Lissie Gercke - A mother of four who has completed the Royal College of Veterinary Surgeons Certificate in Camelid Medicine and Surgery which I was proud to write and develop.

Veterinary Treatment of Llamas and Alpacas

2nd Edition

Graham R. Duncanson

Blackthorn Lodge, Crostwick, Norwich, Norfolk NR12 7BG

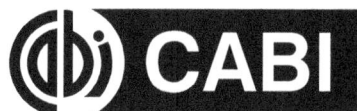

CABI

CABI is a trading name of CAB International

CABI
Nosworthy Way
Wallingford
Oxfordshire OX10 8DE
UK

CABI
200 Portland Street
Boston
MA 02114
USA

Tel: +44 (0)1491 832111
E-mail: info@cabi.org
Website: www.cabi.org

Tel: +1 (617)682-9015
E-mail: cabi-nao@cabi.org

A catalogue record for this book is available from the British Library, London, UK.

Library of Congress Cataloging-in-Publication Data

Names: Duncanson, Graham R., author.
Title: Veterinary treatment of llamas and alpacas / Graham R Duncanson.
Description: 2nd edition. | Wallingford, Oxfordshire ; Boston : CAB International, [2023] | Includes bibliographical references and index. | Summary: "This book provides practical veterinary advice for llamas and alpacas. The new edition covers husbandry, nutrition, examination, vaccines, analgesia, anaesthesia, dermatology and poisons, as well as expanding on zoonotic diseases coverage, biosecurity, handling, and advances in treatment options and surgical techniques"-- Provided by publisher.
Identifiers: LCCN 2023019013 (print) | LCCN 2023019014 (ebook) | ISBN 9781800623552 (hardback) | ISBN 9781800623569 (ebook) | ISBN 9781800623576 (epub)
Subjects: LCSH: Llamas--Diseases. | Alpaca--Diseases. | Llamas--Surgery. | Alpaca--Surgery.
Classification: LCC SF997.5.C3 D86 2023 (print) | LCC SF997.5.C3 (ebook) | DDC 636.2/966--dc23/eng/20230627
LC record available at https://lccn.loc.gov/2023019013
LC ebook record available at https://lccn.loc.gov/2023019014

ISBN-13: 9781800623552 (hardback)
          9781800623569 (ePDF)
          9781800623576 (ePub)

DOI: 10.1079/9781800623576.0000

Commissioning Editor: Alexandra Lainsbury
Editorial Assistant: Lauren Davies
Production Editor: Rosie Hayden

Typeset by Straive, Pondicherry, India

Contents

Foreword

The New World camelids are a collective group inclusive of llamas, alpacas, guanacos and vicunas, all originating in Central America and forming the Camelidae family. I am delighted to be writing the foreword for the second edition of this book, demonstrating our need to keep our veterinary knowledge up to date with the growing popularity of camelids in the UK. While guanacos and vicunas are still scarce in the UK, alpacas and llamas are becoming increasingly popular whether as pets, show animals or farmed for their sought-after fleeces. This unusual book should give the reader the confidence to take on any camelid-related case.

Camelids are of increasing interest not only as farmed or companion animals but because of their unique contribution to science. After an accidental discovery in the 1980s, it became known that members of the camelid family produce a special class of antibody, known as a nanobody. This has allowed scientists to study previously inaccessible body proteins and understand how those proteins malfunction in disease. Structural biologists can select a nanobody to lock in place their protein of interest. This secure bond allows the protein's atomic structure to be tested, allowing more precise drug development than previously with antibodies. Virologists have discovered these nanobodies have the potential to form better receptor bonds with human cells than current HIV vaccines, stimulating further interest into these specialist cells.

While having an extraordinary immune system, camelids too are vulnerable to infectious and non-infectious diseases, which we need to be prepared to diagnose and treat. The zoonotic potential of tuberculosis has become a growing concern in this family of animals, meaning owners and veterinary surgeons need to be armed with the knowledge necessary to recommend precautions for the herd as well as address the individual.

My father can't help but demonstrate his persistent enthusiasm for life which is again captured in this book making it an invigorating read. I continue to admire my dad's dogged commitment to professional development and support of the veterinary community. I hope I have the energy to do half as good a job!

Amelia Shanklin MRCVS

Acknowledgements

———————————

I would like to thank two camelid associations, The British Llama Society (BLS) and the British Camelids Ltd (BCL), for their permission to include their information sheets and forms for agreement of owners.

I am very grateful to my veterinary friend and colleague Bob Broadbent MRCVS for his input on tuberculosis in camelids.

Glossary

Abortion: the premature birth of young.

Annual: a plant that grows from seed, flowers and dies within a year.

Anthelmintics: drugs that expel parasitic worms from the body, generally by paralysing or starving them.

Antigen: a molecule or part of a molecule that is recognised by components of the host immune system.

Awn: a bristle or hair-like appendage to a fruit or to a glume, as in barley and some other grasses.

Bacteraemia: bacteria in the blood.

Biennial: a plant that flowers and dies in the second year after growing from a seed.

Bradycardia: decrease in heart rate.

Bruxism: grinding of teeth.

Calculi: stones formed in the urinary system.

Cerebral: relating to the cerebrum, the largest part of the brain.

Cestodes: parasitic flatworms, commonly called tapeworms, which usually live in the digestive tract of vertebrates as adults and in bodies of various intermediate hosts as juvenile stages.

Colitis: inflammation of the colon, often used to describe an inflammation of the large intestine.

Coma: profound unconsciousness from which the patient cannot be roused.

Congestion: the presence of an abnormal amount of blood in an organ or part.

Contusions: severe bruises.

Convulsion: a violent involuntary contraction of muscles.

Corm: underground bulbous root.

Cria: a young SAC in its first year.

Cryptorchid: rig.

Cystitis: inflammation of the bladder.

Deciduous plants: those that shed all their leaves annually.

Detoxicate: to render a poison harmless.

Distension: the filling of a hollow organ to more than its usual capacity.

Diuresis: excessive urination.

DNA fingerprinting: much like the fingerprint used in human identification, but done with unique DNA characters for each individual animal. Utilizes PCR to replicate small samples.

Drenching: giving an anthelmintic dose by mouth.

Dysentery: an illness characterized by diarrhoea with blood in the faeces.

Dysphagia: difficulty in swallowing.

Dysphonia: hoarseness heard when vocalizing.

Dyspnoea: difficulty in breathing.

Dystocia: difficulty at parturition.

Egg reappearance period: the time taken (usually expressed in weeks) for eggs to reappear in faeces after anthelmintic treatment. Usually this is described for drug-sensitive worm populations at the time of product licensing.

ELISA (enzyme-linked immunosorbent assay): a technique used primarily in immunology to detect the presence of an antibody or an antigen in a sample. Basically, an unknown amount of antigen is bound to the surface of a plastic well, then a specific antibody is added and if specific will bind the antigen. This antibody is linked to an enzyme or is detected by incubation with a second antibody that is linked to an enzyme. In the final step a substance is added that the enzyme can convert to some detectable signal (usually a colour change that is detectable by a spectrophotometer).

Emaciation: excessive body wasting.

Emesis: vomiting.

Emetic: a substance that causes vomiting.

Emphysema: air or gas in the interstices of a tissue.

Enema: rectal injection.

Epidemiology: the study of factors affecting the health of populations and often how diseases are transmitted.

FECRT (faecal egg count reduction test): a test that measures the effect on faecal egg output of anthelmintic treatment. Generally, efficacy is assessed by comparing FECs obtained on the day of treatment with those obtained 14 days after treatment. This is an important tool in detecting anthelmintic resistance in the field.

Gelding: castrated SAC.

Gene mapping: the gene on a given chromosome.

Genome: an organism's entire hereditary information, encoded either in DNA or, for some types of virus, in RNA. The genome includes the genes that code the proteins and non-coding sequences of the DNA.

Genotype: The inherited instructions organisms carry in their genetic code.

Granules: small grains.

Gravid: the pregnant horn of a uterus.

Haematuria: blood in the urine.

Haemoglobinuria: haemoglobin in the urine.

Haemolytic: a substance that causes breakdown of red blood corpuscles.

Helminths: a group of eukaryotic parasites that live inside their host. They are worm-like and live and feed off animals.

Hembra: female SAC.

Hepatitis: inflammation of the liver.

Herbaceous perennials: plants in which the greater part dies after flowering, leaving only the rootstock to produce next year's growth.

Herd: the collective word for a group of SACs.

Iatrogenic: resulting from treatment.

Ileus: failure of peristalsis.

In cria: pregnant SAC.

In vitro: in the test tube.

In vivo: in the living body.

Jaundice: a disease in which bile pigments stain the mucous membranes.

Larvae: juvenile forms that many animals undergo before they mature to an adult stage. Larvae are frequently adapted to environments different to those adult stages live in.

Leucocytosis: increase in WBC in the blood.

Leucopenia: decrease in WBC in the blood.

Linear leaves: those that are long and narrow.

Lumen: the inner space of a tubular structure, such as the intestine.

Macho: entire male SAC.

Markers: a short tandem repeat (STR) that may be used to aid in the identification of a trait.

Melena: dark tarry faeces indicating bleeding high in the intestinal tract.

Metritis: inflammation of the uterus.

Myiasis: fly strike.

Nematodes: roundworms, one of the most diverse phyla of all animals.

Nodule: a small round lump.

Paracentesis: the technique of puncturing a body cavity.

Pathogenicity: the ability of a pathogen to produce signs of disease in an organism.

Pathognomic: a single specific sign of a disease.

Phenotype: any observable characteristic or trait of an organism, such as its morphology, development, biochemical or physiological properties, or behaviour. Phenotypes result from the expression of an organism's genes as well as the influence of environmental factors and possible interactions between the two.

Polydactyly: having an extra limb.

Polydipsia: drinking excessive amounts of water.

Polymerase chain reaction (PCR): a technique to amplify a single or a few copies of a piece of DNA by several orders of magnitude generating thousands to millions of copies of a particular sequence. Polymerase chain reaction relies on cycles of repeated heating and cooling of DNA melting and enzymatic replication of DNA. Primers (short DNA fragments) containing sequences complementary to the target region along with a DNA polymerase (after which the method is named) are key components to enable selective and repeated amplification. As PCR progresses, DNA generated is used as a template for replication, setting in motion a chain reaction in which the template is exponentially amplified.

Polyphagia: eating an excessive amount.

Premix: medicine available in a concentrated form to be added to food.

Primer: several thousand copies of short sequences of DNA that are complementary to part of the DNA to be sequenced.

Ptyalism: excess saliva production.

Purgative: a strong laxative.

Pyrexia: raised rectal temperature.

Recumbency: unable to get up.

Rhinitis: inflammation of the structures in the nose.

Rig: a male in which one or both testicles have not descended into the scrotum.

Rostral: towards the nose.

Rye grass: a commonly grown grass *Lolium perenne*.

Schistosomus reflexus: a deformity of a fetus in which the spine is bent backwards.

Septicaemia: pathogenic bacteria in the blood.

Short tandem reprints (STR): sections of DNA arranged in back to back repetition.

Slough: dead tissue that drops away from living tissue.

Spasm: involuntary contraction of a muscle.

Staggers: an erratic gait.

Stomatitis: inflammation of the mouth and gums.

Stricture: a narrowing of a tubular organ.

Subclinical: when the symptoms are not evident.

Syndrome: a group of symptoms.

Tachycardia: increased heart rate.

Tachypnoea: increased respiratory rate.

Tenesmus: straining to pass urine or faeces.

Teratoma: a developmental embryological deformity.

Tourniquet: an appliance for temporary stoppage of the circulation in a limb.
Tympanic: distended with gas.
Ubiquitous: everywhere.
Udder: mammary gland.
Ureter: the tube connecting the kidney to the bladder.
Urethra: the tube leading from the bladder to outside.
Urethritis: inflammation of the urethra.
Urine scald: inflammation of the skin caused by persistent wetting with urine.
Urolithiasis: the formation of stones in the urinary system.
Vagus: tenth cranial nerve.
Vesicle: a collection of fluid in the surface layers of the skin or of a mucous membrane.
Viraemia: virus particles in the blood.
Volatile: a substance that evaporates rapidly.
Wether: a castrated SAC.
Zoonoses: diseases communicable between animals and man.

Abbreviations

AGIDT	Agar gel immunodiffusion test
AI	Artificial insemination
AST	Aspartate aminotransferase
BAL	Broncoalveolar lavage
BAS	British Alpaca Society
BHB	Beta-hydroxybutyrate
BLS	British Llama Society
BTV	Blue tongue virus
BVD	Bovine virus diarrhoea C Celsius
C1/C2/C3	First, second and third compartments of the stomach
CCN	Cerebro-cortico-necrosis
CL	Corpeus luteum
CLA	Caseous lymphadenitis
cm	Centimetre
CNS	Central nervous system
CRT	Coproantigen reduction test
CSF	Cerebrospinal fluid
CT	Controlled test
cu	Cubic
Cu	Copper
DIC	Disseminated intravascular coagulopathy
DM	Dry matter
DMSO	Dimethyl sulfoxide
DNA	Deoxyribonucleic acid
EDTA	Ethylene diamine tetra-acetic acid
EHA	Egg hatch assay
EHV	Equine herpes virus
ELISA	Enzyme linked immunosorbent assay
EPG	Eggs per gram
EU	European Union
F	Fahrenheit
FAO	Food and Agriculture Organization
FAT	Fluorescent antibody test

FEC	Faecal worm egg count
FECRT	Faecal egg count reduction test
FMD	Foot and mouth disease
FPT	Failure of passive transfer
g	Gram
GGT	Gamma glutamyltransferase
GI	Gastrointestinal
GLDH	Glutamate dehydrogenase
GnRH	Gonadotropin-releasing hormone
Hb	Haemoglobin
HCN	Hydrogen cyanide
IgE	Immunoglobulin E
IgG	Immunoglobulin G
im	Intramuscularly
ip	Intraperitoneally
IU	International units
iv	Intravenously
kg	Kilogram
l	Litre
LDT	Larval development test
LH	Luteinizing hormone
MAP	*Mycobacterium avium* subspecies *paratuberculosis*
MAPIA	Multi-antigen print immunosorbent assay
MCF	Malignant catarrhal fever
MCH	Mean corpuscular haemoglobin
MCHC	Mean corpuscular haemoglobin concentration
MCV	Mean corpuscular volume
mg	Milligram
min	Minute
ml	Millilitre
MRCT	Malignant round cell tumours
NEFA	Non-esterified fatty acids
NSAID	Non-steroid anti-inflammatory
Ov-VH2	Ovine herpes type 2 virus
PCR	Polymerase chain reaction
PCV	Packed cell volume
PELF	Pulmonary epithelial lining fluid
PG	Prostaglandin
pH	Negative logarithm of hydrogen ion activity
PI	Persistently infective
PLR	Papillary light reflex
PMN	Polymorphic nuclear cell
pp.	Pages
ppm	Part(s) per million
PPR	Peste des petits ruminants
PRA	Progressive retinal atrophy
PUBH	Polymerized ultrapurified bovine haemoglobin
RBC	Red blood cell
RNA	Ribonucleic acid
rpm	Revolutions per minute
RVF	Rift Valley fever

SAC	South American camelid
sc	Subcutaneously
sid	Once a day
SNT	Serum neutralization test
spp.	Species
ssp.	Subspecies
TAT	Tetanus antitoxin
TB	Tuberculosis
TBC	Total blood count
TCBZ	Triclabendazole
TDN	Total digestible nutrients
tid	Three times daily
TMS	Trimethoprim-sulfadoxine
UK	United Kingdom
USA	United States of America
v	Volume
VMD	Veterinary Medicine Directorate
VNT	Virus neutralization test
w	Weight
WBC	White blood cell
ZN	Ziehl-Neelsen

1

Animal Husbandry

Introduction

South American camelids (SACs) were a vital part of life in the Andes in the days of the Incas before the arrival of the Spanish Conquistadors. Cattle, sheep and goats took over in the following centuries but now SACs are making a very strong resurgence. The area of greatest rearing of SACs is on the Andean Cordillera in southern Peru, central Bolivia and northern Chile. There are significant populations of SACs in Argentina, Australia, New Zealand, USA, Canada and the UK. Numbers are rising on mainland Europe, particularly in Sweden and Eire.

Evolution

Camelid evolution is traced back to North America 40 million years ago. There were probably several genera. Many became extinct but some crossed the land bridge, which at that stage was across the Bering Strait so North America was linked with Asia. The camelids that evolved in Asia to become the camels we know today are outside the remit of this book. The camelids in North America migrated to South America or died out, leaving the SACs we know today. These are mainly domestic or semi-wild. It is not known whether the wild SACs are feral or whether they are truly wild. Most camels in the old world and Australia are actually feral. The only exceptions are the wild camels of the Gobi Desert found in China and Mongolia. Sadly there are only 600 remaining. Both camels and SACs have the same number of chromosomes and if cross-fertilized can produce fertile young. Obviously, their variation in size prevents natural mating.

SACs evolved from a common ancestor approximately 2 million years ago. There is evidence of domestication 6000 years ago in the central Peruvian Andes at altitudes of over 4000 m. This plateau-type high altitude grassland has extreme variations of daily temperatures. Frosts are frequent as are high winds. The area is extremely dry with very limited rainfall.

Numbers

In 2010 it was estimated that there were 36,000 SACs in the UK. Of these 31,000 were thought to be alpacas and 5000 to be llamas with just a few hundred farmed guanacos and a very small number of vicunas in zoos or private collections. Thirteen years later the numbers have risen to a total of more than 50,000 alpacas and 8000 llamas in the UK. In 2023 there are more than 175,000 SACs in Australia. These all stem from a herd of 250 that was brought into Australia in 1858. In the USA there are over 400,000 SACs

© Graham R. Duncanson 2023. *Veterinary Treatment of Llamas and Alpacas,* 2nd Edition
(G.R. Duncanson)
DOI: 10.1079/9781800623576.0001

after an initial import in 1984. These numbers are very small compared to the 4 million in South America.

Classification

The normal classification is into four types, llama, alpaca, guanaco and vicuna. To be exact the first three are placed in the same genus, *Lama*, making the species *L. glama*, *L. pacos* and *L. guanicoe*. Vicuna are placed in a separate genus, *Vicugna*. This genus is divided into two subspecies, *V. vicugna mensalis* from Peru and *V. vicugna vicugna* from Argentina. They are all classified in the Lamini tribe, which is part of the Camelidae family. SACs are grouped with camels, both the dromedary and the bactrian, in the suborder Tylopoda. Tylopoda and the suborders Cetruminantia, which includes cattle, sheep, goats, water buffalo, giraffe, deer, antelope and bison, and Suinia, which includes pigs and peccaries, make up the order Artiodactyla.

Tylopoda has some important differences from ruminants of the suborder Cetruminantia. Ruminants have red blood cells (RBCs), which are round and 10 microns in diameter. SACs have elliptical RBCs, which are only 6.5 microns in diameter. Ruminants have feet that have hooves, consisting of a horn wall and sole. SACs have toenails and a soft pad. Their second and third phalanges are horizontal, whereas in ruminants the second and third phalanges are nearly vertical.

Both ruminants and tylopods are foregut fermenters, with regurgitation, rechewing and reswallowing. However, tylopods have only three stomach compartments and are resistant to bloat. Ruminants have four stomach compartments and suffer from bloat.

The teeth in SACs cause real confusion whereas in ruminants they are straightforward. Ruminants have no upper incisors or upper canines. On their lower hemi-mandible, they have three incisors and a canine. This canine has migrated rostrally and resembles an incisor. They therefore appear to have four lower incisors. SACs have on their upper hemi-maxilla one canine and one upper incisor, which have migrated caudally and resemble a canine. So, they appear to have two upper canines on each

side. SACs on their hemi-mandible have three incisors and one canine. There are also differences with the cheek teeth. Ruminants have three upper and lower premolars on each side. SACs have one and maybe a second, upper and lower premolar on each side. Both SACs and ruminants have three upper and lower molars on each side.

It is perhaps in the reproductive system where ruminants are at variance the most from SACs. Ruminants have an oestrus cycle, with spontaneous ovulation and no follicular wave cycle. SACs do not have an oestrus cycle and are induced ovulators. They have a follicular wave cycle. Ruminants copulate in the standing position with short and intense ejaculation. SACs copulate in the prone position and have prolonged ejaculation. The male SAC has a cartilaginous projection on the tip of his penis. This is absent in ruminants. SACs have a diffuse placenta, and the fetus is surrounded by an epidermal membrane. Ruminant fetuses do not have such a membrane but have placental cotyledons.

SACs are primarily nasal breathers with an elongated soft palate. Mouth breathing in SACs is an extremely serious sign. Ruminants have a short soft palate and can breathe nasally or orally.

SAC's kidneys are smooth and elliptical. Some ruminants have smooth kidneys, e.g. the sheep, and some have lobed kidneys, e.g. the ox. Female SACs have a sub-urethral diverticulum at the external urethral orifice. Ruminants have no such diverticulum.

There has been less research carried out on parasites occurring in or on SACs than in or on ruminants. However, this is being rapidly rectified as knowledge is constantly being accrued. SACs have unique internal parasites and protozoa as well as sharing other species of parasite with cattle, sheep and goats. The picture with external parasites is confusing. SACs certainly have unique lice. They may also have unique mange mites, but the classification is not yet confirmed.

The author takes issue with camelid owners and veterinary surgeons who maintain that SACs are minimally susceptible to many infectious diseases. The author does not think this is an exact assessment of the situation. SACs were believed to have some resistance to bovine tuberculosis. The situation in the UK in 2023 makes nonsense of this statement where numbers of infected camelid herds are rising monthly. SACs have also been found to be susceptible to human tuberculosis, and they have been found to be a source of infection of bovine and human tuberculosis to humans. SACs are a definite zoonotic danger. Owing to a high-profile single importation of an alpaca from New Zealand, which after arrival had dubious testing results and was subsequently slaughtered, the testing of SACs is in complete disarray.

The author does agree that there is no evidence of bovine brucellosis in SACs; however, SACs are definitely susceptible to foot-and-mouth disease (FMD) and blue tongue virus (BTV). Further examples will be given in Chapter 17.

There are two lines of alpaca, depending on their fleece types. The more common huacaya has an even fine fleece and the less common suri has a fine crimped fleece. In the USA huacaya outnumber suri by nine to one. They may be bred together freely but the results may not be as predictable as desired. For example: a total of 1980 suri × suri matings produced 278 huacaya and 1702 suri offspring; 145 suri × huacaya matings produced 89 huacaya and 56 suri offspring; 19,637 hyacaya × hyacaya matings produced 19,633 huacaya and 4 suri offspring (Sponenberg, 2010). No linkage or other influence of sex was noticed. These results are consistent with a single autosomal dominant gene controlling suri fleece production, with an additional relatively common genetic mechanism that can suppress the suri phenotype in some animals. These results are especially important in cases where the two fleece types are crossed with one another, as they result in a relative underproduction of suri fleeces.

Colours

There are 22 colours recognized for alpacas, ranging from black to white. Some also produce multicoloured fleeces. In fact alpacas can come in a very wide variety of colours. The main colours, though, are brown, black, white, palomino and grey. In the USA the Alpaca Owners and Breeders Association will allow only one or more of 16 standard colours to be registered. The official colours are:

- White;
- Beige;
- Light Fawn;
- Medium Fawn;
- Dark Fawn;
- Light Brown;
- Medium Brown;
- Dark Brown;
- Bay Black;
- True Black;
- Light Silver Grey;
- Medium Silver Grey;
- Dark Silver Grey;
- Light Rose Grey;
- Medium Rose Grey; and
- Dark Rose Grey.

There can also be patterns of several colours.

Llamas are the same, with pinto and appaloosa also being recognized. Guanacos are reddish brown in colour with an under-colouring of white. They often have black marks on the top of their noses and heads. Vicuna are basically a yellowish light brown. There are various bib markings of white.

Terminology

A female SAC is called a hembra and a male a macho. Castrated males are called geldings or wethers. Young animals are called crias.

Fibre

The first SAC fibre known to be imported into the UK was in 1834. Sir Titus Salt found some bales used as ship's ballast on the docks in Liverpool. Being a wool merchant he realized its potential. Importation increased during the next 50 years, particularly after Queen Victoria was given some garments. At the same time in Australia Sir Charles Ledger imported a herd of 250 SACs.

Behaviour and Behaviour Problems

Introduction

The single dominant male controls the family group (Fig. 1.1). He decides its size and its territory and he spends most of his time patrolling and protecting the group. It is because of this trait that male llamas have been used with sheep flocks to protect young lambs from foxes (Fig. 1.2). His period of dominance only lasts until he is deposed by another male. Under him there is a strong hierarchy, with the oldest female in top position with the other females ranking below her. Crias tend to have the rank of their mothers so young weaned animals tend to be at the bottom of the pecking order.

In the wild a group will consist of one male with up to 20 females and their babies. The adolescents are driven away. Young females soon go to join another male's family group. The young males and the deposed males tend to live in large groups of up to 200.

In the wild, groups stay well away from each other and travel great distances (Fig. 1.3). SACs are very aware of their limitations so that they will drive off small predators but run away from large predators or packs of smaller predators. They depend on body language for communication. In the wild the normal age at death is 12, but under domestication they may well live on into their early twenties. There are no toxic plants on the altiplano and so SACs are very sensitive to poisoning.

SACs even in the wild tend to defecate in a pile. This is used by the male to smell for strangers and for receptive females. It is also useful as it is a natural way to reduce intestinal parasites. Overcrowding should be avoided at all costs because all types of disease will flourish. Disease control,

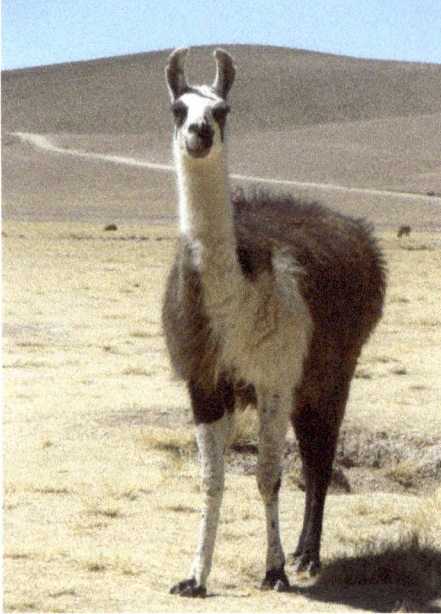

Fig. 1.1. A dominant male on the altiplano.

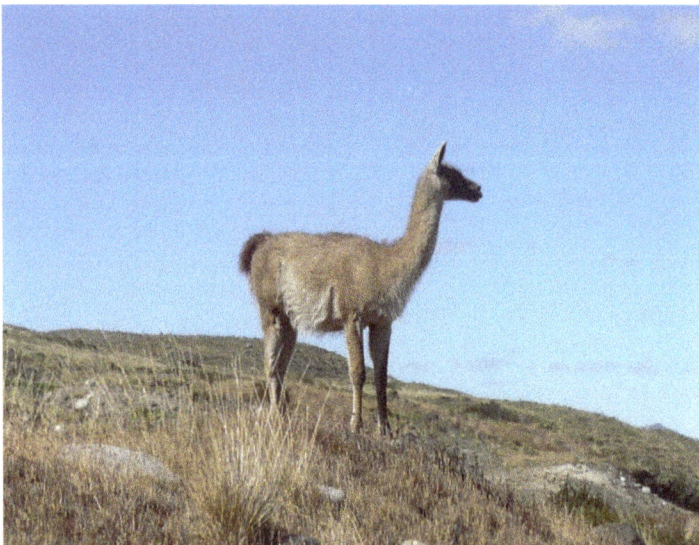

Fig 1.2. A single animal stands guard.

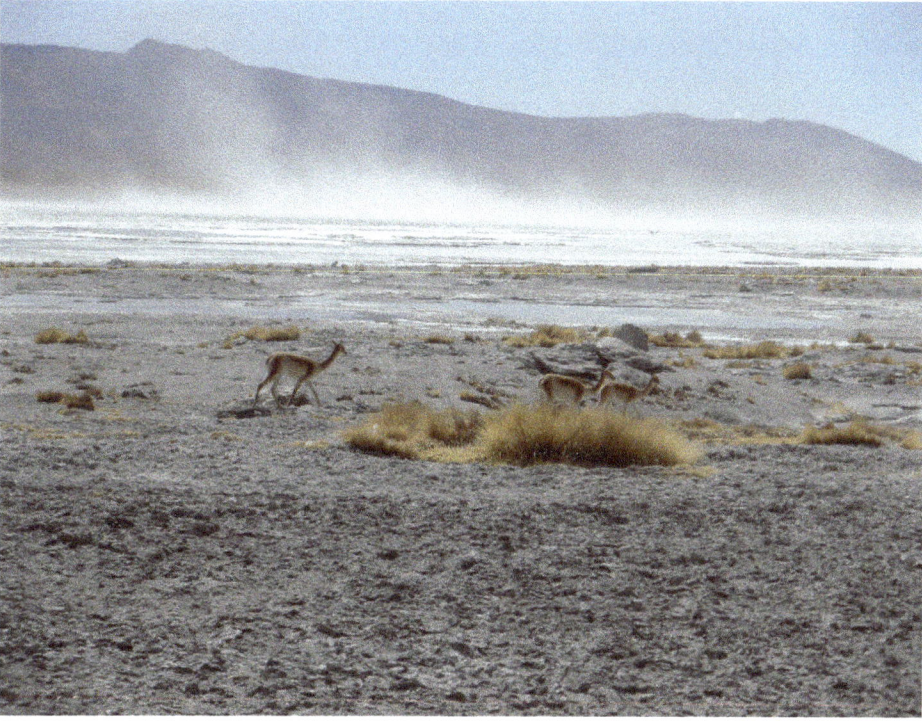

Fig. 1.3. Wild groups travel great distances.

particularly the control of internal and external parasites, will be very difficult if there is overstocking.

Heat stress is a real problem for SACs. Temperatures over 26°C and humidity of over 80% need to be avoided, so fans, shade and ponds need to be provided in hot climates. However, liver fluke is becoming a major parasite in the UK so ponds should be avoided. SACs will also defecate in water and so pollute it and increase the risk of coccidiosis. SACs are excellent swimmers and so ditches, dykes and rivers will not contain them.

Vocalization by humming is the most common sound used by SACs. It is probably used to confirm contact as it will become louder on separation. A lack of humming may be a cause for concern. Groaning or bruxism is a real cause for alarm for the keeper as it indicates pain. Veterinary attention should be sought. Snorting denotes mild aggression. This will turn to screeching in males if being handled or meeting other males. The position of the ears and tail denotes status. Males may spit and kick. They may even charge and bite. Submission will be shown by a drooping of the upper eyelid and imitation mouth breathing. Males make an ogling sound before and during mating.

Behavioural problems

A number of behavioural problems have been found in captive SACs, but to date there has been little research carried out into their causality. The two most common 'vices' are spitting at people and the Berserk Male Syndrome (this syndrome is not actually exclusively in males) where SACs respond aggressively to people.

SACs have a largely unfair reputation for spitting, since they will rarely spit at people unless they have become overfamiliarized. The activity is part of the animal's natural defensive mechanism, and is usually a response to the invasion of personal space. An unwary person can be caught in the cross fire of two spitting animals. An animal that commonly spits at people is extremely rare. The actual contents of the spit can take three forms, food, saliva or stomach contents, the latter is the so-called green spit. Adults and more commonly crias will spit food and/or saliva when they are eating to warn other animals to back off and give them space. The green spit, which is much more unpleasant both to humans and other SACs, is used in more severe confrontations. It is used by SACs to establish dominance. Most animals will pre-warn the challenger by pinning its ears back very tightly and tilting its head back so that the nose is pointing up in the air. If this warning is ignored then the animal will spit.

The more serious problem involving human–camelid interaction is the Berserk Male Syndrome, which, like spitting at people, is likely to have a root cause in overfamiliarization with people at a young age. It is extremely common in orphaned animals that have had to be hand reared. The syndrome may slowly develop until eventually the animal will pace a fence line, screaming and spitting, when anyone approaches. Such animals become highly dangerous and should be destroyed. However, the syndrome can be avoided by not bottle feeding animals unless absolutely necessary and then only handling the animal at feeding time, leaving it with other crias for the rest of the time.

Wild South American camelids

The wild vicuna (*Vicugna vicugna*) in southern Chile were pushed to near extinction by poachers who shot and skinned the animals for their very valuable fleece, until by the 1970s only 6000 were left in the wild. A ban on trade in wild vicuna products has allowed the population to recover to over a quarter of a million. In the 15th century the Incas used a system called 'Chaku' to round up, shear and release the vicuna annually. This system has been revived recently by the Aymara Indians. It involves stretching a rope, decorated with brightly coloured ribbons, up to a mile long, across a hillside and 'walking' the vicuna down. Eventually the animals are driven into a corral which is made like a labyrinth. The vicunas once caught are blindfolded before being shorn and then are released back into the wild.

Restraint

Some practitioners have issues with handling alpacas and llamas. There are some very wide differences in behaviour and hence handling in individual animals and in types of animal varies enormously. Practitioners familiar with cattle should reflect on the differences between handling dairy cattle and suckler cattle that are kept extensively. Alpacas kept in small groups by one quiet kind owner are very different from a large group of semi-wild llamas herded on large areas (Fig. 1.4).

Quiet animals can easily be handled by firmly grasping them around the neck having herded them into a small pen or stable with long ropes (horse lunge-lines are ideal) or long white rods. For injecting animals intravenously the author has found getting an assistant to hold both ears and stretch the neck upwards to be useful. It would appear that grasping the ears acts like a twitch in horses. Certain individuals, usually well known by the owners, will kick if the handler is up close to them. This is of little consequence. It is only if the animal is 3 feet away and the kick of the hindleg lands at its full force that it is serious. Llamas may strike forwards with their front legs. However, this does not seem to be a problem if the handler grasps them firmly around the neck. Many males will bite other males but it is very rare for a human to get bitten when holding an animal firmly.

Both llamas and alpacas will 'kush' when restrained. They can be made to continue in this position of ventral recumbency if they are held firmly around the neck or if they are 'chukkered'. This is when a rope is looped around their abdomen in front of their pelvis in a noose. Their hindlegs are brought forward above their fetlocks through this loop. The noose is then tightened when they are on the ground.

Drug Administration

SACs have an inelastic skin, which is thick. There is little subcutaneous space. Most clinicians

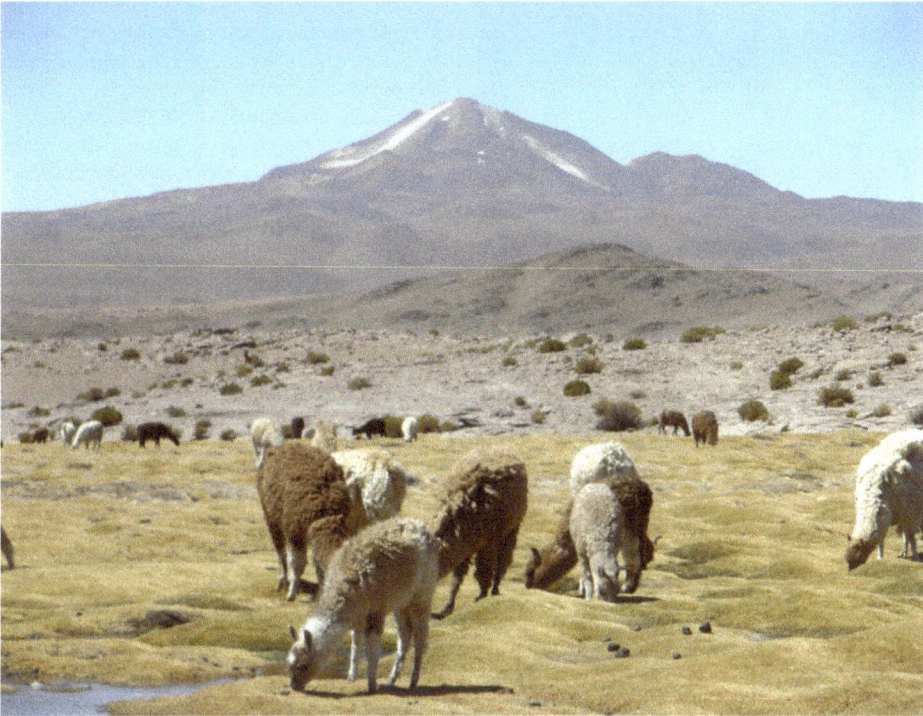

Fig. 1.4. Large groups are herded over a wide area.

favour the subcuticular route for injections as there is little muscular development in SACs. The best sites for subcutaneous injections are in front or behind the shoulder. The author prefers the quadriceps muscle as a site for intramuscular injection. However, the triceps and semitendinous/semimembranous can also be used. Intravenous injection is best carried out into the right jugular vein to avoid any danger of penetration of the oesophagus. In adults the skin is too thick for the raised jugular to be visible (Fig 1.5). Some authors (D'Alterio, 2006) prefer to use the lower part of the neck, using the ventral projection of the transverse process of the fifth and sixth cervical vertebrae (laterally) and the trachea (medially) as landmarks. There is some danger of injection into the carotid artery as the carotid artery runs only just deeper to the jugular vein in this site. Therefore the author prefers higher up the neck between the third and fourth cervical vertebrae, where the carotid is deeper. To carry out catheterization it is easier to cut through the skin with a scalpel rather than trying to place the catheter directly into the vein. The hair should be clipped, local anaesthetic should be infiltrated and the skin should be surgically prepared.

Gastric intubation in SACs can only be accomplished orally. A calf-sized gastric tube or an oral calf rehydration bag and tube is ideal for this procedure. If a soft gastric tube is used the mouth will need to be held open to prevent damage to the tube from the sharp cheek teeth. With good equipment and well-trained staff, SACs can be drenched (Fig 1.6).

Reproductive Anatomy and Physiology

Introduction

The reproductive anatomy and physiology of SACs is quite unique, more closely resembling the horse than the ruminant by having a gestation period of 335–350 days, a diffuse placentation,

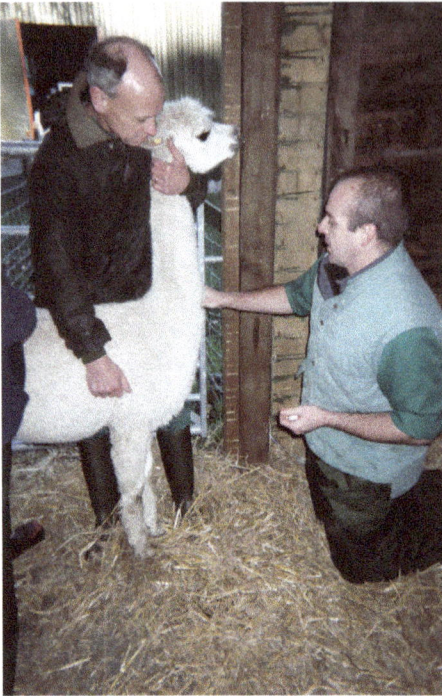

Fig. 1.5. The right side is used for venipuncture.

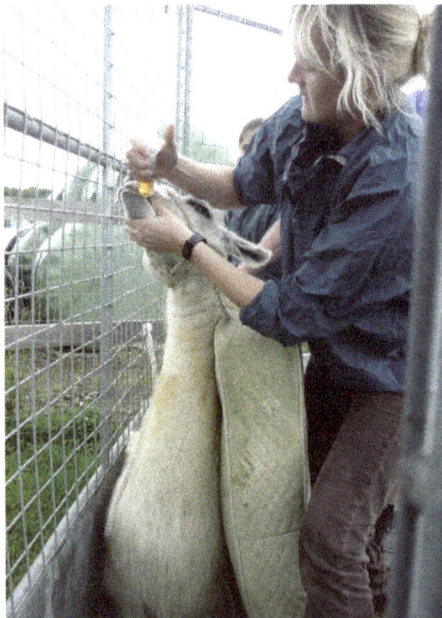

Fig. 1.6. Experienced staff are required for drenching.

the ability to breed back shortly after parturition, and very rare term twinning occurrence. Induced ovulation, which occurs 24 h after copulation in females with a tertiary follicle in excess of 7 mm, is obviously not comparable to the horse.

Males reach sexual maturity at 2.5 years. They have a fibroelastic penis and sigmoid flexure like ruminants. There is an embryonic preputial adhesion (frenulum), which prevents penile protrusion until repeated sexual stimulation occurs. This normally occurs in the animal's third year. In a normal size llama the penis when extended is 40 cm, of which half extends beyond the prepuce. There is a very short cartilaginous process that dilates the cervix during prolonged copulation, which occurs with both animals on the ground. In the relaxed state, the prepuce points caudally and urination is in a caudal direction. When sexually aroused the prepuce is directed cranially by the protractor prepuce muscle.

Testicles are small, averaging 24 g for adult llamas and 20 g for adult alpacas. The males have two small paired bulbo-urethral glands and a small prostate gland. The volume of the ejaculate is 3 ml or less.

The gross anatomy of the female SAC's reproductive tract is very similar to that seen in ruminants. The vagina of a mature female is approximately 25 cm long and 3 cm in diameter. The external os of the cervix protrudes slightly into the vagina. There are two or three rings in the cervix. In the maiden mature female, the uterus has a short body of 2.5 cm × 2.5 cm and two uterine horns of 2 cm × 6 cm. As 98% of pregnancies occur in the left horn this is bigger in the bred female even after involution. The gravid horn is roughly 3 cm × 10 cm and the non-gravid horn 2 cm × 6 cm after involution. Inactive ovaries are roughly 1.5 cm × 1.0 cm × 0.5 cm but will double in size with the development of multiple follicles or a corpus luteum.

From puberty females normally have a 12-day follicular wave pattern with follicles developing alternately on each ovary. Peak sexual activity is reached when the follicles are over 1 cm in size. Ovulation will occur 24 h after copulation, usually due to a luteinizing hormone (LH) surge after the stimulation from the male. The LH surge is not increased by further breeding within 48 h. After ovulation the corpus luteum will develop in a standard cottage loaf form approximately 1.5 cm in size. If the mating is non-fertile it will regress in 13 days with sexual receptivity recurring at 14 to 21 days after the original mating. If the mating is fertile the corpus luteum will remain, as pregnancy depends on the corpus luteum in SACs.

Mating

Mating has been seen in 6-month-old SACs but it is not recommended to breed animals before 18 months. If young females are mated there is a danger of stunted crias and dystocias. There are no significant differences in the reproductive anatomy and physiology among llamas, alpacas, guanacos and vicunas. A non-pregnant sexually mature female will, after a few minutes in the presence of a normal sexually mature male, adopt a sternal recumbent position, called the 'kush position'. The male will straddle the female to allow penile penetration. Initially semen is deposited in the cervix. However, with prolonged copulation the cervix will dilate enough for the semen to actually be deposited in the uterus. If a tertiary follicle is present ovulation will be induced. The time taken for copulation will vary between 5 and 45 min with an average of 20 min. If the female then refuses the male it is likely that ovulation has occurred. This can be confirmed by a blood test 5–7 days later, which will show a progesterone level greater than 1 ng/ml.

Female SACs show extended periods of sexual receptivity, indicating that the association of oestrogens and sexual receptivity is not quite related as it is in spontaneously ovulating ruminants. In ruminants, females are sexually receptive to the male only for a short period of time, in contrast to 1 to 36 days in SACs.

In SACs pregnancy may result from ovulations originating from either ovary; however, implantation occurs over 95% of the time in the left horn of the bipartite uterus. Implantation starts at approximately 30 days after the successful mating and is complete by 90 days.

Pregnancy cannot be readily seen even in the advanced state in SACs. Mammary development may be observable 1 week prepartum with some enlargement of the four teats. Waxing of the teats is rare as is prepartum milk let-down.

Postpartum females are often receptive to the male soon after birth. It is prudent to withhold the male for 2 weeks or longer if a vulval discharge is seen. SACs are reproductively active for their whole lives, which is often over 20 years.

Breeding strategies

Domestic SAC breeders should reflect that wild vicuna and guanaco manage to reproduce very satisfactorily without human interference. Therefore, it is likely that given sufficient area and adequate fencing herds of alpaca and llama will reproduce very well with minimum interference. Often 350 females are run with ten males on a vast area. However, there are some disadvantages to such a management strategy, which is called stud pasture breeding. The management is in the dark as to the pregnancy status of the females, which, because they are not handled, will be more wild and harder to train. If such management is reduced to one male to 35 females there is a danger that without good and early pregnancy diagnosis an infertile or subfertile male will not be found and pregnancies will be missed. If more than one mature male is run with say a group of 70 females there is a danger that the mature males will tend to fight and injure themselves.

The other end of the spectrum is hand mating, where females are bred to a selected stud at a selected hour at various time intervals. The advantages are that the management knows exactly what the breeding record is for each female, progesterone samples can be taken at the correct times and all the stock become easier to handle. Obviously there is considerably more work required but more importantly there is a danger that breedings may be forced and lead to genital tract trauma and infections.

The ideal system if there are good facilities may be a halfway house of stud pen breeding where one stud has one or more females living with him in a confined pen.

The real problems come with very small herds without a stud or with a stud that is related to the females. In these herds either the females have to be transported to a stud or a stud male has to be brought on to the farm. In either case there are considerable disease control issues. These are made worse if studs are just moved from farm to farm. A risk table (Table 1.1) should be completed by practitioners for each

Table 1.1. Breeding activities risk categories.

Activity	TB risk	General disease risk
No animals move on or off farm for breeding		
No animals move on farm for breeding without 6 week quarantine period on arrival at farm (includes males or females visiting farm)		
Females visit farm for breeding (drive-by):		
• Designated area		
• Pasture/management area used by farm for own stock		
Females visit farm for breeding (board on farm):		
• Separate area >3 miles from home herd		
• Separate paddock but fence line contact with home herd		
• Mixed with farm's stock		
Males go out to do drive-by breedings:		
• One out and back visit (one destination, quarantine on return for 6 weeks between visits)		
• One out and back visit (one destination, no quarantine on return)		
• Male visits several farms in one day		
• Several males on trailer visiting multiple farms		
• Male visits multiple farms on different days without quarantine in between: mixes with regular group in between visits		
Males received by farm for drive-by breedings of farm's own females:		
• Designated area		
• Not different from regular breeding area		
Females going out for drive-by breedings on other farms:		
• Quarantine on return		
• No quarantine on return		

The risks should be graded as between 0 and 5: 0 indicates an activity of no risk at all; 5 indicates an activity of high risk.

holding so that owners are made aware of the dangers they face from TB and also from other diseases called 'general disease risk', which would include parasites, BVD, etc. Practitioners should discuss the results of these tables with the owners. Targets should be set. Owners should be made fully aware of the risks they are taking.

Shearing

Shearing during the first or last 60 days of pregnancy is a risk, due to the dependence of SACs on the corpus luteum (CL) for maintenance of pregnancy. Stress results in prostaglandin (PG) production and subsequent luteolysis. However, heat stress could cause worse problems if animals are left until it becomes really hot just because they are pregnant, i.e. the stress of shearing may be less important than more persistent heat stress issues. Additionally, the timing of shearing may depend on many outside factors. If a late pregnant animal is shorn in the last couple of weeks of pregnancy and early parturition occurs, the chances are this will be all right. However, if

parturition is more than 2 weeks early survival is less likely. The main problem of early parturition is that mammary development may not be sufficient to allow adequate colostrum production. The cria may be a candidate for frozen plasma transfer (FPT). The immunoglobulin G (IgG) concentrations of the cria should be checked (see Chapter 4). Clinicians should explain the relative risks and let their clients choose what they perceive to be the best option on the basis of their farm's situation.

Physically shearing alpacas is more labour intensive than shearing sheep where several sheep catchers and wool packers are required for one shearer. The alpaca needs to be secured by ropes and its head is held. It is then held in lateral recumbency. The dorsal surface of the alpaca is shorn first. It is from this site that the fibre sample is taken and examined for quality (Fig. 1.7).

Heat Stress

Heat stress can be a serious problem in tropical and subtropical countries and in temperate

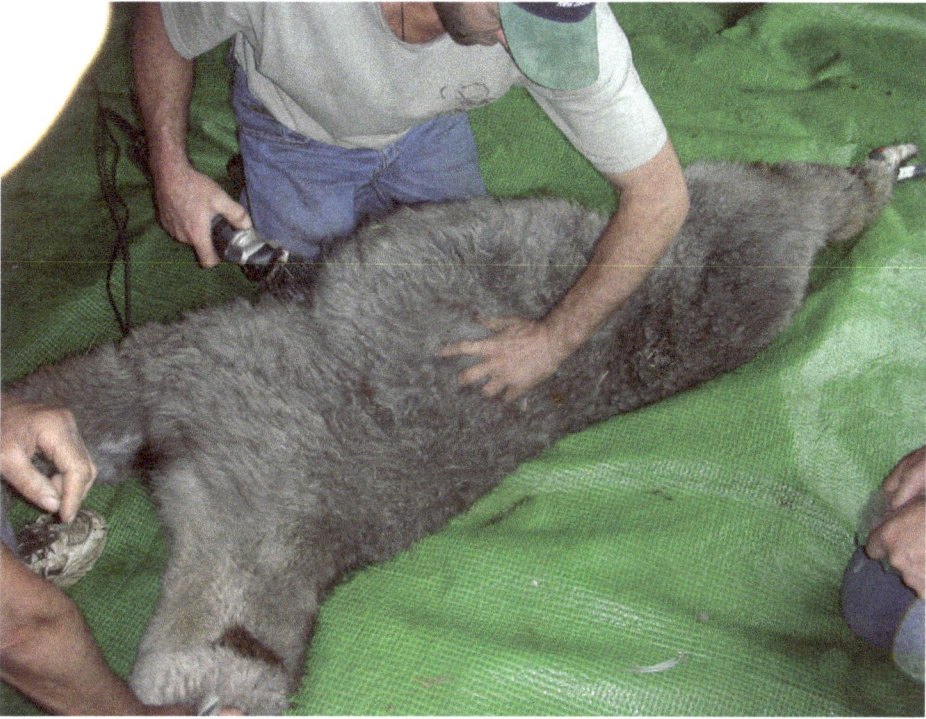

Fig. 1.7. Fibre is taken from this site for quality evaluation.

countries in the summer. However, SACs are well adapted compared to other mammals to maintaining a wide range of body temperature somewhere between 98°F (37°C) and 104°F (40°C). Without a resting temperature in this range the body and organ systems of a SAC can be seriously compromised in their ability to maintain proper function, particularly if the increased temperature is maintained for several days. Normal metabolic functions that generate heat include breathing, walking, eating, digesting, and assimilating nutrients, etc. To prevent heat stress the animal has to utilize mechanisms to dissipate excess heat. If the body of the SAC rises it will shed this heat into the surrounding air by vasodilatation and concurrent increase of blood flow to the skin and periphery. This occurs particularly around the perineum, between the legs and on the ventral abdomen. SACs pant, thus warming the inspired air and cooling the lung fields. This increased air movement into the lungs will cause

evaporation of fluid from the respiratory tract, and cause further cooling down of the animal. SACs also sweat.

The thermoregulatory mechanism begins to fail if the air around the animal becomes stagnant. If the ambient temperature is the same or higher than the body of the SAC, or if the ambient humidity is high enough to decrease the effectiveness of evaporation, then heat dissipation is prevented. The animal's ability to respond to environment changes that predispose it to heat stress are further reduced by exercising, breeding, or working during the hot part of the day. Obesity in SACs is very common and it decreases the animal's ability to effectively deal with excess body heat in the face of high environmental heat or humidity. A long and shaggy, poorly groomed fibre coat is a good insulator and decreases the animal's ability to rid itself of excess heat. Animals sweating excessively become dehydrated, further depressing the body's ability to respond to rising temperatures. The evaporation of fluids from the respiratory tract with panting results in further dehydration. This results in a loss of blood volume and an increase in heart rate.

Signs of heat stress include depression and anorexia. Animals with heat stress will have a rectal temperature of more than 104°F (40°C). They will be panting with a respiration rate greater than 30. There will be frothing at the mouth and a drooping lower lip and a heart rate greater than 100. There is likely to be ventral oedema and oedema of the legs before collapse and death.

The most effective treatment is simply cooling the animal down. This can be achieved by a hose, pouring buckets of cold water over it or standing it in a pond. Once it is drenched the use of a fan is beneficial. Common sense should be used to decide the best methods to be implemented. Dehydrated animals must be allowed to drink or if too weak they should be given cold electrolytes by orogastric tube. If they are very dehydrated they should be put on a drip of polyionic fluids. Non-steroid anti-inflammatory drugs (NSAIDs) are useful. Injectable B vitamins are useful to improve appetite and vitamin B1 will prevent cerebro-cortico-necrosis (CCN) (see Chapter 12). Recumbent animals are likely to have a compromised immune system and should be given antibiotics. Beware of excessive feed on recovery as there is a danger of acidosis from grain overload.

Prevention of heat stress is once again up to common sense, with shearing being carried out at an appropriate time and the provision of shade at all times. Trees are ideal to provide shade as are houses with high ceilings. Breeding should be avoided in the heat of the day. Parturition should be timed to avoid the very hot time of the year.

Diets high in poor quality roughage give off excess heat during digestion, and therefore should be avoided during times when heat stress is a danger. Energy requirements may actually be increased by panting and faster heart rates associated with attempts by the body to maintain temperature in a safe range. Unfortunately, with decreased feed intake, which is commonly associated with heat stress, the intake of nutrients is also diminished. During hotter weather the rate of passage of ingesta through the gut tends to be slower than normal, therefore signs of colic may be seen as impactions may occur. With the association of altered thermoregulatory ability the feeding of fescue infected with endophytic fungus *Acremonium* spp. should be avoided.

In large countries, e.g. the USA and Australia, the movement of animals from a colder climate to a hotter climate should be avoided. Equally, movement from the high altiplano to lowland areas should be avoided in the hottest time of the year. It takes over 6 months for an alpaca or llama to adjust to a new climate. Owners should avoid regrouping animals during hot weather to avoid fighting.

A useful measure to decide if animals are at risk from heat stress is to add together the ambient humidity and the temperature in Fahrenheit. If this number is 120 or less only minimal problems exist. If the number is 150 or more, as many precautions as are available should be taken. But as the number approaches or exceeds 180, extreme caution should be exercised, as animals are at great risk.

Hypothermia

There are two likely times when this is a problem in adults: (i) if they are shorn early and then there is a sudden cold snap; and (ii) if they are left out in severe weather conditions with no access to shelter. Crias are at risk if they are born in the autumn and are faced with cold conditions.

Treatment of hypothermia involves warmth, nutrition and correction of underlying problems, e.g. milk supplements for crias whose dam is not lactating. Critical hypothermia occurs when core body temperature drops below 90°F (32°C). The following actions need to be taken:

1. Protection. Get the animal into a well-insulated, preferably heated area.
2. Warmth. Wrap the animal in heated blankets. Using a heat lamp or a convection heater in a cold stable can be detrimental because the direct heat causes dilation of the surface blood vessels, which can make the heat loss worse particularly if the animal is wet.

3. Time. Avoid too rapid heating.

4. Energy in the form of intravenous administration of electrolytes and glucose are most useful. Syrups can be given carefully by mouth. Glucose in solution can be given per rectum. Fluids should be given at 95–100°F (35–38°C).

5. Oxygen is useful in debilitated critically hypothermic animals.

6. Steroids are controversial. Prednisone at 1mg/kg is preferable to Dexamethazone.

7. Ulcers. Give omeprazole at 2 to 4 mg/kg orally daily to high-risk animals.

8. Nutrition. Encourage them to eat. Also heat the offered water.

9. Stress. Avoid separation anxiety.

10. Recovery. This will take time and animals should be monitored for a minimum of 5 days.

Normal Crias

In many instances practitioners are less aware of normality than are owners. A normal cria will be lively and on its feet within 1 h. It will be sucking within 4 h and have passed meconium within 8 h. Most mothers will not allow suckling until the placenta has been passed. The act of sucking and the ingestion of colostrum encourages the passing of meconium. A cria's rectal temperature will exceed 37°C. The ear tips will be straight and the incisors can be felt. Everything should be done to maintain the maternal bond. There should be no interference if there is no problem. If it is a cold day then the mother and cria should be encouraged into a warmer place, e.g. a shelter or under the trees out of the wind. This should be achieved without stressing the mother.

If all is normal after approximately 6 h, often towards evening, the cria may be quickly checked. The sex can be checked together with the patency of the anus and in females the vulva. The navel can be dressed with iodine or oxytetracycline spray and be checked for an umbilical hernia. The cria can be quickly weighed on bathroom scales in the paddock.

Abnormal Crias

Most problems are associated with premature or dysmature crias (see Chapter 3). There are some other factors relating to the female, e.g. poor teat conformation, poor milk production from very thin maidens or over-fat mature females. There are of course outside factors, e.g. bad weather and overcrowded paddocks.

Mortality of Crias

In the Andes Mountains, alpaca rearing is the main economic activity of many families. One of the factors that affects the economic viability of the breeding activity is the mortality of offspring. An investigation was taken to analyse factors that influence the probability of survival of alpaca crias raised under extensive management conditions in the high elevations of the Andes Mountains in Peru (Gommez-Quispe *et al.*, 2022)

The study involved 100 crias born during a normal calving season that were monitored from birth to 12 weeks of age. Mortality of crias was monitored daily whereas body weight and other variables were recorded weekly. Cria survival was estimated using the Cox proportional hazard regression. Crias that never showed clinical signs of disease had a higher ($P = 0.001$) probability of survival (93.9%) than crias with visible signs of disease (5.6%). Crias with a heavy birth weight (exceeding 7.13 kg) had a greater ($P = 0.001$) probability of survival than those born with a moderate (80.6%) or low (52.6%) birth weight. Survival of crias was not affected by sex ($P = 0.303$) or fleece color ($P = 0.361$). The most important factors that influenced the survival of the crias were clinical health status ($P < 0.001$) and birth weight ($P = 0.001$). These results highlight the importance of cria health care management during the first six weeks of life. More vigilant observation of cria health during this time could reduce clinical disease and improve cria survival, thereby improving the profitability of alpaca producers through the reduction of cria losses.

Appendix 1.1. British Llama Society Trekking Code of Conduct

The British Llama Society prepared a code of conduct to encourage commercial llama trekking establishments to operate to the highest standards of safety and welfare. It is also intended to promote the well-being of the animals themselves and to provide operators with a minimum standard for conducting their business.

This code of conduct establishes that the undersigned member of the British Llama Society, when providing a llama trekking activity, will abide by the following code of conduct and display this page in a public place.

1. To abide by current health and safety legislation regarding the safety of the public.
2. To have adequate Public Liability Insurance.
3. If preparing or providing food, to be within the environmental health regulations and hold a food safety certificate if required.
4. Clear instructions and information must precede every trek regarding handling, leading and behaviour of llamas. Appropriate supervision for the circumstances must be provided whilst trekking.
5. Llamas under two years of age will not be used for trekking or to carry a pack. Young llamas in training for trekking should not be overworked and should only carry packs that are lightly loaded. Llamas of four years or older should not carry packs of more than 25kilos/55lbs. Consideration must be made for smaller llamas, i.e. not overburdened.
6. Llamas used for trekking must be properly trained and of a suitable strength and temperament.
7. Females should not be used for trekking with entire males.
8. All treks should carry a mobile phone and a first aid kit for humans and llamas.
9. Permission from the relevant landowners to trek across their land must be given before the trek takes place.
10. Trekkers should use considerate behaviour to horse riders, dog owners, landowners, etc. that they meet and follow the Countryside Code. Due care and attention must be taken when trekking on roads.
11. Always endeavour to uphold the good name of the British Llama Society and maintain the goodwill of National Parks, The Forestry Authority, Local Authorities and other local organizations. Promote the friendly aspects of llama trekking.
12. Always aim to ensure that the media continue to have a high regard for llamas. Avoid any suggested sequence that might cause llamas undue stress which could be recorded and then published or broadcast.

Members whose names are included in the British Llama Society Enterprise Directory for Llama Trekking, will have formally undertaken to comply with this Code of Conduct for Commercial Llama Tekking.

If it comes to the notice of the British Llama Society that the terms of this Code of Conduct for Commercial Llama Trekking have been breached, the matter should be referred to the Board of Directors of the British Llama Society, who will investigate and take appropriate action.

Declaration:
I, the undersigned, agree to comply with the foregoing British Llama Society Code of Conduct for Commercial Llama Trekking when offering llama trekking as an activity to the public, and to abide by this agreement. I hereby indemnify the British Llama Society from any consequences should I fail to do so.
On behalf of ....Llama Trekking
Signed.........................Date.........
Name..................M'ship No:........
Address...................................
...
...

This is to certify that
Mr A Smith
Membership Number: 12345
of
Peruvian Dream Llama Trekking
Has signed the British Llama Society Trekking Code of Conduct, thereby agreeing to abide by the standards laid down by the Society.

1. To abide by current health & safety legislation regarding the safety of the public.
2. To have adequate Public Liability insurance.
3. If preparing or providing food, to be within the Environmental Health Regulations and hold a Food Safety Certificate if required.
4. Clear instructions and information must precede every trek regarding handling, leading and behaviour of llamas. Appropriate supervision for the circumstances must be provided whilst trekking.
5. Llamas under two years of age will not be used for trekking or to carry a pack. Young llamas in training for trekking should not be overworked and should only carry packs that are lightly loaded. Llamas of four years or older should not carry packs of more than 25kilos/55lbs. Consideration must be made for smaller llamas, i.e. not overburned.
6. Llamas used for trekking must be properly trained and of a suitable strength and temperament.
7. Females should not be used for trekking with entire males.
8. All treks should carry a mobile phone and a first aid kit for humans and llamas.
9. Permission from the relevant landowners to trek across their land must be given before the trek takes place.
10. Trekkers should use considerate behaviour to horse riders, dog owners, landowners, etc. that meet and follow the Countryside Code. Due care and attention must be taken when trekking on roads.
11. Always endeavour to uphold the good name of the British Llama Society and maintain the goodwill of National Parks, The Forestry Authority, Local Authorities and other organizations. Promote the friendly aspects of llama trekking.

This certificate will be displayed only so long as the above-mentioned remains a paid up member of the British Llama Society.

Certificate Issued: Dated ....

Society Secretary

Appendix 1.2.

Welfare of Animal (Transport) Order 1997

Schedule 1

Part I

GENERAL REQUIREMENTS FOR THE CONSTRUCTION AND MAINTENANCE OF MEANS OF TRANSPORT AND
RECEPTACLES FOR ALL MAMMALS AND BIRDS

Avoidance of injury and suffering
1. Means of transport, receptacles, and their fittings shall be constructed, maintained and operated
so as to avoid injury and unnecessary suffering and to ensure the safety of the animals during
transporting, loading and unloading.

Substantial construction
2. Every part or fitting of a means of transport or receptacle which may be exposed to the action
of the weather shall be constructed, maintained and operated so as to withstand the action of the
weather.

Size
3. The accommodation available for the carriage of animals shall be such that the animals are,
unless it is unnecessary having regard to the species of animal and the nature of the journey,
provided with adequate space to lie down.

Floors
4. Any floor on which the animals stand or walk during loading, unloading, of transport shall be –
    (a) Sufficiently strong to bear their weight;
    (b) Constructed, maintained and operated to prevent slipping; and
    (c) Free of any protrusions, spaces or perforations which are likely to cause injury to animals.

Weather and sea conditions
5. Means of transport and receptacles shall be constructed, maintained and operated so as to
protect animals against inclement weather, adverse sea conditions, marked fluctuations in air
pressure, excessive humidity, heat or cold.

Projections and sharp edges
6. Means of transport and receptacles shall be free from any sharp edges and projections likely to
cause injury or unnecessary suffering to any animal being carried.

Cleanliness
7. Means of transport and receptacles shall be constructed, maintained and operated so as to allow
appropriate cleaning and disinfection.

Escape-proof
8. Means of transport and receptacles shall be escape-proof

Noise and vibration
9. Means of transport and receptacles shall be constructed, maintained and operated so as to ensure
that animals are not likely to be caused injury or unnecessary suffering from undue exposure to
noise or vibration.

Lighting
10. – (1) Means of transport and receptacles shall have sufficient natural or artificial lighting to en-
    able proper care and inspection of any animal being carried.

(2) Passageways, ramps and other loading equipment shall be provided with adequate natural or artificial lighting to enable the animals to be loaded or unloaded safely.

(3) Artificial lighting required by this paragraph may be provided using a portable light.

Use of partitions

11. – (1) Partitions shall be used if they are necessary –
    (a) to provided adequate support for animals; or
    (b) to prevent animals being thrown about during transport.

(2) When partitions are used, they shall be positioned so as to prevent injury or unnecessary suffering to animals as a result of –
    (a) lack of support; or
    (b) being thrown about during transport.

Design of partitions

12. Partitions shall be –
    (a) of rigid construction;
    (b) strong enough to withstand the weight of any animal which may be thrown against them; and
    (c) constructed and positioned so that they do not interfere with ventilation.

Special provision of rail wagons

13. Any rail wagon used in the transport of animals shall be marked with a symbol indicating the presence of live animals.

14. Any rail wagons in which animals are carried shall be –
    (a) equipped with a roof ensuring effective protection against the weather;
    (b) capable of travelling at high speed; and
    (c) provided with sufficient large air vents or a ventilation system which is effective even at low speeds.

15. The inside walls of any rail wagon used for the carriage of animals (other than in receptacles) shall be of suitable material, completely smooth and shall have, if necessary, means for tying the animals to the walls.

Special provisions for transport by water or air

16. Animals being transported by water or air shall –
    (a) be accommodated in suitable pens or receptacles unless they are in a vehicle or rail wagon on board a vessel or aircraft; and
    (b) where necessary, be secured to protect them against injury from the motion of the vessel or aircraft.

Additional provisions for transport by water

17. There shall be adequate passageways on a vessel providing access to all pens, receptacles, vehicles or rail wagons in which animals are accommodated.

18. All parts of a vessel in which animals are accommodated shall be provided with adequate drainage and shall be kept in a sanitary condition.

19. – (1) Enclosed decks of a vessel in which animals are transported (whether in vehicles or otherwise) shall be provided with an adequate means of mechanical ventilation.

(2) Vehicles in which animals are being transported in an enclosed deck shall, where possible, be placed near a fresh air inlet.

(3) Where animals are transported in rail wagons on board vessels, adequate ventilation shall be provided for animals throughout the voyage.

20. Where animals are transported by water, there shall be provisions for isolation of ill or injured animals during the voyage and for first aid treatment to be given, when necessary.

21. Where animals are transported in vehicles on board vessels –
    (a) the animals' compartment shall be properly fixed to the vehicle;

(b) the vehicle and the animals' compartment shall be equipped with tying facilities enabling them to be adequately secured to the vessel;

(c) the animals' compartment shall have a sufficient number of vents or other means of ensuring that it is adequately ventilated bearing in mind that the air flow is restricted in the confined space of the vessel's vehicle deck;

(d) there shall be sufficient room inside the animals' compartment (at each of its levels) to ensure that there is adequate ventilation and sufficient air space to allow the air to circulate properly; and

(e) direct access shall be provided to each part of the animals' compartment so that the animals can, if necessary, be cared for, fed and watered during the voyage.

Part II

GENERAL PROVISIONS FOR THE TRANSPORT OF ALL MAMMALS AND BIRDS

Jolting
22. Animals shall not be transported in such a way that they are severely jolted or shaken.

Loading and unloading
23. Animals shall be loaded and unloaded in such a way as to ensure that they are not caused injury or unnecessary suffering by reason of –

(a) the excessive use of anything for driving animals; or

(b) contact with any part of the means of transport or receptacle or with another obstruction.

Emergency unloading
24. Unless an animal can be loaded or unloaded in accordance with the provisions of paragraph 10 (6) or (7) of PART II of Schedule 2 below, a vehicle shall, at all times, carry the means to enable animals to be unloaded without causing them injury or unnecessary suffering at a place where there is no other unloading equipment.

Segregation of animals and goods
25. – (1) Goods which are being transported in the same means of transport as animals shall be positioned so that they do not cause injury or unnecessary suffering to the animals and in particular goods which could prejudice the welfare of animals shall not be carried in pens or receptacles in which animals are transported.

(2) A carcase shall not be carried in the same road vehicle, receptacle, rail wagon or pen as an animal, other than the carcase of an animal which dies in the course of a journey.

Cleaning and disinfection
26. – (1) Animals shall be loaded only into means of transport or receptacles which have been thoroughly cleaned and where appropriate disinfected.

(2) Dead animals, soiled litter and droppings shall be removed from means of transport or receptacles as soon as possible.

Litter
27. Floors on which animals are transported shall be covered with sufficient litter to absorb urine and droppings unless equally effective alternative arrangements are in place or unless urine and droppings are regularly removed.

Labelling of receptacles
28. Receptacles in which animals are transported shall –

(a) be marked or labelled so as to indicate that they contain live animals and the species of those animals.

(b) be marked with a sign indicating the receptacle's upright position; and

(c) be kept in an upright position.

Securing of receptacles
29. Receptacles shall be secured so as to prevent their displacement during transport.

Humane slaughter on vessels and aircraft
30. Vessels and aircraft on which animals are transported shall carry appropriate means for effecting the humane slaughter of the type of animal being carried if necessary.

Attendants
31. – (1) In order to ensure the necessary care of the animals during transport, consignments of animals shall be accompanied by a sufficient number of attendants, taking into account the number of animals transported and the duration of the journey.

(2) At least one attendant shall accompany the animals except in the following cases –

(a) where animals are transported in receptacles which are secured, adequately ventilated and, where necessary, contain enough food and liquid, in dispensers which cannot be tipped over, for a journey of twice the anticipated time;

(b) where the transporter performs the function of attendant; or

(c) where the consignor has appointed an agent to care for the animals at appropriate stopping or transfer points.

Schedule 5

Article 4 (b)

Part I

ADDITIONAL REQUIREMENTS FOR THE CONSTRUCTION AND MAINTENANCE OF MEANS OF TRANSPORT AND RECEPTACLES OF MAMMALS AND BIRDS NOT COVERED BY SCHEDULES 2, 3 AND 4

Ventilation
1. Means of transport and receptacles shall be constructed, maintained, operated and positioned to provide adequate ventilation and air space.

Size and height
2. The accommodation available for the carriage of animals shall be such that the animals are provided with adequate space to stand in their natural position.

Special provision for receptacles
3. Receptacles in which animals are transported shall be constructed and maintained so that they allow for appropriate inspection and care of the animals.

Special provisions for road vehicles
4. Vehicles shall be equipped with a roof which ensures effective protection against the weather.

5. Vehicles shall be equipped, on each floor on which animals (other than marine mammals) are carried (other than in receptacles), with barriers so constructed and maintained as to prevent any animal from falling out of the vehicle when any door used for loading and unloading is not fully closed.

6. Every ramp which is carried on or forms part of a vehicle shall be constructed, maintained and operated –

(a) To prevent slipping;

(b) So that it is not too steep for the age and species of that animal being transported;

(c) So that any step at the top or bottom of the ramp is not too high for the age and species of the animal being transported;

(d) So that any gap between the top of the ramp and the vehicle or at the bottom of the ramp is not too wide for the age and species of the animal being transported; and

(e) In this paragraph, a ramp shall be considered too steep, a step shall be considered too high and a gap shall be considered too wide, if animals using the ramp are likely to be caused injury

or unnecessary suffering by reason of the slope of the ramp, the height of the step or the width
of the gap.

7. In the case of animals which are normally required to be tied, suitable provision shall be made so
that animals may be tied to the interior of the vehicle.

Part II

ADDITIONAL PROVISIONS FOR THE TRANSPORT OF MAMMALS AND BIRDS NOT COVERED BY SCHEDULES 2, 3
AND 4

Loading equipment

8. – (1) Animals shall be loaded and unloaded in accordance with this paragraph.

(2) Save as provided in sub-paragraphs (5) and (6) below they shall be loaded and unloaded
using suitable ramps, bridges, gangways or mechanical lifting gear, operated so as to prevent
injury or unnecessary suffering to any animal.

(3) The flooring of any loading equipment shall be constructed so as to prevent slipping.

(4) Ramps, bridges, gangways and loading platforms shall be provided on each side with protection which is –

(a) of sufficient strength, length and height to prevent any animal using the loading
equipment from falling or escaping; and

(b) positioned so that it will not result in injury or unnecessary suffering to any animal.

(5) An animal may be loaded or unloaded by means of manual lifting or carrying if the animal
is of a size that it can easily be lifted by no more than two persons and the operation is carried
out without causing injury or unnecessary suffering to the animal.

(6) An animal may be loaded or unloaded without equipment or by manual lifting or carrying
provided that, having regard to the age, height and species of the animal, it is unlikely to be
caused injury or unnecessary suffering by being loaded or unloaded in this manner.

Movement from floor to floor

9. – (1) Animals shall be moved from one floor or deck of a vehicle, vessel or receptacle to another
in accordance with this paragraph.

(2) Save as provided in sub-paragraph (4) below, suitable ramps or mechanical lifting gear shall
be used and operated so as to prevent injury or unnecessary suffering to any animal.

(3) Where a ramp or mechanical lifting gear is used it shall be –

(a) provided on each side with protection which is of sufficient strength, length and
height to prevent any animal using it from falling or escaping;

(b) positioned so that it will not result in injury or unnecessary suffering to any animal;
and

(c) of a gradient which is suitable to the age and species of the animals concerned.

(4) Manual lifting or carrying may be used if the animal is of a size that can easily be lifted by
no more than two persons and the movement is carried out without causing injury or unnecessary suffering to the animal.

Segregation of species

10. No animal may be placed in the same undivided pen, receptacle, vehicle or railway wagon as any
other animal unless it is known that they are compatible with each other.

Duties of attendants

11. The attendant or consignor's agent shall look after the animals and, if necessary, feed and water
them.

Notice describing animal

12. Where the means of transport or receptacles contains animals which are wild, timid or dangerous
a notice to that effect shall be fixed to it.

Special provisions for transport by water

13. Vessels used for the transport of animals shall, before sailing, be provided with sufficient supplies of liquid for drinking (unless they are equipped with a suitable system allowing its production) and appropriate foodstuffs, having regard to the species and number of animals being transported as well as the duration of the voyage.

Sedation

14. Sedation shall be given only exceptionally and under the direct supervision of a veterinary surgeon. Written details of such sedation shall accompany the animal to its destination.

Conditioning of animals

15. Where appropriate, animals shall be held for a suitable period prior to transport to prepare them for loading, unloading and transport. During that period they shall, if necessary, be moved gradually into their receptacle.

Appendix 1.3. Code of Conduct for the Sale of Llamas

The purpose of this Code is to help buyers avoid pitfalls in the purchase and sales process. It is also intended to promote the well-being of the animals themselves and to provide sellers with a minimum standard to which they should conduct their sales.

The British Llama Society does not accept advertising, nor will promote in any way, the sale of llamas by anyone who is not a signatory to the code. We advise prospective owners to purchase llamas only from members who have signed the Code.

Signatories to this Code are issued with a dated certificate, which should be renewed every three years by application.

A separate code is available for sale of guanacos.

When selling or offering for sale any llama the undersigned member of the British Llama Society undertakes:

1. To give appropriate advice and information, to the best of their knowledge, to any purchaser on the pros and cons of owning llamas.

2. To offer purchasers after-sales advice, whenever needed, particularly concerning care and welfare.

3. To give full and appropriate advice on choosing the right animal for the purchaser's intended purpose.

4. To declare any known faults in conformation or temperament which could hamper or obstruct the purpose for which the llama is purchased.

5. To knowingly offer cross-bred, in-bred, or infertile stock, or related pairs without declaring them as such.

6. To provide purchasers with a full record of the animal's breeding and veterinary history, including worming, vaccinations, etc. as they are known.

7. To ensure that purchasers understand that, if they have more than one entire male, the males will need to be kept separately if within sight or smell of a female.

8. (a) That crias will not be bottle-fed/hand-reared except in life-threatening circumstances, in which case the fact that an animal has been reared in this way will be declared to a potential purchaser and reasons given.

(b) To explain to all purchasers of camelids which are capable of breeding that, although bottle-fed/hand-reared youngsters are extremely tame and friendly when small, they are very likely to become extremely difficult to manage when they mature.

(c) To explain that any male camelid which has been reared in this way should be castrated at between six and twelve months of age but that castration might not necessarily prevent such problems.

(d) To request all purchasers of animals capable of breeding, to pass on this information (*a-c) to anyone who might buy from them in future.

9. Females sold as pregnant are declared –

Confirmed pregnant: only following a blood test or ultrasound scan and there has been no reason to suspect a miscarriage.

Believed to be pregnant: only when mating has been witnessed and subsequent putting of the male to the female has been witnessed and not resulted in further mating.

Possibly pregnant: where no mating has been witnessed but an adult female has been running with an adult male.

10. (a) To advise purchasers that female camelids should not be intentionally mated until they have attained at least 60% of their likely adult weight or be at least eighteen months of age.

(b) To advise that it is possible for mating and conception to occur at as young an age as nine months, which is detrimental to the well-being of the female. This must be borne in mind if young males and females are to be kept together.

11. To ensure that when declaring that an animal is handleable or halter-trained, the animal can be led and the halter be easily put in place, with minimum stress to animal and/or handler.

12. To ensure suitable transport is provided for the llamas.

Signatories to this code are duty bound to not sell llamas:

- Without ensuring that purchasers understand the long-term commitment;
- As being 'easy-to-keep' without making it clear that all livestock needs daily observation, care and attention, and can be subject to health and other problems; and
- Without making every effort to ensure that the new home offers adequate grazing, shelter, fencing, and fresh water, etc.

Declaration:
I, the undersigned, agree to comply with the British Llama Society Code of Conduct when offering for sale any llama.
Signed:....................................... Date.......................
Name:............................ M'ship No:........................
Address:...
....
....

If any purchaser believes that the terms of this code have been breached, the matter should be referred to the Society Committee, who will investigate and take appropriate action.

Appendix 1.4. British Alpaca Society Code of Conduct for sale of alpacas

All persons wishing to advertise alpacas for sale in *Alpaca* magazine or on the Society website must be current members of the British Alpaca Society (BAS) and have signed this Code of Conduct for the sale of alpacas.

1. To ensure the proper well-being of the alpaca by advising the intended purchaser of the requirements laid down in the Guide to Welfare to avoid selling alpacas which might be kept alone, and to ensure that adequate grazing is available to accommodate the increase in herd size if breeding animals are being purchased.

2. To advise on the long-term commitment pertaining to alpaca ownership.

3. To declare any known faults in breeding ability, conformation, temperament and ancestry, where this relates to the intended purpose of the purchaser.

4. To offer after-sales help and advice whenever needed by the purchaser.

5. To provide the purchaser with proper records of date of birth, breeding history, medical history and last worming and vaccination dates. Also to provide the BAS registration certificate duly completed with change of ownership details.

6. To ensure that the alpaca is in good health, with all routine husbandry completed.

7. To declare a female believed pregnant only when mating has been observed and subsequent putting back to a male does not result in further mating.

8. To declare a female confirmed pregnant only when supported by evidence of an ultrasound scan test, or a blood progesterone assay, or a current veterinary certificate of pregnancy.

9. Not knowingly to sell line bred, or inbred stock, or related male/female pairs without declaring them as such.

10. To ensure the animal you are buying is registered with BAS.

11. To ensure that the animal you are buying is transferred to your ownership on the BAS registry.

12. To recommend membership of the British Alpaca Society.

13. To be honest and truthful in all matters relating to the alpacas being offered for sale.

2

Nutrition and Metabolic Diseases

Introduction

To satisfy the five freedoms – the ethical framework around which the codes of recommendation for the welfare of farmed livestock are presently crafted in the UK – all farm animals must be given access to proper nutrition. SACs are included under this umbrella. This means not just that forage and water must be offered at all times but that the nutrient balance is such that the animals do not suffer from hunger, thirst or malnutrition. In the UK and in the EU there are strict rules regarding the feeding and watering of animals in transit.

The diet of animals must be suitable to their production needs and must overcome any potential dietary shortcomings such as mineral deficiencies, energy shortfall or constituent imbalance. Feeding practice in particular must be good to optimize the health, welfare and productivity of the animals. Judicious use of grazing can be used to satisfy the nutrient demands for a large part of the year for SACs in the UK. The grazing needs to be managed to maintain sward height and ensure that fresh grazing is available to the animals as needed or the animals must be allowed to roam to find new pasture. The roaming may be timed to make best use of the grazing to fit in with the weather or the harvesting of forage for conservation. Great care should be exercised when animals are trekking or are allowed

into gardens on account of the possible ingestion of poisonous plants (see Chapter 16).

In an intensive situation, attention to stocking rates and the monitoring of sward height will allow the best use of grazing with optimal swards of 4–6 cm being maintained. Properly managed grazing patterns coupled with good forage preservation are the goal. Complications to diets start as soon as supplements are introduced. Balanced diets do not need *ad libitum* mineral blocks or powder supplements and indeed either mineral blocks or mineral supplements may cause dietary imbalance by either competing with nutrients in the diet or by indirect competition. An example is the rich red mineral supplement that is often supplied by farm wholesalers, which contains high levels of iron and will effectively lower the adsorption of copper from the gut, possibly leading to marginal or deficient status. Similarly imbalances of calcium, magnesium and phosphates can be precipitated by injudicious use of mineral supplements.

Poor Feedstuffs

Feeding mouldy forage is usually unintentional and occasionally unavoidable. However, the potential disease impact and reduced palatability of spoilt feed mean that this should be avoided if at all possible. Incorrect storage of forages

© Graham R. Duncanson 2023. *Veterinary Treatment of Llamas and Alpacas,* 2nd Edition
(G.R. Duncanson)
DOI: 10.1079/9781800623576.0002

intended for later feeding can result in the ideal conditions for growth of various organisms capable of causing disease in SACs. These include:

- *Listeria monocytogenes* – this organism is associated with various neurological diseases (see Chapter 12).
- Fungal organisms – diseases caused by fungi include placentitis and abortion, so particular care should be taken to ensure pregnant animals are kept away from spoilt feed. These fungi are not zoonotic diseases per se, however humans can be directly infected by the spores. The fungi cause an extrinsic allergic alveolitis, otherwise known as 'farmer's lung'. SACs can develop a similar condition.
- *Bacillus licheniformis* – this organism can cause abortions and stillbirths in SACs.

It is therefore important that feedstuffs are stored correctly. Where areas of mould are seen these should be removed and destroyed carefully. This care should also be exercised with mouldy bedding material.

Nutrition

SACs perform better than ruminants when grazing on poor quality pasture as the gastrointestinal tract is slower for particulate matter. On the other hand it is faster for fluids. This may be due to the larger amount of saliva produced in relation to the volume of the stomach. This is considered to be an adaptive response to the coarse, highly lignified vegetable material that SACs originally grazed on the altiplano. Llamas perform better than alpacas. In the Western world SACs are normally maintained at pasture all the year round but with access to shelter not only to escape the sun and insects in the summer, but also to avoid the wind and cold in winter. Most SACs are given additional concentrate feed except when the pasture is very abundant. Because of this, obesity can be a problem in the Western world. This may cause infertility, dystocia and reduced milk yield. Hepatic lipidosis is never seen in animals kept on the Andes. However, it is often seen in other parts of the world.

Outside of South America it is common practice to feed SACs concentrate feed prepared for horses or, even worse, pigs. Clinicians must advise against this practice. Concentrates specially prepared for SACs are now available and should be fed to the manufacturer's recommendations. In fact non-breeding animals can exist totally on good grass. In the winter in the UK or in northern areas of the USA they require conserved forage, e.g. hay. An adult requires approximately one 30 kg bale of hay every 15 days.

Digestibility studies conducted with SACs on conserved forages have suggested higher digestion coefficients in comparison with true ruminants when fed low- or medium-quality diets. SACs are reported to consume less than true ruminants if live weight is taken into account. However, this may not be the case if they are grazed free-range. The myth that SACs are less efficient than sheep at digesting high quality forage has been proven to be false.

SACs require a maximum dry matter intake of 1.8% of body weight daily. This would appear to be low compared to sheep and goats. SACs have a slower rate of passage through the pregastric fermentation, which allows a greater degree of fermentation of the lower-quality cell wall materials and greater generation of available nutrients. This slower rate does reduce the daily intake. To establish a good feeding programme, daily intake amounts are important. Herd owners should be encouraged to weigh amounts of feed that are being fed daily, for several days, to establish how much of each feedstuff is being consumed daily.

Along with the amount being fed, the nutritive value of each feedstuff must be known. Since most of the diet should be forages, forage analysis is critical to establishing a viable feeding programme. Forages will vary greatly with stage of maturity when they are harvested, handling procedures and soil conditions. It is rare that forage will fulfil all of the nutrient requirements for SACs. There are many useful generalizations that may be made, e.g. meadow hays will be low in calcium. However, after the forage analysis has been carried out the clinician can see what is missing and see what needs to be added to complement the forage. In many cases all that is required is the addition of a trace mineral supplement. On the whole the supplement will need to be energy rich, high in calcium, selenium, vitamins D and A and zinc. As a general rule, if more than 0.25 kg for an alpaca or 0.5 kg for a llama is required then better forage should be obtained.

The basic diet if not grass, i.e. in the winter in temperate countries or in the dry season in hot countries, should be quality grass hay, which will contain 8–10% protein. This should be the basis of the diet. Only certain groups of llamas, e.g. weaners and lactating mothers, will need any supplementation. Alpacas will require slightly more protein. This can be given either as concentrates or as lucerne (alfalfa) hay. Otherwise there is no cause for supplementation except in debilitated individuals. The feeding of excessive protein should be avoided in hot climates as this will result in an increase in water loss as urea excretion will require excessive urination, which is to be avoided if there is a danger of heat stress (see Chapter 1). Protein requirements should be met but not exceeded. Mineral supplementation may be required in deficient areas. Periodic blood sampling of groups for selenium, copper, zinc and iron may be useful.

In summary it should be stressed that on the whole except for conditions in South America, the problem of SAC nutrition is one of overfeeding rather than underfeeding.

Patrick Long DVM from Oregon has prepared useful tables (Tables 2.1 and 2.2) for the dietary requirements of llamas and alpacas.

Owners are advised to buy the best hay available, as SACs thrive on fibre rather than concentrates. If quality hay is not available then lucerne should be brought into the diet rather than just increasing the concentrates.

In the UK pet SACs are a particular problem as they tend to be overweight. This leads to hepatic lipidosis. It is difficult to get these animals to lose weight, especially if they are fed in a group and tend to push others away from the food trough. These animals may have to be fed separately.

Body Conditioning Scoring in South American Camelids

The most commonly used body condition score system used in the UK is a 1 to 5 score. In the USA a 1 to 10 score is used. In both systems 1 is very thin. In the UK 5 is obese but obese in the USA is 10. Body condition in SACs is best assessed by palpating the transverse process of the lumbar vertebrae, areas around the shoulders and over the loins. If the ribs are easily palpated, the condition is usually less than half way in both systems, but if the ribs are difficult to feel and if the loin is bulging and slightly soft, the animal is going to be a 3 in the UK or a 6 in the USA. The lateral aspects of the transverse processes of the lumbar vertebrae should not be sharp, but easily palpable. The shoulder should also be palpable with the bones and joint edges not sharp, but appearing to have slight smoothness. As animals gain weight they begin to lay down fat on the brisket, between the hindlegs, and around the perineum. The pelvic bones can be easily felt. An accurate set of scales will also be useful in aiding the practitioner in herd dietary management. In the northern hemisphere SACs naturally gain weight in spring and early summer and tend to lose weight in the late summer, autumn and winter. If animals are weighed at 2-monthly intervals, those adults who do not show this seasonal pattern but continue to gain weight should be monitored and fed accordingly. Where possible, body weights should be evaluated on a yearly basis, and steps taken to prevent continual and possibly insidious body weight changes, which are difficult to observe on a day-to-day basis.

Table 2.1. Alpaca recommendations.

Nutrient	Maintenance	Lactation
Protein	12%	15%
TDN	55–60%	60–65%
Fibre	25%	25%
Calcium	0.6–0.85%	0.6–0.85%
Phosphorus	0.4–0.6%	0.4–0.6%
Selenium	1 mg/45 kg/day	1 mg/45 kg/day
Copper	10–15 ppm	10–15 ppm
Zinc	80 ppm	80 ppm
Vitamin D	2000 IU/day	2000 IU/day
Vitamin E	400 IU/day	400 IU/day

Table 2.2. Llama recommendations.

Nutrient	Maintenance	Lactation
Protein	10%	12%
TDN	50–55%	55–60%
Fibre	25%	25%
Calcium	0.6–0.85%	0.6–0.85%
Phosphorus	0.4–0.6%	0.4–0.6%
Selenium	1 mg/45 kg/day	1 mg/45 kg/day
Copper	10–15 ppm	10–15 ppm
Zinc	80 ppm	80 ppm
Vitamin D	2000 IU/day	2000 IU/day
Vitamin E	400 IU/day	400 IU/day

Feeding During Pregnancy

Feeding prior to mating is very important. The aim is for the female to have a body condition score of 5–6 (US measurement) at mating and maintain this score throughout pregnancy. Ideally this should be checked and recorded monthly throughout pregnancy. What is even more ideal is for the female to be weighed monthly. With constant monitoring, problems can be recognized early. Early disease states can be treated. Stress-induced weight loss, e.g. when individuals are moved into new groups and bullying occurs, can be recognized quickly. Poor feeding during pregnancy will be picked up at these monitoring sessions. Pregnancy toxaemia will be prevented. Early births resulting in weak underweight crias are less likely to occur. Dams in a good nutritional state will produce ample good quality colostrum. This, together with strong crias, will prevent failure of passive transfer of antibodies. Poor nutrition during pregnancy leads to poor milk production. This will result in poor cria growth rates. Obviously, weighing of crias should be encouraged. Poor body condition score at parturition will result in a delay in breeding and poor conception rates. However, SACs are not like cows and body condition scores are not directly related to breeding performance. Practitioners will have a problem advising clients who have overweight females towards the end of pregnancy. These animals will tend to lack appetite and be lethargic. These signs lead to an increased prevalence of pregnancy toxaemia and dystocia problems. If the parturition is due in late summer, heat stress will make things worse. However, practitioners should not advise owners to starve these obese females or the risk of pregnancy toxaemia is even greater. They should be allowed to hold their weight, obviously not allowing any increase. Then hopefully the lactation will bring about natural weight loss. If these animals have problems at parturition resulting in a dead cria, then after the metritis has been cleared up they should be dieted aggressively.

Maiden females also need to be monitored during pregnancy. Obesity is not normally a problem. They need to be 'fit not fat' so that they have a normal parturition and have sufficient milk.

Cria Nutrition

Normal alpaca crias should weigh a minimum of 5.5 kg and llama crias a minimum of 7 kg. Averages are likely to vary but 7 kg for alpaca crias and 9 kg for llama crias would be the norm. Like most newly born animals, crias will lose weight initially, usually 0.25 kg in the first 24 h. This should be replaced in the following 24 h and from then on they should gain between 0.25 kg and 0.5 kg daily. To do this the cria needs to consume 10% of its body weight daily. This should be colostrum in the first 24 h.

Should a cria be too weak to stand, colostrum may be given with a feeding bottle with a small teat. It will only be possible to milk out approximately 30 ml at any one time from a dam. Ideally this should be repeated at hourly intervals for the first 24 h. Prudent owners will draw off colostrum from milky quiet females and store it in the deep freeze. Proprietary lambs' colostrum is available in powder form, which is suitable for crias if half as much again of powdered glucose is added to the colostrum powder. Cow or goat colostrum can also be used, though once again glucose should be added. The milk from SACs has a higher sugar content, i.e. 6.5%, and a lower fat content, i.e. 2.7%, than ruminants. Colostrum from other species has the danger of being a source of disease. The most dangerous likely diseases are Johne's disease and leptospirosis. Only small quantities, i.e. 60 ml, should be offered at one time, ideally every 2 h to crias. Large quantities should be avoided as they will tend to pool in compartment one of the stomach (C1) rather than go straight to compartment three (C3). Obviously if there is no suck reflex the colostrum will have to be given by stomach tube. This is easily accomplished with a lamb stomach tube. As these are not quite long enough they should be pushed down the oesophagus to their full length and the colostrum should be given slowly. Larger stomach tubes, e.g. foal nasogastric tubes, should not be used as they are too large and will damage the oesophagus.

Creep feeding crias that are running with their mothers is hazardous. There are several dangers: crias may get stuck getting into the creep, small mothers may get stuck trying to get into the creep or mothers with their extremely long necks may find a way to eat an excess of creep and get problems with grain overload.

Trace Element Deficiencies

Vitamin D deficiency and hypophosphataemic rickets syndrome

This is a particular problem in the northern hemisphere in autumn-born SACs. In their first winter their growth rate will slow down. They will play less and appear to have stiff backs. They will show an abnormal gait, which has been described as a bunny hop. Angular limb deformities will develop. This condition is said to be more common in dark-coated animals. If tested, these animals will have normal calcium levels but low phosphorus levels. Vitamin D will also be low. It is this low level of vitamin D that is reducing the uptake of phosphorus and causing the rickets. It is thought that in South America in the Andes where there are large amounts of sunlight, SACs have evolved to require less vitamin D in the diet as it is made in the body. Poor levels of sunlight in the autumn and winter in the northern hemisphere do not allow the young SACs to produce their own vitamin D, leading to rickets. The effect of sunlight on reducing the incidence of rickets is less as crias reach a certain age. Therefore it is critical to ensure adequate vitamin D status in crias at a young age and efforts should be concentrated on nutritional means in order to prevent rickets.

The most sensible preventive measure is to increase the vitamin D in the diet. Oral supplementation of vitamin D can be given but this is difficult to administer and so breeders tend to favour monthly injections of vitamin D in the form of an oily solution of vitamins A, D and E. This should start at 2 weeks of age and continue until the spring equinox. The suggested dose of vitamin D is 1000 IU/kg.

Copper deficiency

Copper is an essential constituent of the diet and is required for harvesting of energy from digested feeds and with iron is required in haemoglobin metabolism. It is required for bone, tendon, and cartilage and melanin production. It is also required by the body for protection against certain toxins. Copper is absorbed into the body from the small intestine and stored in the liver. Beta-carotene is required to aid absorption. Copper availability is depressed when there is an increase in molybdenum, sulfur, iron, zinc, cadmium, selenium and calcium in the diet. Lush growth of forages, particularly those raised on alkaline soils, are lower in available copper than hay and legumes. When evaluating the diet for copper adequacy, the practitioner should try to maintain a copper to molybdenum ratio of between 6:1 and 10:1 (ratios of 15:1 have been implicated in copper toxicity; see Chapter 16). Copper deficiency is more likely to occur on improved grass pastures where lime or molybdenum-containing fertilizers have been applied. If copper content of the pasture is less than 5 ppm on a dry matter basis and/or where molybdenum exceeds 1 ppm and/or sulfur exceeds 2000 ppm, copper deficiency may occur. This will cause signs of ataxia, anaemia, depressed immune function, infertility, loss of hair and skin pigments. It will also cause the growth of abnormal bone, connective and tendon tissue, which will cause lameness and poor growth rate. Production of stringy fibre and excess shedding are normally the first signs observed by the owner. Diagnosis is not as straight forward in SACs compared with sheep as plasma copper levels are less reliable. The ultimate measure is a liver biopsy (see Chapter 4).

Iron deficiency

This deficiency is only seen in crias and yet iron is absorbed more efficiently in younger animals than in adults. Vitamin C, citrate, cysteine, histidine and lowered intestinal pH all serve to enhance the absorption of iron while high dietary concentrations of cadmium, calcium, manganese, phosphorus, zinc, phytates, tannins, tetracycline and heavy parasitism all depress iron absorption.

Clinical signs of iron deficiency in crias include poor growth/chronic weight loss, diarrhoea and a non-regenerative microcytic, hypochromic anaemia. A decreased haemoglobin concentration will be indicative of the condition but the ultimate diagnostic tool is a bone marrow biopsy smear.

Crias do not seem to respond to oral supplementation of iron. Parenteral administration of iron dextran is required. The dose of 600 mg of iron as gleptoferron should be divided into three and injected on alternate days as three injections of 1 ml containing 200 mg.

Selenium deficiency

The minimum daily allowance of selenium is 0.1 ppm on a dry matter basis. The Altiplano in South America and certain areas in the UK are known to have low selenium levels. Selenium deficiency is associated with lameness and acute cardiac death of 'white muscle disease' in crias. It also causes infertility, stillbirths and very weak newly born crias. Diagnosis is straight forward with plasma samples to measure glutathione peroxidase. Heparin is the anti-coagulant required (normally a green-topped vaccutainer). Treatment of selenium deficiency involves oral supplementation or parenteral selenium injections.

Zinc deficiency

Absorption of zinc from the small intestine is inhibited by phytase, oxalates, organophosphates and high dietary concentrations of calcium, cadmium, iron and tin. Zinc absorption is enhanced by vitamin C, citrate, histidine and lactose. On average, legumes are better sources of zinc than grasses. Zinc is poorly available from cereals. The main sign observed is usually in 1–2-year-old SACs as papules or dry plaques of alopecia on the ventral abdomen, inner thighs and the bridge of the nose. The lesions initially are erythemic, but become very thick and eventually crack. Biopsies of the affected skin will show parakeratosis. When evaluating such biopsies, the pathologist is reminded that the cellular infiltrate around the arterioles of the dermis, which may appear to be 'suggestive of inflammation', are normal in SACs. Clinicians are reminded that rubber contains zinc and any blood samples in rubber-topped bottles will not indicate any zinc deficiency.

Treatment is simple, with oral supplementation of 1 g of zinc sulfate daily. It should be stressed that this is a very over-diagnosed disease and other causes of the parakeratosis should be investigated.

Metabolic Disease

Hypocalcaemia

In SACs the condition of hypocalcaemia occurs at peak lactation, i.e. 3–4 weeks post parturition. The camelid will be anorexic and will normally go into sternal recumbency. The rectal temperature will be lowered and the movement of compartment one (C1) of the stomach will stop. The condition can be confirmed on a blood serum sample showing the low calcium level. Treatment with intravenous calcium, normally 100 ml of a 20% solution for an alpaca, will effect an improvement but not as rapidly as in sheep and goats. Also this will not be a 'one off' treatment but will need to be repeated daily until the blood calcium levels adjust. The cria should be left with the mother to encourage her recovery. The cria may need some supplementary feeding. Ideally this should be milk drawn from another mother, although there are special milk powders available. If the worst comes to the worst goat's milk can be used. It is important to avoid over feeding or the cria will start to scour. Often full recovery will take 3 or 4 days. Owners should be discouraged from giving any treatment by mouth as there is a considerable danger of inhalation pneumonia unless an orogastric tube is used (see Fig. 2.1).

The ingestion of certain plants that contain oxalates may cause hypocalcaemia in SACs (see Chapter 16).

Hypomagnesaemia

This condition is extremely rare in SACs. Magnesium, which is readily available in most feeds, needs to be ingested daily and be absorbed daily. If the transit time through the bowel is too rapid then insufficient magnesium will be absorbed. Although lush green grass is a very good source of magnesium, it causes a rapid transit time of ingesta through the bowel and so can provoke the condition. If blood levels of magnesium are low then any stress will cause the signs. These are neurological. Sternal recumbency is rapidly followed by lateral recumbency and convulsions. The heart rate is raised and so is the rectal temperature. There is frothing

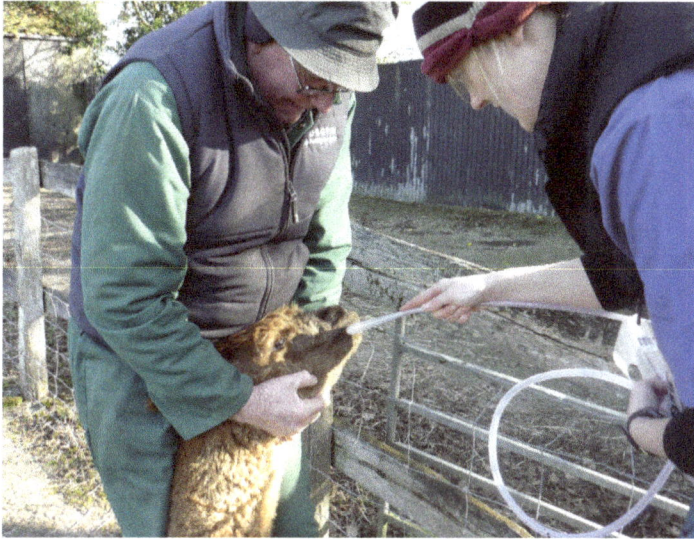

Fig. 2.1. An orogastric tube being used.

at the mouth and rapid eye movement. The legs will paddle. The sex of the animal is not relevant. In temperate climates it is a condition of the spring and autumn. This is due to the likelihood of lush grass at these times and the very changeable weather, which may act as a trigger. Such a situation will not arise for llamas as they will tend to browse as well as graze. Alpacas are principally grazing animals and in the UK are often kept on very lush pastures. However, on the whole SACs do not seem to suffer signs of hypomagnesaemia, probably on account of the slower bowel transit time.

Treatment in SACs is rarely successful if they are convulsing. Although blood magnesium levels can be restored to normal, there is usually irreparable brain damage. Treatment can be attempted. It should consist of a subcutaneous injection of 100 ml of 25% magnesium sulfate. It is important that this drug is given subcutaneously as it will cause death if given intravenously. It is prudent to give other supportive treatment, e.g. a mixture of 20% calcium borogluconate, 5% magnesium hypophosphite and 20% glucose given intravenously, coupled with non-steroid anti-inflammatory drugs (NSAIDs). It should be remembered that these cases are on a knife edge and so any treatment by any route may well cause death.

Hypophosphataemia

This condition, which causes recumbency in cows, does not seem to affect SACs. A deficiency in phosphorus may cause other signs, e.g. generalized lack of calcification of bones and a pica for anything containing phosphorus, like bones. It has been recorded in Australia and South America. However, it is not likely to occur in the UK where real deficiency of phosphorus has not been recorded.

Hyperlipaemia/keto-acidosis

Keto-acidosis in SACs is a complex condition. It can occur at any stage. However, the animals that are most likely to be affected are grossly overweight and then receive a stressful situation, e.g. parturition, a long journey or even husbandry procedures such as shearing, teeth grinding, etc. The animals will immediately become anorexic and will show acute depression. Movement of C1 will cease. The animals are suffering from hyperlipaemia. Fat can be seen in a blood sample. It is vital that the animals are encouraged to eat anything possible. Hand-feeding is useful. Frequent high-energy drenches if given very carefully to avoid inhalation pneumonia are useful. However, ingestion of fibre is important to get movement of C1. Intravenous injections of NSAIDs are useful. If the animal is recumbent, a drip should be set up, initially with normal saline as there is some dehydration and followed by a solution of 5% glucose. All the time every encouragement must be given to the animal to eat. The wall of C3 should be examined by trans-abdominal ultrasound. In this condition oedema of the wall is often seen as a dark line. A small volume of fluid is normal. However, if it is flocculent this may indicate a perforated ulcer. This should be treated accordingly (see Chapter 9).

Pregnancy toxaemia

This is a rare condition in SACs. As in sheep, it occurs in late pregnancy. However, unlike sheep it occurs when there is only a single cria. The aetiology is unclear. It is thought that stress brings about inappetence, which brings on the disease, which is then self-perpetuating. The less the animal eats the worse the condition becomes. Initially, animals appear to be slightly depressed and weak. They then appear to be reluctant to move. They then become ataxic, which will lead to recumbency. There may also be neurological signs. Azotaemia, lipaemia or hyperlipaemia may be shown on a blood sample. There will be an elevated GGT. There will be a ketonuria. The underlying cause needs to be addressed, e.g. parasitism; however, it may be too late, i.e. it may have been caused by transportation or changing of animal groups. Everything must be done to encourage the animal to eat. In severe cases a drip line will need to be established with normal saline, which can then be spiked with glucose and B vitamins. Corticosteroids should not be given as they will abort the fetus, which will result in the death of both fetus and dam. Propylene glycol by mouth is not advisable as there have been reports of toxicity in SACs together with the danger of inhalation pneumonia. Sadly the prognosis for recumbent cases is poor.

Chronic Wasting Disease

Practitioners who are familiar with sheep and goats will have to change their mindsets with SACs. Obviously it is the body condition scores that will need to be examined, as fleeces may deceive the eye. However, it should be remembered that on the whole SACs will feel thinner than sheep or goats.

Practitioners should be on the lookout for tuberculosis with any SAC showing chronic wasting signs. However, there are many other causes that can be ruled out by a careful clinical examination. It should be remembered that Johne's disease in SACs is not usually associated with diarrhoea, neither is chronic liver fluke infection. Lymphosarcoma is the most common tumour seen in SACs. It is usually multicentric. Diagnosis is typically in the terminal stages due to failure to show clear clinical signs earlier. There is often weight loss over a period of months and then lethargy sets in and after showing a reduced appetite the animal becomes rapidly recumbent. Most cases have ascites on abdominal ultrasound. Abdominal masses may be seen to confirm the diagnosis. Peritoneal taps are not helpful as these tumours rarely shed cells. Obviously if the tumour invades the liver, the liver enzymes will be raised. Haemangiosarcomas and adenosarcomas will affect the liver and raise liver enzymes but they are extremely rare.

Liver abscesses are much more common than tumours. There will be a raised white cell count and fibrinogen. The abscess may be visible on ultrasound. Prolonged antibiotic treatment is required, i.e. for 1 month. Liver enzymes may not be markedly affected. On the other hand, with the very rare condition of cholangiohepatitis the liver enzymes will be greatly increased.

3

Examination

Normal Temperature, Pulse and Respiration

The rectal temperature in SACs can vary from 99.0 to 101.0°F (37.4–38.3°C). The thermo-regulatory ability of the neonate is so poor that there can be a much wider range. Although SACs have evolved in harsh cool climates, the insulation ability of their fleece allows a certain tolerance to the sort of heat extremes encountered in the UK and other countries outside of South America where SACs are kept, and the fleece-free underside acts as an area for heat dissipation.

Resting heart rate of an adult SAC varies from 60 to 90/min and is best ascertained by auscultation caudal to the triceps in the fleece-free area medial to the elbow. Very few respiratory sounds will be heard either here or anywhere else unless there is some pathology. Borborygmi are much quieter than in sheep and goats, mostly coming from the major fermentation chamber, C1. This first compartment contracts between 3 and 5 times/min depending on feeding.

Normal Neonates

These animals are particularly precious as they are valuable not only financially but also often emotionally. They have had a long gestation period. History of previous offspring is always important, which should include pregnancy problems, parturition problems and post-parturition problems. It should also include an enquiry for any congenital defects. This is particularly relevant if the previous sire was the same. Also it is important to enquire whether the previous cria grew as well as it was expected to do. The actual rebreeding history of the dam since the last parturition is relevant. Enquires should be made to find out if the afterbirth was retained and whether there was any vulva tearing or any vaginal discharge. It is relevant whether the dam bred successfully within 30 days of parturition or whether the dam was thought to be pregnant and then found to be empty and then re-served.

Obviously some of these enquiries are not applicable to a maiden. However, it would be of interest whether it was difficult to get the maiden pregnant and also the mothering ability of the maiden's dam.

Of course the full history of the dam may be relevant. It would be important to know if she suffered heat stress or any medical condition, e.g. colic, parasitism, diarrhoea or constipation, or if she has had previous surgery, e.g. a laparotomy or Caesarean section, or if she has had any problems with her husbandry, e.g. transport, showing or general mixing in groups. Her body condition score is relevant.

© Graham R. Duncanson 2023. *Veterinary Treatment of Llamas and Alpacas*, 2nd Edition (G.R. Duncanson)
DOI: 10.1079/9781800623576.0003

The recent pregnancy history and gestation length will be relevant. It should be remembered that llamas on average have a longer gestation period by 10 days compared with alpacas. SACs are also capable of an embryonal diapause, i.e. the fetus can appear to hibernate in the uterus with an extension of gestation length, which is absolutely normal and of no detriment to mother or offspring. Neonatal care will be influenced by the delivery whether it was normal or prolonged. It will also be influenced by the birth weight of the cria. Fat mothers tend not only to have crias with lower birth weights but also tend to have more prolonged labour.

Normal gestation lengths are quite variable. The range is from 320 to 360 days. However, a premature or dysmature cria can be born at 350 days. A normal cria should be lively and on its feet within 1 h and drinking within 4 h. Alpaca crias should be in excess of 6 kg and llama crias in excess of 8 kg. Crias should have passed their meconium within 8 h. This is aided by colostrum intake. Their rectal temperature should be in excess of 98°F (37°C). Their ear tips should be straight and their incisors should be felt under the mucosa or already erupted.

A normal cria may lose a few hundred grams in the first 24 h. However, they should gain at least 1 kg in the first week. Normal crias will have doubled their birth weight within 1 month.

It is vital to maintain the maternal bond and so all fussing should be avoided. There should be no interference if there is no problem.

When carrying out a cria check:

- Check the sex;
- Check the anus;
- Dress the navel and check for an umbilical hernia;
- Weigh cria on bathroom scales;
- Check suck reflex;
- Check teeth.

The following characteristics are evidence of prematurity:

- A truly short gestation;
- Low birth weight;
- Soft silky hair;
- Round domed head;
- Unerupted incisors;
- Hoof slippers do not readily peel off;

- Tendon laxity;
- Abnormal vigour (either very lifeless or overactive);
- Droopy ears;
- Congenital defects.

Later signs may also be indicators:

- Failure to try to get up;
- Lying on the side rather than the 'kush' position;
- Abnormal mucous membranes. They should be pink, not bright red indicating septicaemia, or blue indicating heart failure, or purple indicating toxaemia;
- Cold ears;
- Mouth breathing;
- Erratic heartbeat and rate;
- No evidence of sucking;
- No evidence of the passing of the meconium;
- No evidence of urination;
- Broken off short umbilicus;
- Dull eye;
- Rectal temperature below 98°F (37°C).

The more of these signs that are present, the more serious is the problem. Clinicians should be slightly mindful of economic considerations but of course their first consideration must be welfare. Ideally a total blood count (TBC) and biochemistry should be taken, but a packed cell volume (PCV) and a total protein will be very helpful and probably sufficient. An initial blood glucose to compare with a repeat sample after 24 h is very helpful. A measurement of passive transfer of IgG is vital (see Chapter 4) and appropriate plasma transfusion may be required.

The following tests may be helpful if available and economically feasible:

- Arterial blood gas analysis;
- Blood culture;
- Urinalysis;
- Cerebrospinal fluid (CSF) analysis and culture;
- Abdominal fluid analysis and culture;
- Radiographs.

Initial treatments will need to include the following if appropriate:

- Oxygen via nasal insufflation (pure oxygen should not be given for more than 30 min);
- Broad spectrum antibiotics;

- Oral colostrum;
- Plasma intravenously or intraperitoneally;
- Fluids;
- Regular weighing.

If there is no sucking reflex, in a low 'tech' situation goat's colostrum may be given, warmed to blood heat, via a stomach tube. Crias require 5% of body weight in the first 12 h. Obviously the dam's four teats should be checked for patency. Milking dams is a real challenge as 500 ml of colostrum is required.

Cria rejection is rare. It is more common in maidens particularly if their cria is weak. It is also more common after Caesarean section. Failure to pass the placenta may make mothers reluctant to allow the cria to suck.

Emergency intervention is required if a cria is less than 5.5 kg in weight or has a rectal temperature of less than 97°F (36°C). Intervention is required if the cria is lying on its side, not in the 'kush' position, and has laboured breathing. Treatment should be to warm the cria but keeping it with its mother. Infra-red lamps can be a fire risk so hot water bottles are preferable. An intravenous drip line should be set up so plasma can be given (see Chapter 11). If a drip line is not possible the plasma can be given intraperitoneally.

Warm glucose can be given as an enema. A dose of 20 ml of 20% glucose should be given. This can be repeated in 30 min. Giving colostrum is difficult; it is not only difficult to collect but also rarely is it given in sufficient quantities. If the cria is below 97°F (36°C) no IgG will be absorbed. Equally if the cria is over 24 h old there will be little absorption. Cow and goat colostrum has been tried with varying results, with the added danger of spreading diseases between species. Remember a normal cria requires in excess of 0.5 l of good colostrum within the first 24 h of life.

Examination of the Head of Neonatal Crias

Mild ectropion of the lower eyelid can be normal and should not be confused with either congenital or acquired ectropion. The whole eye should be examined. There will be seen a large dorsal and a small ventral granula iridica nigrum of unknown function but of no clinical significance. Occasionally an absence of pigment will be observed. It will be seen that there is no fovea or tapetum but a pronounced vascular pattern to the retina. The nasolachrymal duct will be easily seen at its origin from the medial canthus. Its termination will be observed within the nares on the cutaneous side of the mucocutaneous border, 1 cm dorsal to the floor of the ventral meatus on the lateral wall over the ridge formed by the pre-maxilla.

The inside of the ears cannot be examined easily without sedation. However, ear problems are extremely rare. In older crias ear infections can often produce a secondary facial paralysis, and laceration of the pinna can be a common sequel of fighting. The canines and the incisors can be examined by curling back the lips (see Chapter 9). Malocclusion is common. Capillary refill can be determined using areas of non-pigmented gingival mucosa.

Examination of Adults

Animals may have to be examined for various different purposes. These may include for insurance, for purchase, for entry into another country or for fibre value. The forms shown in Appendices 3.1–3.3 will be helpful for practitioners to act as an aid to memory.

Appendix 3.1. Physical Examination Screening Checklist for South American Camelids

(Disqualifying traits are indicated by asterisks)
Name of Import _____ Date of inspection _____
Lot No. _____ Ear Tag No. _____ Microchip No. _____ Date of Birth _____
Male _____ Female _____ Age _____ _____

Head   Disqualifying trait present? Yes ___ No___
Normal (Y / N)
Face: wry face___ slight (<2°) ___, moderate (between 2° & 5°)* ___, severe (>5°)* ___
Nostrils: air movement in both nostrils ___
Ears: long___, short___, gopher* ___, frostbitten___, curled* ___
Eyes: entropian* ___, ectropion ___, laceration ___, tearing (evidence of blocked tear ducts) ___,
corneal opacity ___, cataract* ___, dilated pupil ___, constricted pupil___, evidence of blindness*
___, persistent papillary membrane* ___
Teeth: superior brachygnathism* (undershot jaw, with central incisors protruding more than 0.3 cm
beyond the dental pad)___ or inferior brachygnathism* (parrot mouth, overshot jaw, with dental pad
protruding more than 0.3 cm beyond the lower incisors) ___, retained deciduous incisors ___,
canine teeth erupted ___
Comments: _____

Neck and Body   Disqualifying trait present? Yes___ No___
Normal (Y / N)
Throat latch: swelling ___
Cervical spine: symmetrical___, scoliosis* ___
Movement of neck
Thoracic and lumbar spine: scoliosis* ___, lordosis* ___, kyphosis* ___
Tail: twisted* ___ (must be straight, no bends or kinks)
Comments: _____

Front limbs   Disqualifying trait present? Yes___ No___
Normal (Y / N)
Front view: base wide ___, base narrow ___, carpal valgus: slight (<5°) ___, moderate (between 5°
and10°) ___, severe* (>10°) ___; bowed out at carpus ___, splay footed ___, pigeontoed ___, polydactyly* ___, syndactyly* ___
Side view: camped forward ___, camped behind ___; angulation: OK ___, too straight ___, too flexed
___; buck kneed ___; calf kneed: slight (<175°) ___, moderate (170–175°) ___, severe*(<165°) ___;
pastern angles: cocked ankle* (>90°) ___, down in the fetlock* (<30°) ___
Comments: _____

Rear limbs   Disqualifying trait present? Yes___ No___
Normal (Y / N)
Rear view: base wide ___, base narrow ___, cow-hocked: slight (<5°) ___, moderate (between 5° and
10°) ___, severe *(>10°) ___; bowed out at hock ___, splay footed ___, pigeon toed ___, polydactyly*
___, syndactyly* ___
Side view: camped forward ___, camped rearward ___; angulation: post legged ___, too much flexion
___, sickle hocked: slight (hock angle <135°) ___, moderate (hock angle 135–125°) ___, severe*
(hock angle <125°) ___; cocked ankle* (>90°) ___, down in the fetlock* (<30°) ___, luxating patellas* ___
Comments: _____

Reproductive   Disqualifying trait present? Yes___ No___
Normal (Y / N)
Male
___Testicles: both testicles not in scrotum* ___, cryptorchid* (one testicle) ___; size* (length>3 cm)
___; consistency*: hard ___, too soft ___; scrotal oedema___
Female
Position of vulva
Clitoris enlarged* (evidence of intersex)
Comments: _____

Cardiovascular   Disqualifying trait present? Yes___ No___
Normal (Y / N)
Heart: murmur* ___
Comments: _____

Miscellaneous defects   Disqualifying trait present? Yes___ No___
Normal (Y / N)
Teats: Must have normal anatomical placement of not more than, nor less than, 4 normal teats*
Hernias: umbilical* (>1 cm) ___, scrotal* ___
Toenails: elongated ___, curled ___, abnormal horn ___
Other defects: Screening panel members are obligated to report any other serious defects that are
present and that should, in the veterinarian's professional opinion, result in disqualification.
Comments: _____

Having conducted an examination of this alpaca, the undersigned verifies that the animal is
[ ] Disqualified for the above-noted defect(s).
[ ] found to be free of the listed defects within the limitations of this field examination done without
laboratory assistance. This verification does not constitute a guarantee that the animal is free from all
congenital or genetic defects.
Signature: _____ Date: _____
Signature: _____ Date: _____

[A second signature is generally necessary only for disqualification.]

Appendix 3.2. Alpaca Phenotype Characteristics Evaluation Form

A total of 55 or 60 points is available on this portion of the evaluation. An alpaca receiving a combined (phenotype and fibre) score of 80 points will be accepted for registration if it otherwise qualifies.

Name of Import _____ Date _____
Height (32 in (80 cm) @ withers Minimum) _____ Weight (105 lb (48 kg) Minimum) _____
Colour _____ Ear Tag _____ Microchip _____ Male _____ Female _____

Please circle the appropriate score, deduct total faults for each section from maximum points, and record points scored.

CHARACTERISTIC		POINTS SCORED
1. Shape of Head, Muzzle and Ear	**10 points maximum**	_____
a. Head and Muzzle		
1. Normal	0	
2. Llama like	−10	
3. Moderately large	−2	
4. Fragile face or roman nose	−2	
Scored on degree of fault		
b. Ear		
1. Normal, spear shaped	0	
2. Asymmetric spear	−2	
3. Rounded	−2	
4. Banana shaped	−15	
5. Pancake ear or other anomalies	−15	
2. Body Score	**15 points maximum**	_____
a. Excessive thinness (emaciated)	−20	
b. Thin	0	
c. Optimum	0	
d. Somewhat overweight	0	
e. Obese	−15	
3. Conformation and Balance	**15 points maximum**	_____
a. Leg conformation		
1. Correct leg conformation	0	
2. Buck kneed or knee sprung		
• Moderate	−5 (per front leg)	
• Normal	0	
3. Calf kneed or sheep kneed		
• Moderate	−7 (per front leg)	
• Normal	0	
4. Sickle hocked		
• Mild	−3	
• Moderate	−10	
5. Cocked ankle		
• Present	−20	
• Normal	0	
6. Down on the pasterns		
• Present	−5 (per pastern, possible −20)	
• Normal	0	
7. Post legged in rear or straight legged in front		

CHARACTERISTIC   POINTS SCORED

    • Present front   −2
    • Present back   −5
    • Normal   0
  8. Front view
    • Knocked kneed
      Mild   −3
      Moderate   −10
    • Pigeon toed   −5
    • Base narrow   −3
    • Base wide   −3
    • Bow legged   −3
    • Normal   0
  9. Rear view
    • Cow hocked
      Mild   −3
      Moderate   −10
    • Pigeon toed   −5
    • Bow legged   −3
    • Base narrow   −3
    • Normal   0
 b. Balance or correct proportion of
  legs, body and neck
  1. Normal   0
  2. Long legged   −5
  3. Short legged   −5
  4. Short neck
    • Out of proportion   −5
    • Normal   0
  5. Long neck
    • Out of proportion   −5
    • Normal   0
  6. Tail set
    • Normal   0
    • High (llama like)   −5
  7. Sway backed or hump backed
    • Normal   0
    • Abnormal   −5
  8. Locomotion
    • Normal   0
    • Excessive winging   −7
    • Crossing mid-line   −7

Fleece Density (Huacaya)   **15/20 points maximum** _____
 a. Light fleece   −10
 b. Average   −3
 c. Dense   0
 d. Very dense   +5

Lustre and Curl (Suri)   **15 points maximum**   _____
 a. Absence of lustre   −7
 b. Absence of curl   −8

TOTAL POINTS of 55 or 60 _____ (60 points possible with very dense fleece)
Pheno Screener Signature_____ Date_____
Pheno Screener Signature_____ Date_____

Fibre Characteristics Evaluation Form
The points for fibre on this form are the results of a sample taken by the screener.
The tests are done by Yocom-McColl Testing Laboratories.
The points are determined by Yocom-McColl according to a computer program developed
exclusively for the Alpaca registry.

CHARACTERISTIC	POINTS AVAILABLE	POINTS SCORED
Huacaya fibre characteristics		
a. Micron count (deduct 10 points or fraction thereof for every micro over the 26-micron maximum)	15	_____
b. Standard deviation (deduct 5 points or fraction thereof for every 0.5 micron over maximum)	15	
17 or less max.std. deviation = 3.5		
17.1–19 max.std. deviation = 4.0		
19.1–21 max.std. deviation = 4.5		
21.1–23 max.std. deviation = 5.0		
23.1 and up max.std. deviation = 5.5		
c. % of fibre over 30 microns (deduct 5 points for every % point in excess of 5% of fleece – i.e. 7% of fleece over 30 microns would result in loss of 10 points)	15	
Suri fibre characteristics		
a. Micron count (deduct 10 points or fraction thereof for every micro over the 27-micron maximum)	15	
b. Standard deviation (deduct 5 points or fraction thereof for every 0.5 micron over maximum)	15	
17 or less max.std. deviation = 3.5		
17.1–19 max.std. deviation = 4.0		
19.1–21 max.std. deviation = 4.5		
21.1–23 max.std. deviation = 5.0		
23.1 and up max.std. deviation = 5.5		
c. % of fibre over 30 microns (deduct 5 points for every % point in excess of 5% of fleece)	15	
Total Points	45	

Signed: _____   Date: _____

Appendix 3.3. Certificate of Camelid Veterinary Examination

For alpacas aged 60 days or over
Date: _____
Owner: _____ Address: _____
_____
Animal I.D.: Colour: _____
Ear Tag: _____ Microchip No: _____
Sex: _____ D.O.B.: _____ (or) Estimate of Age: _____
This is to certify that I _____, have today examined the animal described above,
and my opinion at the time of examination is as follows:

DETAILS OF EXAMINATION

1. Limbs and Locomotion:
    Lameness: YES/NO   Comment: _____
    Limb deformities: YES/NO   Comment: _____
    Feet/Cleats/Pads: Normal/Abnormal   Comment: _____
    Joints: Normal/Abnormal   Comment: _____
2. Lymph Glands:
    Normal /Abnormal   Comment: _____
3. Condition:
    Poor/Lean/Good/Overweight
    (*Note*: Lean condition in camelids is not necessarily abnormal)
4. Eyes:
    Visual Assessment: Normal/Abnormal   Comment: _____
    Examination with   YES/NO
    magnification in a dark area:
    Cornea: Normal/Abnormal   Comment: _____
    Lens cataracts observed: YES/NO
    Persistent papillary membrane: YES/NO
    Further observations: _____
5. Teeth:
    Are incisors level with hard pad: YES/NO
    Are incisors Normal/   If Undershot or Overshot, state by how much e.g. < or >
    Undershot/Overshot   5mm............
    Number of incisors present: _____
    Structure of incisors: Very good/Good/Poor
6. Mandible Palpation: Normal/Abnormal   Comment: _____
7. Cardiovascular System   Normal/Abnormal   Comment: _____
    Auscultation:
8. Respiratory System   Normal/Abnormal   Comment: _____
    Examination:
9. A) Male
    Both Testicles present: YES/NO
    Measurement: Left: Length: _____ cm   Width: _____cm
                                       Right: Length: _____ cm   Width: _____cm
    (*Note*: Average length 4 cm, width 3 cm in an adult Alpaca at approximately 3 years of age.)
    Penis examined: YES/NO   Normal/Abnormal
    (Note: The prepuce can be adhered to the penis up to 2 to 3 years of age in some males. Normal
    finding.)

B) Female   External genitalia and   Normal/Abnormal
                             mammary glands:
10. Comments
    Other comments / detected abnormalities / or relevant information regarding examination:

    _____
    _____
    _____ Signed: _____
    Address: _____ Print name _____
    _____ Qualifications _____

                      THIS SECTION TO BE COMPLETED BY OWNER

1. **Breeding history:** _____
2. **Female – History of Dystocia:**   **YES/NO**
   Last mating recorded: _____
   Tests done to support pregnancy status and dates: _____
   _____

3. **a) Vaccination History**
   Last reported date of vaccine:_ _____
   Vaccine used: _____
   b) Worming History
   Last herd worm egg count: _____
   Including liver fluke examination: YES/NO   Present/Absent
   Including coccidian examination: YES/NO   Present/Absent
   Last date of worming and product used: _____
   Signed _____ Date _____
   PRINT NAME _____

4

Sample Taking and Simple Diagnostic Tests

Introduction

Many textbooks assume that the parameters for samples are the same the world over. This is not necessarily very helpful. This chapter will give a very broad range so that the reader can adapt this book by adding narrower ranges for the environment of the individual's practice and from the laboratory available. The term 'reference range' is now widely used, rather than normal range. Classically a normal animal is said to be within 95% of the normal range. By definition 5% of normal animals will not appear to be normal. Thus if 20 tests are carried out every animal is likely to have one value outside of the normal range. Therefore there is a strong argument for only carrying out specific tests for the parameters in which the clinician is particularly interested. Laboratories on the whole do not like this arrangement as they favour a blanket approach, which they find easier and cheaper. Clinicians are urged therefore to work closely with their particular laboratory so that a compromise regarding cost and relevance is reached.

The author is well aware that getting samples to laboratories will not be easy or quick in many parts of the world. High temperatures are likely to be a problem. The logistics should be considered with the laboratory. Fresh samples are likely to be the most difficult, so swabs for bacteriology in transport medium should be taken.

Bacteria can be plated out and grown in the field. Only then can they be submitted for identification. Equally smears can be made and microscopic evaluation can be made in the field after appropriate staining. These slides then can easily be referred to a more experienced pathologist. Antibiotic sensitivity testing can well be carried out in the field. Relevant antibiotic testing discs can be used. There is little point in knowing the sensitivity of an isolated organism to an antibiotic that is not available or not useful in SACs. Serum samples after centrifugation can be submitted rather than whole blood. Packed cell volumes (PCVs) can be measured easily with a bench hand-driven centrifuge. Thick and thin blood smears can be used to look for protozoal infections. Dung samples can be examined for bowel worms, lungworms and liver fluke eggs. Coccidia oocysts can be included in this screening. Their size can be evaluated, which is particularly important in SACs (see Chapter 9). Fungi can also be grown. To help, practitioners can submit photographs of post-mortems to referral pathologists. If e-mail is available this can be carried out throughout the world. Obviously histological samples will be extremely helpful in tropical climates, as they will withstand higher temperatures. Care should be taken when packing these, as any contamination from the formalin on to bacteriological samples will be disastrous. Vital signs will vary from climate to climate like normal

© Graham R. Duncanson 2023. *Veterinary Treatment of Llamas and Alpacas,* 2nd Edition
(G.R. Duncanson)
DOI: 10.1079/9781800623576.0004

values and will show a similar bell-shaped distribution curve. Clinicians will obviously routinely carry out a full clinical examination. They will build up their own range of normal values. Experience will show how the climate variations in temperature, air movement and humidity will affect these values. Naturally the physical attributes of the SAC will have a marked effect, for example type, age, gender, pregnancy, etc. The state of the individual, e.g. stressed, recently transported, etc., will cause variation.

Collecting Blood Samples

When collecting blood samples it is important to collect into the right anticoagulant for the type of analysis required. The correct volume of blood for the amount of anticoagulant in the bottle is also important. Blood should be collected from the jugular vein with as little excitement as possible, although this may be difficult with certain individuals. Needles and syringes must be clean and not contaminated with medicines. It should be remembered that the carotid artery lies just deep to the jugular in the caudal aspect of the neck in SACs so this area should be avoided, i.e. the jugular should be entered in the neck nearer to the head. Ideally, less experienced practitioners should blood sample

SACs on the right hand side to lessen the danger of damaging the oesophagus (see Fig. 4.1). For haematological samples the anticoagulant required is EDTA (these bottles often come with a lilac-coloured stopper). Haematological samples will give measures of the haemoglobin and the number of red blood cells. It should be remembered that if a haematocrit tube is not filled from the top of the sample immediately before it is allowed to stand the haematocrit will have a lower reading, i.e. there will seem to be fewer red blood cells in the sample than in reality. Anaemia may then be misdiagnosed. Even in profound cases of anaemia, normoblasts are seen very rarely in the peripheral blood. The number of platelets will be reported. The total number of white blood cells will be given, which is then broken down into the total number of neutrophils, eosinophils, basophils, lymphocytes and monocytes. These can be shown as a percentage, but this may be misleading. Total numbers are a better figure to be studied.

Normal Haematological Values

Erythrocyte parameters

The function of red blood cells (RBCs) is to carry oxygen to the tissues at pressures sufficient to

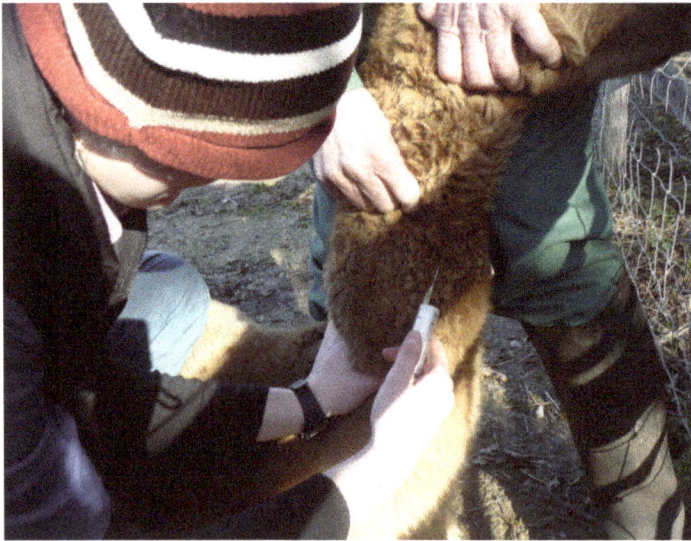

Fig. 4.1. Taking a blood sample from a SAC.

permit rapid diffusion of oxygen. This is particularly important for SACs in the Andes. The carrier molecule for oxygen is haemoglobin. This is a complex molecule, formed of four haem units attached to four globins. Iron is added in the last step by the ferrochelatase enzyme. Interference with the normal production of haem or globin leads to anaemia. Causes include copper or iron deficiency and lead poisoning. In the healthy animal, red cell mass, and thus oxygen-carrying capacity, remains constant. Mature RBCs have a finite lifespan; their production and destruction must be carefully balanced, or disease occurs. However, if animals are moved to higher altitudes the red cell mass will increase over a period of 3 weeks. This is a normal physiological process. Pulmonary hypertensive heart disease, often called 'high-mountain disease' (HMD) is recorded in cattle but not in SACs.

Erythropoiesis is regulated by erythropoietin, which increases in the presence of hypoxia and regulates RBC production. In SACs, the kidney is both the sensor organ and the major site of erythropoietin production, so chronic renal failure is associated with anaemia. Erythropoietin acts on the marrow in concert with other humoral mediators to increase the numbers of stem cells entering RBC production, to shorten maturation time, and to cause early release of reticulocytes. Another factor that affects erythropoiesis is the supply of nutrients, e.g. iron, folic acid and vitamin B12. Chronic debilitating diseases and endocrine disorders, e.g. hypothyroidism or hyperoestrogenism, will suppress erythropoiesis.

A decreased RBC mass (i.e. anaemia) may be caused by direct blood loss, haemolysis or decreased production. In acute blood loss, mortality is usually related to loss of circulating volume, rather than actual loss of RBCs. Iron is the limiting factor in chronic blood loss. Haemolysis may be caused by toxins, infectious agents or congenital abnormalities. Decreased RBC production is very rarely a primary bone marrow disease in SACs. It is much more commonly seen from other causes, e.g. renal failure, toxins or veterinary drugs.

SACs have developed at high altitudes, therefore they have high haemoglobin values. SACs have small ellipsoid erythrocytes, which circulate in larger numbers. This results in a lower PCV. The ellipsoid RBCs in SACs orientate with the long axis in the direction of the blood flow. This makes it possible to traverse small capillaries. Thus there are fewer problems of haemoconcentration when the viscosity of the blood increases during dehydration. This is helpful to the SAC living at altitude. The normal mean corpuscular volume (MCV) of SACs is low because of the smaller erythrocyte size. Normal haemoglobin levels in SACs are high and the PCV is low, so the mean corpuscular haemoglobin concentration (MCHC), which measures the ratio of the weight of haemoglobin to the total volume of the erythrocytes, is high. Normal mean corpuscular haemoglobin (MCH) values in SACs are low as their erythrocytes are small, as seen in Table 4.1.

Leucocyte parameters

The leucocytes consist of the granulocytes (neutrophils, eosinophils and basophils) and the agranulocytes (lymphocytes and monocytes). Although they are traditionally counted by determining each as a percentage of the total leucocyte white blood cells (WBCs) population, meaningful interpretation requires that the absolute number of each type be calculated by multiplying the total white cell count by the fraction attributable to the individual cell type. An increased percentage that is due to an absolute decrease in another cell type is not an increase at all.

Leucocytosis is an increase in the total number of circulating WBCs; leucopoenia is a decrease. Changes in WBC counts and morphologic appearance of various leucocytes are evaluated by comparison with reference ranges for each of the three species. The leucocyte count is higher in SACs. In neonates the total WBC count is more variable and often higher than in adults.

Unsegmented neutrophils do not normally appear in peripheral blood. If they are reported it is an indication of a shift to the right, i.e. their presence indicates that the neutrophils are young and therefore there is an extra usage of neutrophils. This is likely to be a bacterial infection.

The granulocytes are produced in the bone marrow from the myeloblasts. Neutrophils are the most numerous and in the peripheral blood are normally mature, i.e. segmented. Morphological changes in neutrophils cytoplasm, including toxic

Table 4.1. The haematological parameters of adult SACs in the UK.

Parameter	Normal
Erythrocytes × 10^9/l	13.8
Size (μm)	3.2 × 6.5
Lifespan in days	60–225
Haemoglobin (Hb) (g/dl)	15.5
PCV (%)	25–46.5
MCV (fl/cell)	26
MCH (pg/cell)	11.2
MCHC (g/dl)	43
Leucocytes/μl	16,200
Granulocyte/agranulocyte ratio	1.54

granulation, may occur during systemic bacterial infections or severe inflammation and are referred to as toxic changes. Although all circulating WBCs are exposed to the same systemic diseases, only neutrophils are evaluated for toxic changes. Toxic change is graded subjectively as mild, moderate or marked, based on the number of affected neutrophils and the severity of toxic change. Clinical significance is reflected by the type of toxic change and its severity. Toxic granulation is identified by the presence of pink to purple intracytoplasmic granules within neutrophils; these granules represent primary granules of the neutrophils that have retained their staining affinity. Diffuse cytoplasmic basophilia and cytoplasmic vacuolation frequently occur together. The cytoplasmic basophilia is due to persistent ribosomes, and the cytoplasmic vacuolation possibly due to autodigestion of the cell.

The magnitude of neutrophilia induced by inflammation is a function of the size of the bone marrow storage pool of granulocytes, hyperplastia of the marrow, and rate of WBC migration into the tissues. The storage pool is quite large in SACs. Neutrophilia, often the cause of leucocytosis, generally characterizes bacterial infections and conditions associated with extensive tissue necrosis, including burns, trauma, extensive surgery and neoplasia. Extreme leucocytosis is seen in blood-borne protozoal infections and closed cavity infections, e.g. abscesses. The wall of these inhibits the migration of neutrophils into the site of infection, but does not impair the release of leucocyte chemotactic substances. The net effect is a high peripheral neutrophils count, which often includes an increased number of band neutrophils (regenerative left shift).

Eosinophils contain enzymes that modulate products of mast cells or basophils released in response to immunoglobulin E (IgE) stimulation. For example, histamine released by basophils or mast cells is modulated by histaminases in eosinophils. The cytoplasmic granules of eosinophils contain proteins that are involved in parasite killing. Eosinophilia is induced by substances that promote allergic responses and hypersensitivity (e.g. histamine and allied substances) and by IgE. Eosinophils increase in response to parasitic infections, especially those that involve tissue migration, due to the contact of parasite chitin with host tissues. Eosinophilia also may occur with inflammation of the gastrointestinal (GI), urogenital, or respiratory tracts, or of the skin.

On the whole the eosinophil counts are high in SACs. However, it should be noted that it is easy to confuse the eosinophils of SACs with the neutrophils. Careful attention to detail should be taken when counting is being carried out manually. If electronic counting is carried out there may well be some strange results. Usually the number of eosinophils will appear high as a percentage of the total number of granulocytes. If in any doubt the sample should be recounted manually. Eosinopaenia is commonly reported with corticosteroid-induced (stress) conditions.

Basophils are rare in SACs. A basopenia has no diagnostic significance. The granules in basophils contain histamine and heparin, as well as mucopolysaccharides. Although basophils and mast cells have similar functions and enzymatic contents, basophils do not become mast cells and there is no proof of a common precursor cell.

Lymphocytes originate from a marrow stem cell and mature in lymph nodes, spleen and associated peripheral lymphoid tissues. Mature lymphocytes consist of two subpopulations, B cells and T cells. B cells are the precursor of plasma cells and produce antibodies for humoral immunity. T cells engage in cellular immunity. A lymphocyte in tissue may return to the vascular bed and recirculate. Some lymphocytes are long-lived compared with other WBCs and may survive weeks to years. Care should be taken when evaluating a peripheral lymphocytosis as it may be physiological. However, it may be as a result of immune stimulation associated with chronic inflammation. Lymphopenia is a common finding. It is commonly associated with stress or viral disease. However, clinicians should be aware that the administration of corticosteroids will cause a lymphopenia.

Monocytes are formed in the bone marrow and enter the peripheral blood for a day and then exit into the tissues. They tend to be fixed or migrate to sites of inflammation. Monocytosis is associated with chronic inflammation and when there are bacteria in the blood stream, e.g. in an endocarditis. Granulomatous and fungal conditions will also cause a monocytosis. Occasionally there will be a monocytopenia; however, it is of no diagnostic significance.

The ratio of granulocytes to agranulocytes is high in SACs and the response to a bacterial infection is also high.

High neutrophils and protein concentration are indicators for surgery in colic cases. The only differential would be a peritonitis, which should give a high rectal temperature.

Indications for a Complete Blood Count

1. Discolouration of mucous membranes:
   - Pale;
   - Icterus.
2. Signs of sepsis:
   - Injected mucous membranes;
   - Congested mucous membranes;
   - Cold extremities;

- Depression;
- Unable to suckle (crias);
- Abnormal behaviour (crias).
3. Suspicion of gastric compartmental ulcers:
   - Cranial abdominal pain on palpation;
   - Melena;
   - Faecal occult blood;
   - Anorexia;
   - Vague colic signs.
4. Lymphadenopathy.

Questions asked from a complete blood count

1. Is there anaemia – if so what type? (see Table 4.2)
2. Is there inflammation? (see Table 4.3)
3. Is there infection? (see Table 4.2)
4. Are there any changes within the leucocyte population that can guide antimicrobial decisions, e.g. lymphocytosis, neutrophilia or band neutrophilia?
5. Are there any reasons to do further tests, e.g. fibrinogen, haptoglobin, biochemistry (particularly iron concentrations? (see Table 4.4)

Collection

When using vacutainers it is important to take a sufficient sample (anticoagulant:blood ratio). If multiple tubes are being collected the order of collection should be: sodium citrate (light blue top), plain (red top), lithium heparin (green top), EDTA (purple top), sodium fluoride (grey top).

Table 4.2. Blood loss.

Disease	RBC parameters	Type of anaemia	Comments
Mycoplasma haemolamae	PCV 23%	Signs of regeneration Macrocytic hypochromic Reticulcytosis	In some cases aclinical but carrier animals do not have remarkably different PCV/HB/RBC
Fasciola hepatica	Low PCV, RBC, Hb (total protein)	Macrocytic hypochromic Reticulcytosis	Increased liver enzymes
Haemonchos contortus	Low PCV, RBC, Hb (total protein)	Signs of regeneration	Associated very high faecal egg count (high parasitic fecundity)
Acute haemorrhage	Normal PCV (Low total protein)	Signs of regeneration	

Table 4.3. Reduced or defective erythropoiesis.

Disease	RBC parameters	Type of anaemia	Comments
Iron deficiency	Low PVC	Microcytosis Hypochromic	Low serum Fe, low sulfur sat transferrin, lower total blood count
Chronic disease/ inflammation	Low PCV (normal total protein)	Normochromic Normocytic	
Aplastic anaemia	Low PCV (normal total protein)		Pancytopaenia (thrombocytopaenia, leucopaenia)
Kidney disease	Low PCV (low total protein (Albumen))		Normal to higher neutrophil/platelet counts (uraemia + hypoalbuminaemia)

Table 4.4. Accelerated erythrocyte destruction.

Disease	RBC parameter	Type of anaemia	Comments
Haemolytic anaemia (red maple, copper and nitrate toxicity)	Low PCV (normal total protein)	Reticulocytosis is seen in Haemolytic anaemia Hyperchromasia is a sign seen in toxicities Heinz bodies, parasites, spherocytes, poikilocytes are all seen in various haemolytic anaemias caused by other causes	Haemoglobineamia (red plasma) Haemoglobinuria Hyperbiliruminaemia (icterus)

An unstained air-dried blood stain should be made within quarter of an hour. Samples should be stored in a refrigerator.

Good reference ranges can be found at https://icinfo.vet.ohio-state.edu/content/normal-reference-ranges (accessed 14 June 2023).

Leucogram

The leucogram formula in camelids predominates in neutrophils followed by lymphocytes (ratio 1.5:1.0) The ratio is reduced with age.

Neutrophilia

Mature no band neutrophils is associated with:

- Physiological stress;
- Exogenous corticosteroid administration;
- Inflammation; and
- Lymphosarcoma.

Neutropaenia

Typical of:

- End stage inflammatory status; and
- Prematurity in crias.

Lymphocytes

- Granular lymphocytes comprise up to 30% of total lymphocytes.
- Some labs report 'reactive lymphocytes' as large lymphocytes with basophilic cytoplasm occur with antigenic stimulation.
- It is normal for young animals to have higher lymphocyte proportion compared to adults.
- Lymphopaenia occurs with stress (usually accompanied by monocytosis and eosinopenia) and with sickness with a neutrophilia.
- Lymphocytosis occurs with chronic inflammation and viral antigens and is not necessarily seen in lymphoma cases.

Monocytosis

There is a circulating macrophage pool. Monocytes will increase with stress and inflammation.

Eosinophophilis

Numbers are higher than in ruminates. They are higher in juveniles compared with adults and also higher in llamas than in alpacas. There is an eosinophila with endo and ecto parasites. Corticosteroids cause eosinopaenia.

Basophils

These are rarely seen in normal smears. Raised numbers are seen in hypersensitivity reactions and parasitic infections.

Platelets

Ellipsoid RBCs may be confused as platelets by some counting machines. There will be a thrombocytosis in myeloid leukaemia cases, stress, acute inflammation and iron deficiency. There will be a thrombocytopaenia with sepsis and severe coagulopathies.

Obtaining Cerebrospinal Fluid Samples

Collection of cerebrospinal fluid samples (CSF) can be carried out at the atlantooccipital space, but most practitioners use the lumbosacral space as this can be accomplished without a general anaesthetic. It should be remembered that SACs have seven lumbar vertebrae and so the site is caudal to L7. The sample should be collected in the 'kush' position. Light sedation with xylazine is helpful in all but the quietest of animals. The dorso-spinous process of L7 is easy to locate as it is much higher than the dorsal processes of the sacrum. A 3.5 inch 18G needle will be required. After careful skin preparation of the site a small bleb of local anaesthetic with a 23G needle should be placed under the skin half an inch caudal to the spine of L7 in the midline. The site for collection is half an inch long and over an inch wide. It should be entered vertically. Once through the skin the needle will pass through the lumbo-dorsal facia and the interarticulate ligament and suddenly less resistance will be felt.

Analysis of Cerebrospinal Fluid Samples

General

CSF is commonly analysed in SACs with suspected neurological disease because of the ease of collection and characteristic findings associated with certain diseases. The number of neutrophils per microlitre is low in most conditions, less than three, and is associated with decreased odds of short-term survival in SACs (Bennett *et al.*, 2022).

Bacteriology

The sample should be cultured and a smear prepared. This should be examined after Gram stain under the oil emersion on the microscope.

Protein concentration

In a normal CSF sample this should be very low, i.e. <0.4 g/l.

White cell concentration

The normal number of cells in CSF is low, i.e. $<0.012 \times 10^9/l$. A differential count is useful. The macrophages should be examined carefully as phagocytosed RBCs will indicate subarachnoid haemorrhage. A large number of eosinophils will indicate meningeal worm infection. The actual worm is unlikely to be seen.

Important Principles for All Laboratories and Samples

It is important with all laboratory tests that practitioners apply two important principles. Each test should have a known 'test sensitivity' and 'test specificity'. Sensitivity is the percentage of diseased animals that test positive and specificity is the percentage of non-diseased animals that test negative. Ideally all tests would be 100% sensitive and 100% specific. However, this is very rarely the case although normally tests have sensitivities and specificities in the high 90%s. Practitioners should be aware of test limitations.

No practitioner should be without minimal facilities for initial screening and processing of samples for dispatch. Inevitably no practitioner will have the wherewithal to provide all the specialist tests that might occasionally be required. A compromise has to be reached depending on the availability of trained technical staff, likely throughput of samples, etc. Here are some specific hints (MacDougall, 1991):

General (internal or external laboratories):

- DO take samples before any therapy.
- DO examine samples as soon as possible.
- DO dispatch samples as soon as possible.
- DON'T dispatch samples which are unlikely to be diagnostic.

Internal (practice) laboratory:

- DO keep any surplus samples in suitable conditions in case further tests are required.
- DON'T delay in preparation of samples.

External (specialist) laboratory:

- DO ensure all samples are adequately labelled accompanied by full case details and correctly packaged.
- DO be aware of the test's limitations.
- DON'T send sharps with the material.

Safety in the Laboratory

Unlike large organizations with appointed safety personnel, small businesses such as veterinary practices cannot readily dedicate a large amount of time and manpower to health and safety. However, equally high standards of safety must be maintained. The most efficient means of achieving them is to spend some time identifying all safety hazards. These can be categorized as being due to infection, chemicals or equipment. This should be done by a senior member of the practice who should be designated as 'practice safety officer'. An accident book should be kept

for the purpose of recording all injuries, diseases (see Chapter 17) and dangerous occurrences in, or associated with, the work of the laboratory.

Anthrax Smears

These are normally blood smears but they may be taken from swellings around the throat. Two microscope slides are required. A drop of blood or fluid is put on the end of one slide. The other slide is just dipped into this drop and drawn down the length of the slide to make a thin smear. This is then dried in the air. The smear is fixed to the slide by passing the slide through a flame with the smear downwards towards the flame. Once cool the slide with the smear is turned upwards. McFadyeans stain (old methylene blue) is poured on to the slide and left for 30 s. The slide is then rinsed under a running tap. Once dried, the slide can be examined under the oil emersion power of a microscope to check for anthrax bacilli. These will take up the stain and have a characteristic purple capsule.

Abdominocentesis

This should be performed under ultrasonographical guidance. Pockets of fluid will be found on the medial or lateral side of C3 at sites a few centimetres right of the midline or close to the right costo-chondral junction. Clip the area and prepare it aseptically. Instill 2 ml of local anaesthetic under the skin and into the muscle. Make a very small incision through the skin and then push a teat cannula through the peritoneum.

High neutrophils and protein concentration are indicators for surgery. The only differential would be a peritonitis, which should give a high rectal temperature.

Analysis of First Gastric Compartment Fluid

Fluid from compartment 1 (C1) of the stomach can be collected from SACs via an orogastric tube or via percutaneous paracentesis. The results are similar. However, unlike cattle, SACs strongly resist the passing of an orogastric tube and therefore percutaneous paracentesis is the method of choice. Percutaneous paracentesis can easily be performed with a 7.5 cm 16G needle in the left abdominal region caudal to the ribs, which should be clipped and surgically prepared. The best position is 20 cm caudoventral to the costochondral junction of the last rib. The needle can be guided ultrasonographically. It should be pointed in a dorsocraniomedial direction, perpendicular to the contour of the body wall and pushed through the skin and abdominal musculature for its full length into the lumen of C1. Fluid can be aspirated with a 20 ml syringe.

The results can be useful in distinguishing different types of gastrointestinal disturbances and to facilitate the diagnosis of subacute acidosis of C1 on a herd basis. Microbial activity can be measured using the methylene blue reduction test as follows: 1 ml of a 0.3% solution of methylene blue is added to 20 ml of rumen fluid or less on a pro rata basis. The percentage of protozoa that stain with iodine can be measured, which will give an indication of carbohydrate depletion. This should be performed immediately on sampling or an erroneous low result will be obtained.

Bronchoalveolar Lavage Technique

This rather specialized technique can be used to diagnose viral and bacterial lower airway disease. The animal should be restrained in the 'kush' position. The area 5 cm caudal to the larynx should be clipped and surgically prepared. Local infiltration of local anaesthetic solution should be carried out before a further surgical preparation. A 12G 52 × 2.7 mm intravenous catheter should be introduced at 45° to the skin so that the point of the needle is between two trachea rings. A smaller tube of polyethylene with a needle mount is then passed down the catheter for roughly 180 cm. Then 30 ml of sterile isotonic saline is introduced, which is withdrawn in 5 to 10 s. Normally 5 ml will be recovered.

Caseous Lymphadenitis Test

The 'gold standard' caseous lymphadenitis (CLA) test is culture from pus from a lesion. The

internal wall of the abscess should be scraped if possible as the organism *Corynebacterium pseudotuberculosis*, which is fairly straightforward to grow, is more likely to be isolated than just culturing the pus. There is no ELISA test available for SACs.

Coccidiosis Oocysts in Faeces Tests

Modified McMaster technique

The oocysts are floated in a saturated sodium chloride solution (specific gravity 1.20) before light microscopic examination; this method is suitable for detecting small coccidia, for example, *Eimeria alpacae*, *E. lama* and *E. punoensis*.

Improved Modified McMaster technique or saturated zinc sulfate technique (also called the modified Stoll technique)

The oocysts are floated in a saturated zinc sulfate solution (specific gravity 1.36) before light microscopic examination; this method allows the detection of larger coccidia, for example *Eimeria ivitaensis* and *E. macusaniensis*.

Two further modifications of the McMaster technique

Saturated sugar solution is used in this technique. It is prepared by dissolving 454 g of sucrose in 335 ml of hot water.

Method 1

Macerate 4 g of faeces with a little water and leave in a refrigerator overnight. Add 26 ml of the saturated sugar solution and filter. Fill both sides of the McMaster slide and wait for 15 min. Count both sides and multiply by 25. This will give you the number of eggs per gram.

Method 2

Liquefy 2 g of faeces in 98 ml of saturated sugar solution and then centrifuge 10 ml at 1000 rpm for 5 min. Discard the liquid and re-suspend the solids in 10 ml of saturated sugar solution and re-centrifuge. Fill the tube with more saturated sugar solution to create a meniscus. Place a cover-slip and leave for 10 min. Count the eggs and multiply by 5. This will give you the number of eggs per gram.

Both these methods are suitable for the examination of faeces for finding large oocysts.

Determination of Passive Immune Status in Neonates

In order to provide young mammals with passive immunity against disease for a considerable period after birth, immunoglobulin, principally immunoglobulin G (IgG), is transferred from the dam *in utero* and/or by colostrum intake after birth. This immunoglobulin transfer is necessary for protection and survival of the newborn since IgG activates the complement cascade which triggers an immune response. In humans, IgG is transferred directly to the baby through the thin-layered haemochorial placenta. However, SACs have a thick-layered epitheliochorial placenta, which prevents transfer of IgG and thus must obtain passive immunity by intestinal absorption of immunoglobulins in colostrum. Colostral intake of neonates can be influenced by a wide variety of intrinsic and environmental factors. However, it would appear that failure of passive transfer is a serious problem in SACs and has been reported to be a major cause of neonatal deaths (Garmendia, 1987). Assessment of passive immune status of compromised SAC neonates is thus essential to enable prompt remedial action to be instigated, particularly if there has been complete failure of passive transfer.

The most reliable and easy test available to the practitioner is the zinc sulfate turbidity (ZST) test. When zinc sulfate is added to a serum sample it dehydrates the proteins in the serum causing them to precipitate and thus the sample becomes turbid. The degree of turbidity can be directly related to the protein content of the sample. It is a crude but effective precipitation method for measuring plasma immunoglobulin levels and results can be obtained quickly.

Should values be low then measures need to be taken to raise immunoglobulin levels.

Faecal Worm Egg Count

Massive high faecal worm egg counts (FECs) are seen in adults with *Haemonchus contortus* infestation worldwide. With thin animals clinicians should be aware that old SACs with Johne's disease will also show high counts.

Care must be taken using the McMaster technique as this test has a very low sensitivity for eggs from *Capillaria* spp. and *Trichuris* sp. The eggs can easily go undetected, and yet are capable of causing extensive intestinal damage. The presence of these parasites irrespective of the number in the FEC warrants aggressive anthelmintic treatment. The eggs are easier to find using a modified Stoll technique. For a single worm egg count only 6 g of faeces are required but for a combined fluke and worm count 40 g of faeces are required. For pooled worm egg counts 10 × 3 g samples should be submitted separately and pooled in the laboratory. For a pooled fluke egg count 10 × 5 g samples need to be submitted.

When submitting faeces samples for the laboratory it is useful to send them in bags which can be sealed and have the air removed. This will preserve the diagnostic integrity for up to 5 days.

Fluid Therapy

SACs are very used to dealing with dehydration and so estimating fluid deficit is difficult. Tenting of the skin cannot be used and so clinicians have to rely on the mucous membranes to look for dryness or tackiness. Checking urination is useful. Any SAC that does not urinate within 8 h should be suspected of being dehydrated. Hospitalized SACs are often reluctant to drink. Clinical pathology is not easy as SACs often show haemoconcentration and hyperproteinaemia. Water requirements seem to vary between 2 and 10% of body weight. A 5% figure for maintenance would seem approximately correct. Fluids must be given slowly, ideally with a bolus of no more than 2%. Aminoglycosides and non-steroid anti-inflammatory drugs (NSAIDs) should be avoided in dehydrated patients. Acidosis is rare in sick SACs but alkalosis is common, so a plain balanced electrolyte solution is best with an additional supplement of potassium. Most hospitalized gastrointestinal patients are cachexic and will require partial parenteral nutrition. An ideal solution would be 5000 ml of acetate containing electrolyte solution with 1000 ml 8.5% amino acid solution and 20 ml of B vitamins, together with 500 ml of 50% dextrose and 130 mEq potassium as KCl. This solution should be given at 2 ml/kg/h. As the amino acids and B vitamins are light sensitive it should be maintained warm in a black polythene bag. Triglyceride levels are useful to monitor the situation.

Johne's Disease Test

The 'gold standard' test for Johne's disease in SACs is the identification of the causal organism *Mycobacterium avium* subsp. *paratuberculosis* (MAP) following faecal culture. The main limitation of the test is the timescale. Standard cultures take up to 12 weeks. There are modified liquid cultures that will give strong positive results in 3 days. However, there is reduced specificity.

There are polymerase chain reaction (PCR) tests available that give more rapid results and claim similar high sensitivity and specificity but these must be viewed with caution.

Faecal smears can always be examined after staining with Ziehl-Neelsen staining but these will only show acceptable sensitivity values very late on in the course of the disease.

Laboratory Evaluation in Colic Cases

Lymphopenia is the response shown by SACs to stress. There will be a normal or high neutrophil count with no immature cells. Fibrinogen levels will be normal. If fibrinogen levels are up, bacteria involvement is likely. This may be sepsis or gut compromise. Potassium is always low in colic cases. A drop in sodium and chloride is not really significant. However, if the drop in chloride is more marked it is suggestive of an obstruction between the pylorus and the ileocaecal junction. The lower the chloride, the higher up is the obstruction. Low albumen will indicate gastric ulceration. High albumen will indicate dehydration. High liver enzymes will indicate hepatitis and a high amylase will indicate pancreatic disease.

In summary, the most important signs are when two samples are taken 1 h apart and the values are seen to be deteriorating. This is an indicator for surgery.

Liver Biopsy

Hepatic diseases reported in SACs include primary and metastatic neoplasia, ketoacidosis/ fatty liver syndrome and fluke infections. A liver biopsy will aid the clinician in making an accurate diagnosis and prognosis of the case. A biopsy will also help in toxicological problems as well as deficiencies of iron, copper, selenium and zinc. Clinicians should be aware of the dangers of the procedure, which are: haemorrhage at the site; initiation of a systemic inflammatory response; and initiation of hepatic inflammation and cholestasis.

The site for biopsy is 20–30 cm from the top of the back on the right side between the 8th and the 9th rib or the 9th and the 10th rib. The area should be surgically prepared and local anaesthetic should be infiltrated. A small skin incision should be made and a 14G Tru-Cut Biopsy needle should be inserted. Using ultrasound guidance the needle is directed medially and caudally through the edge of the diaphragm. The liver is in direct contact with the diaphragm, and so a biopsy can be obtained after the needle has only been inserted 3 mm through the diaphragm. The skin is closed with a single non-absorbable suture. The animal and the biopsy site should be examined daily.

Liver Enzymes

Alkaline phosphatase (APL)

This is present in the musculoskeletal system and so will be higher in growing animals. It is also an indicator of cholestasis but is not as reliable as gamma glutamyl transferase (GGT) (see below).

Aspartate aminotransferase (AST)

Aspartate aminotransferase (AST) will be raised in liver disease, but it is not liver specific and so will also be raised as a result of muscle cell damage.

Creatininekinase (CK)

This increases after transport and in intense exercise. It will be raised in uterine torsion and downer camelids because of the myositis. It is also raised in vitamin E and selenium deficiencies.

Gamma glutamyl transferase (GGT)

Gamma glutamyl transferase (GGT) is specifically raised in liver disease. Although there are high levels in the kidney it is excreted straight into the urine and does not get into the blood.

Glutamate dehydrogenase (GLDH)

Glutamate dehydrogenase (GLDH) is raised in acute fluke infections and is the most reliable liver enzyme to detect this condition.

Sorbital dehydrogenase (SDH)

This has a limited reliability because it is unstable after blood collection (declines in 24 hours).

Ill-Thrift Panel

Biochemistry can be useful in cases of ill thrift or in any sick camelid to rule out underlying disease. It should be associated with a faecal sample and a good physical examination to rule out dental disease. At the same time the diet and other animal husbandry aspects should be considered. See Table 4.5.

Kidney Function Picture

You require serum or plasma for biochemistry and urine for Specific Gravity. Normal: 1.013–1.048. See Table 4.6.

Kidney function biochemistry

Prerenal causes

- Dehydration;
- Shock.

Renal causes

- Toxicities (acorn, maple tree, clostridia);
- Prolonged NSAIDs;
- Aminoglycosides;
- Vitamin D overdose;
- Renal insufficiencies:
  1. Infections (tuberculosis, leptospirosis)
  2. Pyelonephritis
  3. Abscesses
  4. Cysts.

Postrenal causes

- Imperforated valves in crias;
- Urolithiasis;
- Traumatic post parturition swelling.

Glucose and Lipid Metabolism

- Glucose is higher in camelids compared to ruminants: 4.5–10 mmol/l.
- Sick camelids are hyperglycaemic.
- Hypoglycaemia will be seen in severe hepatic disease, sepsis and in crias post-anaesthesia/sedation.
- Camelids have a weak insulin response to hyperglycaemia.
- There is poor glucose clearance (C. Cebra, personal communication) because cells uptake glucose more slowly and lipolysis is not suppressed in hyperglycaemic states.

Fatty Liver Tests

- Hyperglycaemia + hypernatraemia = hyperosmolar syndrome.
- Severe cortisol response leads to hyperglycaemia >>>glycosuria >>> free water diuresis >>> dehydration and hypernatraemia.
- Usually neonates, but can also occur in adults in severe hyperglycaemia with poor or inadequate access to water leading to dehydration.
- Occurs in premature crias, septic conditions and after steroid administration.
- Glucose will be 0.33 mmol/l and serum sodium will be >160 meq/l.

See Table 4.7.

Table 4.5. Tests for ill-thift.

PCV/MCV/MCHC	To rule out anaemia
Blood smear	To rule out Mycoplasma haemolamae
Leucogram	To rule out inflammation/infection
	Neutrophilia is likely to indicate acute inflammation
	Neutropenia is likely to indicate sepsis with chronic depletion, high tissue demand seen in end stage pneumonia and enteritis
Eosinophils	Check age specific concentrations
	Higher numbers compared to ruminants
	High: parasites, allergies, inflammation
	Females < males; juvenile < adults; llamas > alpacas
Beta-hydroxybutyrate (BHB)	Secondary > 0.1 mmol/ml risk of fatty liver
Non-esterified fatty acids (NEFA)	>600 µmol/l lipid mobilization/fatty liver
Creatinine	Usually low in cachexia, high in prerenal/renal/postrenal
Urea	Low in general lack of amino acid supply or hepatic dysfunction
	High in prerenal/renal/postrenal injury
	If high despite low creatinine suspect gastric ulcers
Potassium	Low in anorexia
GGT	High cholestasis/rule out liver fluke
GLDH	High in liver parenchyma issue/rule out fatty liver/liver fluke/sepsis
Bilirubin	High: liver impairment, cholestasis
Total protein	High in dehydration
	Low: rule out endo and ecto parasites
Glucose	High in stress, lipidosis and sepsis
	Low in liver dysfunction
Albumen	High in dehydration
	Low in parasites, renal loss, liver dysfunction, lymphoma/lymphosarcoma
Globulin	High in antigenic response
Copper	High: toxicocis
	Low: rule out high molybdenum, rule out iron deficiency
Phosphorous	High is rare, seen in excessive supplementation/excess of vitamin D
	Low in hyperparathyroidism, primary and secondary vitamin D deficiency
GSH-Px	Low in poor diet or in starvation

Table 4.6. Tests to measure kidney function.

Blood urea nitrogen (BUN)	Creatinine	Condition	Comments
High	High	Prerenal/renal/postrenal causes	BUN increases much more than creatinine in prerenal and azotaemia. Creatinine increases more than BUN in renal causes. In renal there is also hyponatraemia, hypocalcaemia, hyperkalaemia and hyperphosphataemia
Normal	Low	Emaciation, poor muscle mass	
Normal	High	Newborn	Normal: swimming in creatinine!
High	Normal	Dehydration together with emaciation/poor muscle mass. Ulcerations with digestion of RBC	Check PCV

Electrolytes

Potassium

- Low in anorexia, may cause muscle weakness.
- Hyperkalaemia in acidosis will be increased, but may be masked by anorexia, so supplementation needs to be cautious.

Sodium

- Hypernatraemia, usually with hyperchloraemia (leading to osmolar syndrome) can be caused by loss of free water, decreased water intake, corticosteroid administration or increased sodium in the diet.
- Hyponatraemia/hypochloraemia can occur with GI losses, hypoaldosteronism, renal losses or the dilution effect of uroperitoneum.

Chloride

- Normal sodium with severe hypochloraemia suggests a proximal GI obstruction.

Calcium and magnesium

- May be low in chronic rickets.
- Hypocalcaemia, hypokalaemia, hypophosphataemia and hypomagnesaemia are all potential causes of recumbency.

Phosphorous

- Hypophosphataemia is a crude indication of hypovitaminosis D, which can be secondary to hyperparathyroidism.
- Phosphorous will be low in stemmy forage diets.
- Low phosphorous will be seen in primary hyperparathyroidism, which is very rare.

Lungworm Tests

Normally lungworms eggs will not be seen on the standard FEC. However, in cases of Johne's disease there will be such high levels that eggs will be seen. Normally lungworms are looked for as larvae using the Baermann technique. A sieve and some gauze are positioned in a funnel connected to a tube and a tap. Faeces and some water are placed in the funnel and left for 48 h. The larvae migrate through the gauze and settle in the neck of the funnel. The water in the neck of the funnel is then drained off carefully. This sediment can then be examined under the high power of the microscope to look for first stage lungworm larvae. A minimum of 50 g of faeces is required for the test.

Paired Samples for Serology

These are useful for retrospective diagnosis for a variety of diseases.

Tests for Cerebro-Cortico-Necrosis

Blood test for transketolase estimation

A blood sample in a heparinized tube (green top) is required to test for cerebro-corticonecrosis (CCN).

Faeces test for thiaminase

A total of 30 g of faeces is required.

Triclabendazole Resistance Test

Researchers have found (Flanagan et al., 2011) that a coproantigen reduction test (CRT) protocol can be used for the diagnosis of triclabendazole (TCBZ) resistance using the BIO K201 ELISA. They suggest that the resampling time is 14 days after treatment (with the inclusion of positive and negative coproantigen samples as controls), and that samples be stored in a fridge or freezer before processing.

Tuberculosis Testing

Skin testing procedure

Equipment required

1. Avian and bovine tuberculin.
2. Disposable 1 ml syringes graduated to 0.1 ml.

Table 4.7. Tests to show a fatty liver.

Parameter	Concentrations in fatty liver
GGT	>50 IU/l
GLDH	>30 IU/l
ALP	>14 IU/l
AST	>400 IU/l
NEFA	>600 µmol/l
BHB	>0.1 mmol/l
Triglycerides	>500 mg/dl
Albumin/total protein	May decrease over time >25 g/l/<50 g/l
Bile acids	>20 µmol/l
Ammonia	>5 µg/ml

3. Short 25G needles.
4. Vernier callipers.
5. Marker pen.

Test technique

1. 0.1 ml of avian tuberculin is injected intradermally into a prior marked injection site on the right thoracic cage in the axilla.
2. The intradermal pea-sized swelling is felt and measured to the nearest 0.5 mm.
3. 0.1 ml of bovine tuberculin is injected intradermally into a prior marked injection site on the left thoracic cage in the axilla.
4. The intradermal pea-sized swelling is felt and measured to the nearest 0.5 mm.
5. In the event of the pea-sized swelling not being felt on either side a further intradermal injection should be made on the same side 8–10 cm away.
6. The fold of skin on the same site should be re-measured after 72 h.

Reading and interpretation

SACs are considered potentially infected (reactors) if a positive reaction (i.e. >2 mm increase or detectable oedema) is observed at the bovine tuberculin injection site 72 (68–76) h after injection and the skin thickness at the bovine site exceeds that measured at the avian injection site.

The skin test is claimed to be 100% specific, i.e. if they are positive they almost always have tuberculosis (TB). However, the sensitivity is in the order of 20% and so four out of five diseased animals are going to be missed by the test.

Tuberculosis blood tests

At the time of writing there are three possible blood tests that might be fully developed in time. However, the skin test is the only acceptable test for the UK government.

Chembio Rapid Stat Pak test

This test uses the principle of detecting certain proteins in the blood, which show the animal has mounted an immune response to TB. It appears to be more sensitive than the skin test but less specific.

Camelid Specific Gamma Interferon test

This test is an adaptation from the cattle interferon test, which does not work in SACs. The camelid specific test uses camelid proteins instead of bovine ones. It appears to be promising.

Multi-Antigen Print Immunosorbent Assay test

The multi-antigen print immunosorbent assay (MAPIA) test uses many proteins in an array to detect evidence of immune response to TB. It appears to be more accurate than the other two blood tests. However, it may be too cumbersome to use on large numbers of animals.

Ultrasonography of the Eye

This can be a useful technique in SACs to assess the eye. It is best to use a transpalpedral approach without a stand-off in a horizontal plane. The retrobulbar space can be evaluated to establish the cause of any swellings. Any fine-needle aspirates can be guided by ultrasonography. Tumours and abscesses can be found in this space.

Urine Tests

Normal urine is clear and pale to yellow. Cloudy urine indicates inflammation. The likely causes are:

- Urethral rents or trauma;
- Pyelonephritis;

- Cystitis;
- Urolithiasis;
- Urethritis.

Urine may change colour after it is voided due to the presence of oxidizing agents. Pigments in the urine may also stain bedding a red colour. This may be misleading and give the impression that the urine itself is discoloured.

Discoloration may be caused by:

- Haematuria – erythrocytes in the urine;
- Haemoglobinuria – haemoglobin in the urine, secondary to haemolysis;
- Myoglobinuria – myoglobin in the urine secondary to nutritional muscular dystrophy and in certain plant poisonings resulting in muscle necrosis.

A free catch urine sample is the most appropriate sample to collect. Catheterization in male animals is not possible and in female animals may cause trauma and give a contaminated sample. After a gross visual examination some urine should be retained in a sterile container for bacterial culture.

The urine should be tested with dipsticks. These reagent strips vary and therefore it is important to read the instructions carefully or a false result may be obtained. Most sticks will give an indication of whole blood or the presence of pigment, either haemoglobin or myoglobin. They will give an indication of the presence of protein. The likely cause of this will be inflammation. However, the inflammation may be occurring anywhere from the kidneys down to the urethral orifice. The presence of sugar indicates a clostridial infection (see Chapter 9). However, sedation with xylazine will also cause glycosuria.

The specific gravity will range from 1006 to 1015. The average is 1010. However, rises in the specific gravity must be viewed with caution as it may just indicate the presence of pigments in the urine.

Centrifugation of the urine and examination of the supernatant may help. It will be clear if red cells are in the sediment. However, if there is haemoglobinuria the supernatant will remain pink after centrifugation. This should be carried out at 1000 rpm for 5 min ideally within 30 min of collection. The sediment can be made into smears and examined either immediately or after staining with methylene blue. Cells, crystals and bacteria may be seen. Sperm are a normal finding in urine of sexually active males.

Uterine Biopsy

Uterine biopsy may be performed to evaluate reproductive failure. The endometrium of SACs contains fewer endometrial glands than that of mares, and biopsy results when examined by an equine pathologist will be considered abnormal. An intramuscular injection of 2 mg of oestradiol cypionate given 24 h before the biopsy will allow the cervix to dilate and facilitate passage of the biopsy instruments. There is rarely a need for sedation or an epidural. Before performing the procedure the tail should be bandaged and the perineum washed. A small mare's speculum can be used to visualize the cervix. A pair of endometrial biopsy forceps should be passed through the cervix. Unless the SAC is very large and a rectal examination can be performed the sample will have to be taken 'blind'. The sample should be preserved in 10% formol saline and sent to the laboratory.

Ideally a clinician with small hands should carry out this procedure using copious amounts of lubricant. The owner of the animal should be warned of the risks involved.

Uterine Culture

Uterine culture can be performed in SACs with a commercially available guarded culture swab in a similar manner to uterine biopsy. Frequent pathogens isolated are *Streptococcus* spp., *Staphylococcus* spp., *Escherichia coli*, *Pseudomonas* spp. and anaerobes.

Uterine Lavage

Uterine lavage can be performed in SACs using a 12G Foley catheter. Placement of the catheter is performed in a similar manner as the uterine biopsy forceps. The procedure is made much easier with a piece of wire in the catheter to guide it through the cervix. It can then be removed when the cuff is inflated. A volume of 1 l of isotonic saline should be instilled by gravity and then sucked back out by lowering the plastic giving bag. This should be repeated until the returning liquid appears to be visibly clean. Then a 5 mega crystalline penicillin vial diluted in 20 ml of water for injection and 10 ml of 10% franomycetin should be instilled before the Foley catheter is removed. Penicillin can be injected intramuscularly for 5 days.

5

Veterinary Equipment

Equipment for Handling

- Small halter.
- Lunge line is useful for herding.
- 5 × 1 m lengths of soft 1 cm diameter rope are required to help with restraint during Caesarean section.

Equipment for Diagnosis

- Blood slides and coverslips.
- Blood tubes are required with different anticoagulants.
- Biopsy punches of the small 8 mm disposable type are useful for skin biopsies. There are sophisticated biopsy gadgets available, which are vital for certain biopsies, e.g. liver biopsies.
- A digital camera is important so that the clinician has the ability to download the photographs, label them, store them, and send them as attachments to e-mails.
- Faeces sample bottles of sufficient size are required. Clinicians should be aware that quite large amounts of faeces are required for certain examinations. At least 70 g should be collected.
- Haematocrit centrifuge tubes can be used without a centrifuge to get a quick idea of a packed cell volume (PCV). However, a mini-centrifuge is useful and relatively inexpensive. A hand-driven centrifuge for larger tubes is very cheap and can give adequate results.
- Labels, notebook and a pen are all required for recording cases and sample taking.
- A magnifying glass is useful in skin examination.
- A 'McMaster' slide is required for carrying out faecal worm egg counts. Great care should be taken when handling the cover slip (with the squares), as they are delicate and expensive.
- A microscope is a delicate piece of equipment. I do not recommend that one be carried in the vehicle as a routine. However, the use of a microscope at one's base is vital. It needs to be equipped for oil emersion. 'Diff quick' slides are useful. Gram stain, Giemsa and methylene blue are important.
- Sample bottles containing formalin are required for preserving biopsy material. They should be stored separately from swabs required for bacteriological sampling.
- Small strong polythene bags are useful for skin samples and for double sealing various other samples, e.g. faeces sample bottles.
- Stethoscope is the second vital piece of diagnostic equipment after the clinical thermometer. Ideally it needs to be slim so that auscultation is possible under the muscles caudal to shoulder. Also ideally both a

© Graham R. Duncanson 2023. *Veterinary Treatment of Llamas and Alpacas*, 2nd Edition
(G.R. Duncanson)
DOI: 10.1079/9781800623576.0005

bell and a diaphragm should be present. Obviously there are sophisticated stethoscopes available, e.g. 'Litmans'. However, the inexpensive models are quite adequate.

- A thin stomach tube is required with a rectangular piece of wood to act as a gag, with a hole to pass the tube through. This is useful for giving large volumes of liquid.
- Various types of swab are required. Some should have transport media and some plain. Sometimes a very narrow swab will be required.
- A clinical thermometer is vital. The traditional glass thermometers will last for years if kept carefully in a plastic case. They are hard to acquire in the UK because of the mercury content. However, there are digital thermometers available. The clinician needs to choose whether the thermometer reads centigrade or Fahrenheit. It is just a matter of with which the clinician is happy.
- Urine dip sticks are useful occasionally.

Equipment for the Feet

Gutter tape

A roll of this tape is very useful for making bandages waterproof in the hoof area. It is also useful for covering poultices.

Small, sheep-size hoof clippers

These should be kept well oiled.

Equipment for the Limbs

Oscillating saw

This might be considered not to be essential as a hand-held plaster saw can be used. However, with modern plastering materials it is seriously hard work to remove casts. An oscillating saw is quick and accurate.

Splints

Where funds are tight there is no need for sophisticated splints. Smooth lengths of wood

and plastic guttering are quite adequate. Any sharp ends can be rasped smooth and covered with gutter tape.

Equipment for the Eyes

Catheters

1 mm × 10 cm to cannulate the nasolachrymal duct.

Fluorescein strips

These are inexpensive and vital not only for revealing the presence of deep corneal ulcers but also for testing the patency of the tear ducts. It should be remembered that it takes up to 30 min for the fluorescein to reach the nasal end of the tear ducts in llamas and alpacas after instillation in the eye.

Lacrimal irrigation needle

A 22 gauge is required.

Ophthalmoscope

This is an expensive piece of equipment but is important to the clinician. Much can be found out by examining the eyes carefully with a bright small torch and a magnifying glass. Sadly, however, without a good ophthalmoscope some pathological conditions will be missed. Although a slit-lamp is very useful for examining dogs' eyes, it is not required for llamas and alpacas.

Equipment for Dentistry, Including Equipment for Sinoscopy

Dental elevators

As used for removing wolf teeth in horses are helpful.

Dental picks

These should be strong to allow the practitioner to pick out the food matter compacted between the teeth in diastemata.

Dental rasps

A small diamond-covered rasp is required.

Headlight

There are some extremely bright torches available with heavy battery packs. These are not really required and a light, which is easily taken on and off, is preferable.

Molar extraction forceps

Two pairs are required. They should be 20 cm long, one should be straight and the other should have the extracting jaws at right angles.

Molar spreaders

A small pair 20 cm long is required.

Mouth-washing syringe

A catheter tip 60 ml syringe is adequate.

Small ruminant gag

These are hard to obtain. Figure 5.1 shows a gag adapted by the author.

Equipment for Stitching

These items are self-explanatory. I will list them for completeness. The clinician can manage with very few.

Artery forceps

These can be straight or curved. Several pairs are required.

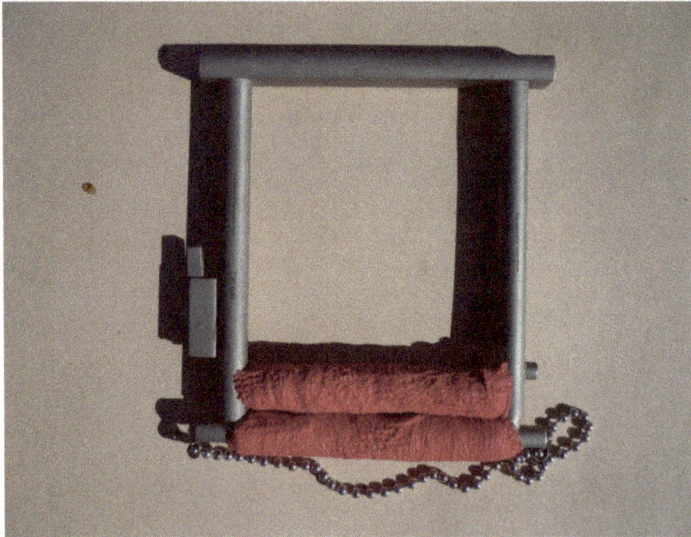

Fig. 5.1. An adapted gag.

Clippers

These are a luxury. However, they make stitching and wound management so much cleaner and easier. The ideal is the rechargeable battery type.

Drapes

A single sterile drape is required as a tray cloth by the ambulatory clinician. However, drapes will be required for other surgery.

Dressing forceps

The ends of these forceps are important: they can be flat or 'rat-toothed'. A pair of each would be required.

Dressing scissors

A pair of curved, blunt-ended scissors needs to be readily available for trimming hair. However, a straight pair with pointed ends is required for a stitch-up kit. There are various different sizes.

Needle holders

There are various types. The most convenient for stitching up wounds is the combination of cutting and holding type called 'Gillies'.

Scalpel blades

These come in different sizes and shapes for different procedures.

Scalpel handle

It is important that the scalpel handle is the same size as the blades.

Stitch-cutting scissors

These small scissors need to be available for removing sutures.

Suture material

This may be absorbable or non-absorbable. It may also be either monofilament or braided. On the whole monofilament non-absorbable will be required for skin wounds.

Suture needles

These come in various shapes. They are also either cutting or non-cutting. On the whole cutting needles will be required for the skin and non-cutting for soft tissue.

Tissue forceps

These forceps are for lifting tissue. A minimum of two pairs is required.

Towel clips

These are not normally required by the ambulatory clinician unless surgery is going to be performed under a general anaesthetic.

Swabs

Sets of sterile swabs are required for a variety of tasks.

Equipment for the Reproductive System

Vaginal speculum

These can be disposable and used with a small hand torch. The small duck-billed type affords the very best visibility.

Equipment for Post-Mortem

These articles are not normally carried by an ambulatory clinician (see Chapter 15).

Specialist Equipment

I have included these items for completeness. It would be very useful to have the use of some of these items of equipment. However, within the scope of this book a full description would not be worthwhile.

- Blood analyser;
- Centrifuge;
- Gaseous anaesthetic machine;
- Operating table;
- Refractometer;
- Ultrasound scanner;
- X-ray machine.

6

Veterinary Medicines

Introduction

There are no medicines licensed for use in SACs in the UK. The owner's consent should always be sought before any drugs are administered to SACs, and the use of a consent form is recommended by one authority (D'Alterio, 2006). Clinicians will need to use their judgement, as drugs licensed for sheep and cattle can be used on the cascade principle. There are a very few drugs that are useful for use in SACs which are only licensed for humans. These may be used using the cascade principle provided there is no similar drug licensed for animals.

Correct storage of medicines is very important. Practitioners should always follow the instructions on the data sheets. The practice medicine store, the practice refrigerator, the in-car refrigerator and the car itself should have their temperatures monitored constantly. Medicines should never become too hot or too cold. Freezing may lead to the active ingredient coming out of suspension. If this previously frozen product is used subsequently the amount of active ingredient given may not be consistent, which could lead to both under- and overdosing. This problem is particularly acute in the winter in temperate climates when products are stored in unheated buildings.

Antibiotics in General

Although SACs are not ruminants, they do have fermentation chambers in their foregut. It is very important that owners are instructed not to give oral antibiotics to adult SACs under any circumstances. They can only be given to young crias.

Before deciding on an antibiotic it is relevant to consider that it can only be given by injection. The owner's ability must be carefully considered. If the antibiotic needs to be given daily, unless the clinician is entirely confident in the owner's ability the clinician must return to repeat the injection every day. In order to decide on a course of action, the clinician might choose to watch the owner actually carrying out the injection after instructing them. On the whole it is prudent to use an injectable antibiotic that can be given subcutaneously to make it easier for the owner. Another alternative is to use an antibiotic that is long-acting and therefore does not have to be injected daily.

Sadly antibiotic therapy is not always successful. There are many reasons. There may be poor compliance by the owner. The clinician can prevent this to some degree by good communication skills. Obviously if an incorrect diagnosis has been made or the wrong antibiotic has been

© Graham R. Duncanson 2023. *Veterinary Treatment of Llamas and Alpacas,* 2nd Edition (G.R. Duncanson)
DOI: 10.1079/9781800623576.0006

selected therapy will be unsuccessful. Clinicians should make sure that the dosage, route and frequency are correct. Obviously, known drug interactions should be avoided. Similarly, the clinician cannot help if the patient has a depressed immune system. Every effort must be made to avoid the use of an antibiotic to which the bacteria are resistant.

Injectable Antibiotics Licensed for Other Species in the UK

Amoxicillin

This antibiotic is available as two separate intramuscular preparations: (i) containing 150 mg/ml for daily administration; and (ii) containing 150 mg/ml for injection every 48 h. The dose for the normal preparation is 2.5 ml/50 kg and for the long-acting preparation it is 5 ml/50 kg. Although this antibiotic is licensed for intramuscular injection in sheep, it is licensed for subcutaneous use in dogs and so can easily be given subcutaneously to SACs. However, in many infections in SACs there is no evidence of resistance problems to procaine penicillin and therefore the use of amoxicillin is not justified.

Amoxicillin with clavulanic acid

This is available as an intramuscular suspension containing 35 mg/ml of clavulanic acid and 140 mg/ml of amoxicillin. This should be injected daily at a dosage of 1 ml/20 kg. Great care is required when drawing up this suspension from the bottle. The syringe and needle must be completely dry or the suspension solidifies. Rarely is the use of this antibiotic justified in SACs. The exception to this is in cases of mastitis, which are rare in SACs. SACs will suffer from pyoderma as a result of secondary staphylococcal infection. Amoxicillin with clavulanic acid might be justified in these cases provided the underlying cause of the skin condition has been treated (see Chapter 14). Practitioners would be wise to carry out bacteriology and sensitivity testing *before* antibiotic therapy is started. Subcutaneous injection of this antibiotic is unwise in SACs as serious skin reactions have been seen.

Ampicillin

This is available in two preparations. There is a 15% suspension, which should be injected intramuscularly daily at 7.5 mg/kg. This works out at 1 ml/20 kg. There is also a so-called 'long acting' preparation containing 100 mg/ml, which should be injected intramuscularly every 48 h at 7.5 ml/50 kg. There is no real justification for this product in SACs. Skin reactions have been reported after subcutaneous use.

Cefquinome

SACs are not kept for milk. So there is little need for this product for use in SACs, particularly the ready-to-use suspension containing 25 mg/ml that needs to be injected intramuscularly at a dosage of 1 mg/kg daily. This is supplied by injecting 2 ml/50 kg. There might be a possible use in SACs for the intravenous soluble preparation, which is supplied as a vial containing 1.35 g of cefquinome as a powder and 30 ml of solvent. The dose is 1 mg/kg, which is supplied by injecting 1 ml/45 kg.

Ceftiofur

This can be given intravenously or intramuscularly and has excellent tissue penetration. Practitioners should avoid the 'ready to use' preparation in SACs. The soluble form, which is supplied as a powder for reconstitution, is more suitable. It is supplied in 1 g or 4 g vials. The small 1 g vials are suitable for SACs. They are reconstituted by adding 20 ml of sterile water for injection. This makes a solution containing 50 mg ceftiofur/ml. A dose of 2 ml is required for a 50 kg animal.

Danofloxacin

This antibiotic is available in two formulations. One contains 180 mg danofloxacin/ml and is suitable for subcutaneous and intravenous injection every 48 h. The dosage of 6 mg/kg can be attained by injecting 1 ml/30 kg. The other contains 25 mg/ml and is suitable for intramuscular or intravenous injection every 24 h. The dosage of 1.25 mg/kg is achieved by giving 1 ml/20 kg. This product is licensed for cattle and could be used in SACs. However, there are few indications and so the likely need is very limited.

Enrofloxacin

This is available in three different strengths: 2.5%, 5% and 10% solution for daily subcutaneous injection. The dosage is 2.5 mg/kg. This can be achieved by injecting 1 ml/5 kg of the 5% solution. There is a fourth preparation for a single long-acting subcutaneous injection of 7.5 mg/kg. This can be achieved by injecting 3.75 ml/50 kg. It can be used safely during pregnancy. It is advisable to double the dose if treating *Escherichia coli* mastitis. This product can also be given intravenously. This is a very useful drug in SACs. It can be given daily or by using the long-acting formulation, which is useful in skin disease. The 2.5% strength is very suitable for crias and small alpacas.

Florfenicol

This is available as a ready-to-use solution containing 300 mg/ml. It can be given intramuscularly every 48 h at 10 mg/kg or at a double dose (20 mg/kg) subcutaneously, which needs only to be given every fourth day. This is the ideal drug for treating apical tooth abscessation in SACs. The 4-day injection period is useful. There is a more concentrated formulation containing 450 mg/ml. There is no reason to use this preparation in SACs.

Framycetin

This is available as a 15% injectable solution suitable for intramuscular injection at a dosage of 5 mg/kg to be given twice daily. This works out at 1 ml/30 kg twice daily. There is no realistic usage for this antibiotic in SACs as it is short acting and needs to be given intramuscularly. Some practitioners have found it useful when included in large volumes of warm saline for uterine washouts.

Gamithromycin

This is a macrolide licensed for use in cattle in the UK against bacteria causing respiratory disease. The single dose is 6 mg/kg, which is equivalent to 1 ml/25 kg if the solution containing 150 mg/ml is given subcutaneously. The author has no experience of its use in SACs. However, it has been reported to have a long-acting effect and appears to be safe. A study was performed to determine the disposition of gamithromycin in plasma, peripheral blood polymorphonuclear cells (PMNs), pulmonary epithelial lining fluid (PELF) and bronchoalveolar lavage (BAL) cells in alpacas (Gordon *et al.*, 2022). No injection site reactions occurred. One alpaca developed colic but no other adverse reactions were noted. Overall, gamithromycin was highly concentrated in white blood cells and pulmonary fluids/cells. Gamithromycin should be used with caution in alpacas until further investigation of potential for colic.

Gentamicin sulfate

This antibiotic should not be used in SACs. It has a very narrow safety margin and it is nephrotoxic. The damage to the kidneys will be shown as uraemia on a blood test. Clinically the animal will be anorexic and drooling. On examination of the oral mucosa, ulcers will be seen. By this stage treatment is unlikely to be successful and so euthanasia is indicated.

Lincomycin

This is available as a sterile solution for intramuscular injection. The dose is 22 mg/kg, which can be achieved by injecting 1 ml/4.5 kg daily. This product is particularly useful for treating abscesses, infected wounds and purulent dermatitis in pigs, for which it has a licence in the UK. There are other more suitable antibiotics available for use in SACs.

Marbofloxacin

This antibiotic is available in a 2% solution and can be given intramuscularly or subcutaneously daily at 2 mg/kg. There is also a 10% solution available but this is not recommended for SACs. There is little advantage in using this antibiotic when compared to enrofloxacin.

Neomycin

This is only available as an injectable solution suitable for intramuscular use when it is combined with procaine penicillin G. The contents of 1 ml of the solution include 100 mg of neomycin sulfate and 200 mg procaine benzyl penicillin. This antibiotic has no real use in camelid medicine.

Oxytetracycline

This is a very useful antibiotic in SACs. This can be given intravenously, intramuscularly or subcutaneously. Depending on the dosage, longer treatment interval levels can be achieved. The normal daily dose is 20 mg/kg. The solutions are supplied in various strengths of 100 mg/ml, 200 mg/ml and 300 mg/ml. The more concentrated solutions are more painful and should be avoided in young animals.

Penicillin-Na G crystalline penicillin

This can be given intravenously or intramuscularly. It needs to be repeated ideally every 6 h. It is really only suitable for hospital use when an intravenous catheter is in place. Dosage is 22,000–44,000 IU/kg. It is normally supplied in 3 g vials (5,000,000 IU), which can be reconstituted into 10 ml of water. Each 1 ml will contain 500,000 IU. A 50 kg animal will require 4 ml. In the UK this product is only licensed for horses. However, it can be used intravenously in SACs under the cascade principle.

Procaine benzyl penicillin

This preparation contains 300 mg/ml of procaine benzyl penicillin. In cattle it is licensed for intramuscular and subcutaneous use at 20 mg/kg. This equates to 1 ml/kg and it is claimed to give cover for 72 h. It is a very useful antibiotic in SACs, is long acting and can be given by subcutaneous injection.

Procaine penicillin G

This is often given in combination with streptomycin. In the preparations containing penicillin alone the dosage is 10 mg/kg. It is normally supplied in a suspension of 300 mg/ml, so the dosage is 1 ml/30 kg. It is claimed that given at double this dosage blood levels are maintained for 72 h. When supplied with streptomycin it is in a suspension of 200 mg/ml with 250 mg/ml of dihydrostreptomycin. A suitable dosage is 1 ml/25 kg. This is a very useful antibiotic combination for use in SACs. It can be given subcutaneously.

Spectinomycin

This is available as an aqueous solution for intramuscular injection. The dosage is 30 mg/kg, which can be achieved by injecting 3 ml/10 kg daily. In the UK this product is only licensed for calves and it is not widely used. It has no specific use in SACs.

Streptomycin

This antibiotic is available on its own in an intramuscular formulation containing 150 mg streptomycin sulfate and 150 mg dihydrostreptomycin sulfate/ml. The daily dose is 10 mg/kg, which is attained by giving 1 ml/30 kg. This product is very useful for treatment of *Actinobacillosis* spp. and *Actinomycosis* spp. in SACs. Its disadvantage is that it has to be injected daily and usually for prolonged periods.

Tilmicosin

This antibiotic has an extremely narrow safety margin in SACs and should not be used.

Trimethoprim-sulfadoxine

Trimethoprim-sulfadoxine (TMS) can be given intravenously or intramuscularly. However, there have been fatalities recorded when the intravenous route has been used so perhaps this risk is best avoided. The dosage is 30 mg/kg. There are several 24% injectable solutions available. The standard clear solution contains 40 mg of trimethoprim and 200 mg of sulfadiazine/ml. This gives a dosage of 1 ml/16 kg. There are two cream-coloured suspensions available, which can only be given intramuscularly: one has a similar concentration of ingredients and is used at the same dosage as the standard clear solution; and the second contains twice the concentration of antibiotic and has a dose rate of 1 ml/32 kg. There is a use for potentiated sulfonamides in SAC medicine to treat infections and for treatment of coccidiosis. Their disadvantage is that they need to be given daily.

Tulathromycin

This new antibiotic has a very long half life in the tissues and neutrophils and gives effective antibiotic cover for 14 days. It is licensed for cattle and has been used safely by the author in SACs. It is a macrolide and should not be given at the same time as another macrolide or lincosamide. It is effective against bacteria in a similar manner to other macrolides. It is supplied in a ready-to-use solution of 100 mg/ml, to be injected subcutaneously. The dosage is 2.5 mg/kg, which is equivalent to 1 ml/40 kg. It is particularly useful because of its long action.

Tylosin

This antibiotic is available as an intramuscular injection for a dosage of 4 mg/kg, which can be achieved by injecting 1 ml/50 kg. The solution contains 200 mg tylosin/ml. Larger doses, up to 10 mg/kg, are licensed for cattle. This antibiotic can be used in SACs but it must be injected daily.

Injectable Antibiotics in Combination with Injectable Non-steroidal Anti-inflammatory Drugs

These products are available and licensed for use in cattle in the UK to treat pneumonia. They can have other uses in SACs as they are useful for owners to inject. Owners should be instructed carefully on the dosages to be given and the frequency of injections.

Florfenicol and flunixin

This is available as a solution containing 300 mg/ml of florfenicol and 16.5 mg/ml of flunixin meglumine. The dose is 2 ml per 15 kg. This combination is very useful in SACs as it can be given subcutaneously and gives 4 days of antibacterial activity.

Oxytetracycline and flunixin

This is available as a solution containing 300 mg/ml of oxytetracycline and 20 mg/ml of flunixin meglumine. The dosage is 1 ml per 10 kg. The disadvantage is that it has to be injected intramuscularly and only gives up to 36 h of anti-inflammatory activity. However, it does give 5–6 days of antibacterial activity and therefore does have some uses in SACs.

Oral Antibiotics

These preparations must only be given to young crias. There are many antibiotic tablets prepared for dogs and cats and there are also boluses prepared for calves. However, antibiotics in these forms are very difficult to administer to crias and should be avoided. Practitioners should use the liquid oral preparations prepared specifically for lambs with a pump. These are much easier to administer to crias. Once again it should be stressed that oral antibiotics should *not* be given to adult SACs.

Practitioners are urged to submit faeces samples for bacteriology and sensitivity before antibiotic usage. Many diarrhoea cases in strong healthy crias are self limiting and antibiotic usage is not useful or appropriate.

Neomycin

This is available combined with streptomycin as an oral solution with 1 ml containing 70 mg neomycin sulfate and 70 mg streptomycin sulfate. The dose is 1 ml/5 kg daily. This product is licensed for lambs in the UK. It is useful in SACs for treating secondary infections following rotavirus infections.

Spectinomycin

This is available as a viscous liquid containing 50 mg/ml. The daily dose for a lamb is one measure of 1 ml from the doser. This product is licensed for lambs in the UK. The dose is 2 ml daily for a cria.

Streptomycin

This is available combined with neomycin as an oral solution with 1 ml containing 70 mg neomycin sulfate and 70 mg streptomycin sulfate. The dose is 1 ml/5 kg daily. This product is licensed for lambs in the UK.

Other Antibiotic Preparations

These include topical antibiotics, which are available as creams, gels, powders and aerosol sprays. The most usual ingredient in aerosol sprays is 2% chlortetracycline hydrochloride. Antibiotics are also available as intramammary formulations licensed for cows. These should not be used in SACs on account of their small teat orifices. Antibiotics are also available in ear and eye preparations. One of the most common preparations is eye ointment containing 1% chlortetracycline hydrochloride, which needs to be applied repeatedly, ideally every 6 h. Cloxacillin benzathine 16.67% w/w eye ointment has a longer duration of action up to 48 h. Only one application of cloxacillin benzathine may be sufficient to control contagious ophthalmia in SACs.

Antifungal Agents

Griseofulvin

This is a very effective treatment for *Trichophyton* spp. These are normally caught from cattle. However, it is banned for use in food-producing animals in the UK. SACs should be given 5 g of a 7.5% powder/50 kg in their feed daily for 7 days. Griseofulvin is not very effective against *Microsporum* spp. Care should be taken by pregnant ladies when handling griseofulvin as it is teratogenic. It should be remembered that ringworm, particularly *Trichophyton* spp., is a zoonosis (see Chapter 17). Vigorous scrubbing and strong disinfectants, which damage the skin, should be avoided. Normal washing with soap is preferable. Ladies and children are particularly susceptible.

Miconazole

This is a good topical treatment for *Trichophyton* spp. and *Microsporum* spp. It should be used as a shampoo twice weekly.

Natamycin

This is also a good topical treatment for *Trichophyton* spp. and *Microsporum* spp. It comes as a powder to be re-suspended. The suspension is then sponged or sprayed on to the affected area every 4–5 days.

Virkon S

This is actually a broad-spectrum virucidal disinfectant. It is a very effective disinfectant and also can be used to treat *Microsporum* spp. It should be made up as a 1% solution, i.e. a 50 g sachet in 5 l water. This solution can be used as a spray or sponged on to affected areas every 48 h. This use is not licensed in the UK but is widely used off licence.

Antiprotozoal Drugs

Coccidiostats

Amprolium

This is available as a 9.6% oral solution. Crias need to be treated daily for 5 days with 3 ml/5 kg. It is not licensed in the UK for ruminants.

Decoquinate

This is available as a 6% premix to add to creep feed to treat crias. A weight of 1.67 kg of the premix can be added to 1 t of feed to provide the recommended concentration of 100 mg/kg. This can be used as a treatment or a prophylaxis during a coccidial challenge. Treatment should be carried on for 4 weeks. It is also available as an individual treatment pack for calves, which can be used in SACs. This allows individual SACs to be treated in the food. Careful weighing of the animal and the complementary feeding stuff is required so that it is fed at the correct dosage.

Diclazuril

This is available as a 0.25% aqueous oral suspension, which is licensed for use in lambs. It can also be used in SACs. The dose is 1 mg/kg by mouth, which is equivalent to 1 ml/2.5 kg. A single dose should be given and repeated if indicated in 3 weeks. It can be used as a preventative as well as a treatment, i.e. it can be given 10 to 14 days after movement of susceptible stock on to pasture known to be infected with oocysts. It is safe in crias from 1 week of age.

Toltrazuril

This is available as an oral suspension containing 50 mg/ml of toltrazuril. It is licensed in the UK for the prevention of clinical signs of coccidiosis and reduction of coccidia shedding in lambs on farms with a confirmed history of coccidiosis caused by *Eimeria crandallis* and *Eimeria ovinoidalis*. It can be used in crias as a single oral dose of 20 mg toltrazuril/kg. This is equivalent to 0.4 ml of the oral suspension/kg. To obtain the maximum benefit the crias should be treated before the expected onset of clinical signs, i.e. in the pre-patent period.

Trimethoprim-sulfadoxine (TMS)

This antibiotic is also effective against coccidia. It needs to be given at 30 mg/kg for 3 days.

Drugs used to treat other protozoal parasites

Diminazene aceturate

This is the most hazardous of this group of drugs. It is extremely effective against *Babesia* spp. However, as less dangerous drugs are available to treat this protozoan they should be considered. On the other hand it is the most effective drug to treat trypanosomiasis available. This includes *Trypanosoma brucei* (Surra), *T. vivax* (acute 'fly'), *T. congolense* (chronic 'fly') and *T. evansi* (camel 'fly'). The first three trypanosomes are only spread by tsetse fly. Therefore they will only be seen in a tsetse area. *T. evansi* is spread by biting flies and therefore can occur outside of tsetse areas. As SACs are not kept in tsetse areas they are not likely to become infected. *T. evansi* has not been reported in SACs either; however, if one did become infected diminazene aceturate would be the drug of choice. It is supplied in 1.05 g sachets for reconstitution in 12.5 ml of water to make a 12.5% solution. This is the normal dose for an adult cow weighing 500 kg. The author has only had experience using it on a pro rata dosage for camels. It would be reasonable to use it on a pro rata basis by weight for treating *T. evansi* in SACs.

Imidocarb

This is the drug of choice for treating *Babesia* spp. These protozoan parasites are spread by ticks. Imidocarb is supplied in a 12% solution in a 100 ml multidose vial. The risk of abscessation is much less than with diminazene. The dose for SACs is 1.2 mg/kg by deep intramuscular injection on two separate days (this is only 1.0 ml for a 100 kg SAC).

Metronidizole

This drug can be used to treat protozoal diseases. However, its principal use in SACs is to treat anaerobic bacteria. These may be in the alimentary system or in wounds or infections in the feet. The best method of administration is by mouth at the rate of 15 mg/kg every 8 h. The drug is supplied in 500 mg tablets. It is also supplied as a 20 mg/kg solution in 50 ml sachets. This solution is best used topically on wounds or hoof infections. However, some workers have used it intravenously at 20 mg/kg every 24 h for 3–5 days to treat clostridial enteritis and peritonitis. The drug per se can cause diarrhoea, so this side effect is very worrying in animals with existing enteric problems. The author would advise against intravenous use. It is useful for treating *Giardia* spp. in immature SACs.

Pyrimethamine

This drug can be used to treat toxoplasmosis and to lessen the rate of abortion in SACs. There is a synergism between pyrimethamine and potentiated sulfonamides and so the two drugs are often given together. Pyrimethamine should be given by mouth at 0.1–0.2 mg/kg daily. Sulfonamides should be given at the normal dose rate of 15 mg/kg. This regime may be given from 2 months after service until parturition.

Anthelmintics

Introduction

In the 1960s and the 1970s there was the development of broad-spectrum anthelmintics in ruminants. These products, the benzimidazoles, the imidazothiazoles/tetrahydropyrimidines (levamisole and morantel) and the macrocyclic lactones greatly improved global sheep production. They also improved goat production worldwide and SAC production in South America. Sadly there has been rather rapid resistance built up to these products. Benzimidazole resistance was first reported in the UK in 1982. Levamisole resistance was reported in 1994 and macrocyclic lactone resistance was reported in the UK in 2001. These reports have been mirrored elsewhere throughout the world. It is vital that effective strategies to combat these resistances are put in place and that farmers should not rely on the recent manufacture of a new class of anthelmintic, monepantel, an aminoacetonitrile derivative.

It is important for clinicians to realize the difference between anthelmintic failure and anthelmintic resistance. Anthelmintic failure occurs due to:

- Insufficient anthelmintic dose due to underestimation of animal weight;
- Failure to follow manufacturers' instructions;
- Poor maintenance of dosing equipment;
- Re-introduction of animals on to heavily contaminated pasture;
- Use of incorrect drug for target worms.

In other cases of apparent failure, anthelmintic resistance should be suspected.

There are two anthelmintic resistance detection methods available *in vivo*: the Faecal Egg Count Reduction Test (FECRT) and the Controlled Test. The FECRT is the most commonly used field assay for all anthelmintic groups. It has a low sensitivity as there are many false negatives. On the other hand there are false positives with levamisole. It requires two visits per farm and there is a seasonal variability. The Controlled Test is a comparison of parasite burdens in treated and non-treated animals that have been artificially infected with worms suspected of being either (i) susceptible or (ii) partially resistant; these two groups are then divided at random into medicated and non-medicated groups. After 14 days the animals are killed and the worms are counted on post-mortem.

There are two anthelmintic resistance detection methods available *in vitro*: the Egg Hatch Assay (EHA) and the Larval Development Test (LDT). These are both cheap and highly sensitive but they are not universally standardized or accepted. Farm visits are not required as submissions can be sent by post. There is a seasonal variability and they are not generally predictive in terms of clinical disease. EHA can only be used for benzimidazole anthelmintics and LDT is not satisfactory for avermectins.

There are various factors that influence the rate of development of anthelmintics resistance. Farm management and husbandry factors can be affected by keepers. These include stocking rates, mixed grazing, grassland management and anthelmintic usage, e.g. frequency, choice, etc. The climate with its seasonal range of temperature and rainfall is a very important factor. The parasitic species, i.e. its biotic potential and its proportion in refugia, is an important factor to be considered.

Modes of action of anthelmintic groups

- Benzimidazoles – this group includes fenbendazole, mebendazole, oxyfendazole, albendazole and ricobendazole. They bind to the parasite's tubulin, leading to inhibition of glucose uptake, which then leads to glycogen depletion and death.
- Probenzimidazoles – this group includes netobimin and acts in the same manner as the benzimidazoles.

- Imidazothiazoles – this group includes levamisole. They are cholinergic agonists, which cause a rapid and reversible paralysis.
- Tetrahydropyrimidines – this group includes morantel and pyrantel. They act in the same manner as the imidazothiazoles.
- Avermectins – this group includes abamectin, doramectin, eprinomectin, ivermectin and selamectin. They open invertebrate-specific glutamate chloride channels in the post-synaptic membrane, leading to flaccid paralysis.
- Milbemycins – this group includes moxidectin and acts in the same manner as the avermectins.
- Salicylanilides – this group includes closantel and oxyclozanide. They uncouple oxidative phosphorylation, decreasing the availability of high energy phosphate compounds.
- Substitute phenols – this group includes nitroxynil. They act in the same manner as the salicylanilides.
- Amino-acetonitrile derivatives – this group includes monepantel. They are cholinergic agonists, which act on a novel site on the receptor, resulting in spastic paralysis of the worms.

New classes of anthelmintics

The relatively new classes of anthelmintics, which have no recorded resistance problems, should be used with considerable care. Naturally they may be used as a quarantine dose at the *correct* dose rate and also where triple resistance has been proven. They should *not* be used for routine worming.

Anthelmintics combined with trace elements

There are available benzimidazoles, which have added cobalt sulfate and sodium selenate. Clinicians should guide their owners carefully on the need for such additives as areas requiring them are not common. On the whole such drenches are best avoided for SACs.

Long-acting injectable products

Certain injectable moxidectin products will give a sustained persistency against helminths in sheep. Persistence of 44 days for *Trichostrongylus colubriformis*, 97 days for *Teladorsagia circumcincta* and 111 days for *Haemonchus contortus* is claimed from a single injection of the correct dose. This same preparation claims efficiency against sheep scab for 60 days. Other intestinal nematodes controlled are the adults of *Trichostrongylus axei*, *Nematodirus spathiger*, *Cooperia curticei* and *Chabertia ovina* and the third stage larvae of *Gaigeria pachyscelis* and *Oesophagostomum columbianum. Dictyocaulus filaria* and *Oestrus ovis* are also controlled by the same product. It should not be used in crias weighing under 15 kg.

Flukicides

An injection of 34% w/v nitroxynil is licensed for use in the UK as a treatment by subcutaneous injection for *Fasciola hepatica* in sheep at 10 mg/kg. It is claimed to be effective against mature and immature flukes. However, the age of the immature flukes is not stated. The drug is probably not effective for the control of acute fascioliasis in SACs in the autumn in the UK. However, no resistance has been reported and therefore it is a very useful medicine to use if triclabendazole resistance is suspected. It is also effective against *Haemonchus contortus*. However, it is not a broad-spectrum anthelmintic and should not be used as such. *H. contortus* and *F. hepatica* are both parasites that cause severe disease and deaths in adult SACs. Therefore it is an extremely useful product. It can be used at the same time as, but in different sites to, levamisole to provide broad-spectrum capability in sheep but not in SACs on account of the danger of toxicity. It has some dangers. The solution contains no preservative so great care must be taken not to introduce a bacterium into the solution. The discard time after broaching of 28 days should be strictly adhered to. It will stain the fibre so very careful injection technique is required. It can be used in pregnant animals but naturally they should be handled with care. In the event of accidental overdose the symptoms are pyrexia, rapid respiration and increased excitability. Patients should be kept cool, and dextrose saline should be given as a drip. In the normal course of events nitroxynil should be repeated within 49 days. Nitroxynil can cause pain on injection. Clinicians are in a 'lose–lose' situation with treating SACs for fluke. Nitroxynil causes pain, fleece damage and has a narrow safety margin. Triclabendazole is a very safe drug in SACs but has the risk of causing choke. The dose rate of triclabendazole is 10 mg/kg in SACs.

Combination fluke and worm products

The liver fluke *F. hepatica* requires the presence of a water snail as the secondary host. Diagnosis is not easy and relies on raised liver enzymes in a serum sample and then very careful floatation of faeces to find the eggs. The presence of one egg is significant. For sheep the following licensed drugs are available: triclabendazole at 10 mg/kg; albendazole at 7.5 mg/kg; closantel at 10mg/kg; and nitroxynil at 10 mg/kg. There is now a plethora of fluke and worm combination products on the market for use in sheep. Naturally there is going to be a demand for products for SACs. Although convenient they should only be used if there is a need to target both fluke and worms. This is a very rare occurrence. Therefore they should not be used without considerable thought. This will not only save owners money but will also lower the risk of drug resistance developing. Combination products undergo extensive testing to ensure that the two components mix evenly and work properly together. It is not acceptable to take two products and mix them together on farm. The greatest danger to SACs from fluke infection is from acute cases. Not all fluke products will kill immature flukes. It is vital that SACs are treated early in the course of the disease with a flukicide which will kill immature flukes at the critical time. This is in early autumn in the UK. A second treatment should be given 2 months later to kill any more recent immature or mature flukes that were not killed by the first dose. It takes 10–12 weeks for 2 mm immature flukes to develop into 2–3 cm adult flukes in the liver. These are the only flukes that will be killed by most flukicides. Therefore these products should only be used in the late winter or early spring in the UK. It is unlikely that SACs will require worming in the autumn unless FECs indicate a high burden. Therefore it is unlikely that combination products will be required.

Anthelmintics as individual drugs

Albendazole

This oral drug is in the same class as fenbendazole but it is not so safe in SACs. It should never be given in the first trimester of pregnancy or to young crias. If possible it should be avoided in pregnancy. A routine dosage is 10 mg/kg. Some authors (Lopez, 2021) advise 20 mg/kg. It is only available in liquid form.

Avermectins

Because of their injectable formulation and because they treat mange mites these drugs have been used constantly in SACs. Resistance is extremely common. The efficacy should be regularly tested. They are obtainable in pouron formulations but these should not be used in SACs as there is poor absorption and there is a danger of skin damage. The only exception to this is if they are diluted 50:50 with dimethyl sulfoxide (DMSO) and are painted on to chronically mite-infested skin lesions. The oral formulations should also not be used in SACs as they are not as active for as long as the injectable formulations. A routine dosage would be 300 mg/kg, which is the equivalent of 1 ml of a 1% solution/33 kg. They should be injected subcutaneously.

Fenbendazole

This oral drug is generally safe and can be given to pregnant females and young crias with confidence at a routine dosage of between 10 and 20 mg/kg. It is available in paste, liquid and granular form.

Levamisole

This drug has a very low safety margin in SACs. Its use should be avoided if possible and should be reserved for multiple nematode resistance problems. Accurate weighing is vital. The oral preparation can be given at 8 mg/kg. The injectable formulation should be given at a lower dosage of 6 mg/kg.

Moxidectin

This drug has an extremely narrow safety margin in SACs. Really accurate weighing is vital. Its use should be restricted to multiple resistance problems. It is only available as a paste. The dose is 400 mg/kg.

Organophosphorus drugs, diethylcarbamazine, morantel and pyrantel

These drugs should not be used in SACs.

Ectoparasiticides

Alphacypermethrin

This is marketed to control nuisance flies, when applied every 14 days. It will control head fly for 4 weeks. Blowfly strike can not only be prevented but also treated by the pour-on preparation. It will give 8–10 weeks cover. It will also help to control mange mites, ticks and lice.

Amitraz

This is available as a clear emulsifiable concentrate for dilution and topical application containing 5% w/v amitraz for treatment of demodectic and sarcoptic mange. A volume of 100 ml should be diluted in 10 l of water. After the animal has been washed in warm water to remove any dirt it should be bathed in this solution. It should then be removed without rinsing and allowed to dry naturally in warm air. It should not be allowed to drink or lick any of the solution. This should be repeated after 1 week. As there have been reports of toxicity it is safer to wash only half the animal at weekly intervals. Obviously the halves should be alternated.

Benzoyl peroxide

This acaricide can be used to treat mange.

Benzyl benzoate

This acaricide, which is a lotion, is very effective against mange mites if applied daily to all the affected areas.

Coumaphos

This so-called louse powder is not very effective. It needs to be applied every 5 days to increase its effectiveness. However, to avoid toxicity it should not be applied sooner than every 14 days in SACs. It has no effect on mange mites.

Cypermethrin

This is marketed as a concentrate for dilution to a solution, which can be sprayed on with a knapsack sprayer or sponged on. It will control nuisance flies and lice. It is also marketed as a pour-on for treating and preventing blowfly strike. It gives 6–8 weeks protection, but only in the area of the pour-on sweep. It also gives protection against lice, ticks and head flies.

Cyromazine

This is marketed as a blowfly strike preventative but not as a treatment. It will last for 10 weeks.

Deltamethrin

Deltamethrin is prepared in a 1% w/v solution as an ectoparasiticide for the topical treatment and control of ticks, lice, keds and established blowfly strike. For prevention, it should be used as a single spot-on between the shoulders after parting the fibre. It may be used by direct application to a maggot-infested area in established blowfly strike.

Dicyclanil

This is a pour-on product to prevent blowfly strike in sheep. It can be used in SACs. It is available as a 5% solution, which offers 16 weeks protection. However, it is also available as a 1.25% solution, which protects for 8 weeks.

Diethyltoludine

This midge repellent is extremely effective. However, sadly it is washed off by rain and even in dry conditions is rarely effective for more than 6 h. It is rarely used in SACs.

Fipronil

This ectoparasiticide is not licensed for ruminants in the UK. However, it is extremely effective against mange mites when the spray is applied to all the affected areas every 14 days. It can be used in the UK under the cascade principle. It is very useful in SACs. However, it is very expensive. The direct environmental impact of fipronil in SACs is unquantified. It is prudent to advise owners of the environmental impacts and how to minimize these. One 100 ml bottle typically dispensed for topical application to ten alpacas contains 0.25 g fipronil – enough toxic doses to kill 40 million bees. It would be prudent to take measures to minimize contamination to both the immediate environment as well as water sources.

Ivermectins and moxidectin

These drugs, which are covered under anthelmintics, do have an ectoparasitic action when given by injection. They do not appear to have any ectoparasitic action when given by mouth.

Piperonyl butoxide

This can be used to control lice if applied every 14 days. However, if it is required to control midge irritation it needs to be applied to the affected areas daily.

Dipping of SACs

The dangers of injury, organophosphate toxicity and inhalation pneumonia make the dipping of SACs extremely hazardous and it is not recommended. However, it has been carried out in Belgium with a specially constructed cage to aid immersion, using an organophosphate compound, phoxim.

Steroidal Anti-Inflammatory Drugs

There is a definite usage for steroids in SACs. An injectable solution of 2% dexamethasone can be used at 0.1 mg/kg by intramuscular or intravenous injection. This is quite safe in SACs except of course in pregnant animals. SACs do not get laminitis. However, they do get hyperlipaemia so care must be used with prolonged treatment. Some authorities think prednisolone at 1 mg/kg is a useful potent short-acting steroid. The author has not found this and certainly it is not effective by mouth.

Non-Steroidal Anti-Inflammatory Drugs

Non-steroidal anti-inflammatory drugs (NSAIDs) need some careful evaluation in SACs, not only because they are very prone to gastric ulceration but also some useful NSAIDs used in horses (e.g. phenylbutazone) have a very short half-life (under 2 h) (Table 6.1). Flunixin meglumine at 1 mg/kg, ketoprofen at 2 mg/kg and meloxicam at 0.5 mg/kg all can safely be used by subcutaneous or intravenous injection. The length of action is not known. However, meloxicam is thought to give 48 h action where the other two are unlikely to give as long as 24 h. Sadly, although they are

Table 6.1. The dosages of both NSAIDs and opiates for injection in other species, which can be used as a guide in llamas and alpacas.

Agent	Dose	Route	Duration (h)
Pethidine	1 mg/kg	im	2
Butorphanol	0.5 mg/kg	sc or iv	4
Buprenorphine	10 µg/kg	sc or iv	8
Flunixin meglumine	2.2 mg/kg	iv or im	24
Carprofen	1.4 mg/kg	sc or iv	24
Meloxicam	0.5 mg/kg	sc or iv	24
Ketoprofen	3 mg/kg	iv or im	24
Tolfenamic acid	4 mg/kg	iv	24

widely used orally, it is extremely unlikely that they are effective unless given at very large doses.

Other Useful Drugs

Cloprostenol

This prostaglandin can be used for luteolysis in SACs. The ideal dosage is 1 ml repeated in 24 h.

Donperidone

This drug is said to help milk let-down. It is available in paste form in the USA and as 10 mg tablets in the UK. The dose of the paste is 1.1 mg/kg twice daily for 2 days then once daily for 5 days.

GnRH

This hormone is useful in SACs to stimulate ovulation (remember they are induced ovulators). The dose is 1 ml given intramuscularly.

Lignocaine local anaesthetic

SACs are very sensitive to the toxic effects of local anaesthetic. Local blocks (e.g. for Caesarean section) should be given with care. You should not exceed the maximum recommended dose of 4 mg/kg. For epidural anaesthesia, 1 ml is quite sufficient.

Oxytocin

Oxytocin is vital to aid the third stage of labour and milk let-down. The dose is 10–20 IU given intramuscularly. If it is given intravenously it must be diluted with at least 20 ml of water or the animal will show quite severe colic. Remember that it should be transported in a car fridge.

Sodium pantoprazole

There is a high incidence of gastric ulcers in SACs. These occur in the caudal third compartment of C3. The normal sign is low-grade colic. Diagnosis may be aided by trans-abdominal ultrasonography. On being faced with a possible acute ulcer liable to perforate, a human drug sodium pantoprazole should be injected intravenously after dissolving the 40 mg powder in the vial with water for injection. Pain can be controlled with NSAIDs but these should be discontinued as soon as appetite is re-established.

Tetanus Antitoxin

Tetanus antitoxin (TAT) should be kept in the fridge. The dose is very empirical. However, the author would recommend 3000 IU for an adult given subcutaneously and 1500 IU for crias. Some authorities regard TAT in SACs as dangerous, although there is no factual basis for this. SACs will certainly get tetanus. The author has seen tetanus in a male llama that had untreated wounds from fighting.

Trace Element and Vitamin Injectable Products

Cobalt/Vitamin B12

Cobalt can be given orally either separately or with an anthelmintic. Vitamin B12, cyanocobalamin, can be given subcutaneously or intramuscularly. It is supplied in a solution containing 1000 mg in 1 ml. The dose is 2 ml per adult. It can be repeated in 7 days. It is also available at a quarter of this strength in a 0.025% w/v solution. The dose is 1 ml for crias.

Selenium

There is a long-acting preparation licensed for use in sheep in the UK, which lasts for 12 months. It is supplied in an aqueous suspension containing 50 mg/ml of selenium (175 mg/ml barium selenate). It should be given by subcutaneous injection. The dose is 1 ml/50 kg, so normally an adult llama will need 3 ml and an alpaca 2 ml. Owners should be warned that in some instances a small nodule will be left at the injection site.

Vitamins B and C

There is a licensed preparation of four B vitamins and vitamin C available for sheep in the UK. It can be used in any deficiency related to these five vitamins including cerebro-cortico-necrosis (CCN; see Chapter 12). Each 1 ml contains 35 mg thiamine hydrochloride (vitamin B1), 0.5 mg riboflavin sodium phosphate (vitamin B2), 7 mg pyridoxine hydrochloride (vitamin B6), 23 mg nicotinamide (vitamin B3) and 70 mg ascorbic acid (vitamin C). The dose is 5–10 ml, which can be given subcutaneously, deep intramuscularly or slow intravenously. It is suitable for llamas and alpacas. Thiamine injection on its own can also be used to treat CCN. The dose is 15 mg/kg given either intravenously or subcutaneously daily for 5 days.

Vitamin D

Rickets is a real problem in SACs in the UK because of the lack of sunlight. Dosages vary; however, 1000 IU/month for crias between November and March will give protection. Products containing Vitamin D3 normally also contain Vitamin A and E. They tend to come and go on the market and often have to be imported from the EU under licence. At the time of going to press the products shown in Table 6.2 below were available (C. Whitehead, personal communication).

Table 6.2. Dosages of available products in 2022.

	Belavit AD3E (per ml)	Hipravit ADE (per ml)
Vitamin D (cholecalciferol)	100,000 IU	75,000 IU
Vitamin A (retinol palmitate	300,000 IU	500,000 IU
Vitamin E (alpha tocopherol acetate)	50.00 mg	50.00 mg
Recommended prophylactic dose for camelids at 1000 IU/kg (repeat every 2 months October–April)	0.1ml per 10kg body weight	0.13ml per 10kg body weight
Recommended treatment dose, at 2000 IU/kg (repeat after one month)	0.2ml per 10kg body weight	0.26ml per 10kg body weight

Injectable Medicines to be Carried by the Practitioner

Table 6.3. Veterinary drugs to be carried by veterinary surgeons carrying out work with SACs.

Drug	Trade name	Dosage	Comments
Acepromazine	ACP injection 2%	0.02–0.05 mg/kg iv or im	For milk let-down and urethral relaxation
Butorphanol	Torbugesic	0.1 mg/kg iv or im	Analgesia
Cloprostenol	Estrumate	1 ml im	Repeat in 24 h
Dexamethasone	Colvastone	0.1 mg/kg im or iv	Not in pregnant alpacas
Diazepam	Valium	0.1 mg/kg	Useful in crias
Enrofloxacin	Baytril	5 mg/kg sc	Double dosage for 48 h
Florfenicol	Nuflor	10 mg/kg sc	Double dosage for 48 h
Flunixin meglumine	Finadyne	1 mg/kg sc or iv	Oral not effective
Ketamine	Ketaset	Various im	Anaesthesia
Ketoprofen	Ketofen	2 mg/kg sc or iv	NSAID for pain relief
Lidocaine 2%	Willocaine	4 mg/kg max dose	1 ml epidural
Oxytetracycline	Various	Vary im and iv	Higher dosage for longer action
Oxytocin	Various	10 IU im	Dilute for iv
Pantoprazole	Protium	4 ml iv	Ulcer treatment
Penicillin	Procaine im; crystapen iv	22,000–44,000 IU/kg	Often with strep
Thiamine	Various	15 mg/kg sc or iv	Every day for 5 days
Vitamin D	Duphafral ADE	1,000 IU im	Winter months
Xylazine	Rompun 2%	0.3 mg/kg iv; 0.6 mg/kg im	Sedation

Table 6.4. Extra veterinary drugs to be carried by the ambulatory clinician.

400 ml 20% calcium
400 ml 20% calcium with added 5% magnesium, phosphorus and glucose
400 ml 25% magnesium sulfate
400 ml 40% dextrose solution
2 × 100 ml barbiturate euthanasia solution
2 × 50 ml somulose solution: 400 mg/ml quinalbarbitone, 25 mg/ml cinchocaine hydrochloride
Coloured antibiotic aerosol spray
Obstetrical lubricant
'J Lube' lubricant powder
Dopram drops: 20 mg/ml doxapram hydrochloride
Powdered oral electrolyte
Vaccutainers coloured red, purple, green and grey, with needles and holder
Diclazuril solution
Triclabendazole solution
An oral anthelmintic
Doramectin injectable solution
An oral antibiotic with a dosing pump for crias
A pour-on to kill fly-strike larvae

7

Vaccines

_____

Introduction

The availability and the need for vaccination against an individual disease will vary between countries and species. As a rule of thumb, vaccines prepared for viral diseases tend to be more effective than vaccines prepared for bacterial diseases. Equally, live vaccines that have been stored and used correctly tend to be more effective than dead vaccines. It should be remembered that if a live vaccine has been used it would be difficult for a serum sample to differentiate between a vaccine titre and that of active disease, unless the vaccine is a 'marker' vaccine. However, 'marker' vaccines are becoming more common, and polymerase chain reaction (PCR) testing has become more sophisticated so these tests can differentiate between reactions to vaccines rather than active disease.

Storage of vaccines is extremely important. It is not only live vaccines that have to be stored at controlled temperatures. Practitioners should read the data sheets carefully for storage instructions before reconstitution of the vaccine and after reconstitution. Vaccines that require reconstitution with a diluent normally have a very short life after reconstitution. This period should be strictly followed. Refrigeration storage should be monitored with maximum and minimum temperatures recorded on a regular basis. It should be stressed that it is vital that expensive vaccines are stored and used in the correct manner, as not only will they be ineffective but also they may cause reactions in the animal. It is also important that the correct technique is used for administration.

Most vaccines are required to be given subcutaneously, so a short needle can be used e.g. 5/8 of an inch. The gauge of the needle is important. In essence the smallest gauge (e.g. 23G) is best especially for small young animals. However, a larger gauge (e.g. 21G or 19G) will be more appropriate for adults. Practitioners should be aware that small gauge needles are more likely to break at the hub. Immediate retrieval of the broken needle is vital. Contamination of the vaccine container must be avoided. Only a clean sterile needle should be used to draw out the dose of vaccine. A different needle should then be used to inject the animal. It is quite reasonable for an assistant to be drawing up doses of vaccine using the same needle in the bottle of vaccine. The same second needle can be used to vaccinate a number of animals. However, this needle should be changed at regular intervals. The use of multidose syringes is widespread and should be encouraged in large herds as on the whole there is less contamination. However, it is important that they are calibrated for the correct dose of vaccine. Once again, the needle should be changed at regular intervals.

© Graham R. Duncanson 2023. _Veterinary Treatment of Llamas and Alpacas,_ 2nd Edition
(G.R. Duncanson)
DOI: 10.1079/9781800623576.0007

It is also important to consider the animals to be vaccinated. They should not be unduly stressed. This is particularly important for pregnant animals. Often there is a need for careful timing of vaccination in pregnant animals so that the risk to the pregnancy is kept to a minimum but the level of immunity in the colostrum is at a maximum. The practitioner should give careful advice to the owner on the timing of vaccination in young crias. If the dam has not been vaccinated then quite young crias can receive their first dose of vaccine. On the other hand if the dam has received a booster during her pregnancy the first vaccination should be delayed. There is no harm in vaccinating crias too early, it is just that the first dose may be ineffective and so an extra dose will need to be given. Having vaccinated the female animals it is important to remember to vaccinate the male animals at the correct time so their immunity is maintained.

In general wet animals should not be vaccinated as there is a much greater risk of needle contamination. It is worthwhile stressing that dates of vaccination and groups of animals should always be recorded carefully.

There are various types of vaccine. Live modified vaccines usually stimulate high levels of solid immunity from a single inoculation. Inactivated vaccines usually contain weaker antigens and require an initial course of two doses. Vaccines often use multiple antigens. There is no evidence to suggest that there is diminution in the individual antigen protection or less protection in the face of field challenge. These vaccines are more economical to produce and also mean that animals have to be handled less frequently.

Most vaccines are licensed to be given subcutaneously. An ideal place is over the ribs behind the shoulder. Data sheets should always be consulted as some vaccines need to be given intramuscularly. The triceps can be used.

With most vaccines circulating antibodies fall to apparently non-protective levels fairly quickly. However, they are rapidly raised by a challenge in the field. Most inactivated bacterins and toxoided vaccines require annual boosters in sheep for which they were specifically prepared. In SACs there is some confusion as the sheep vaccines are not licensed for these species and there is no data sheet available. To make sure these animals are adequately covered most

clinicians give boosters twice a year. The practice of giving twice the dose only once a year is unlikely to be sensible.

To allow the mother time to produce adequate colostral antibodies, booster doses need to be given a minimum of 2 weeks prior to parturition. There is little information available to advise clinicians on the extent of the period of maternal or so-called passive immunity. It is likely to be about 3 months but this period will vary with the vaccine. Therefore if clinicians are in any doubt it is prudent to give vaccines earlier and give an extra dose later. Most vaccines prepared for sheep are relatively inexpensive so that cost is not an issue with SACs, only the handling problems and the fact that many are kept in small groups and therefore some vaccine has to be discarded.

Clinicians may be consulted when there appears to be a failure of vaccination. Careful detective work together with great tact will be required. There are a large number of factors that need to be considered:

1. Incorrect storage. Obviously this can occur at any place along the chain from manufacturer to wholesaler to merchant to owner to animal. As a veterinary surgeon one hopes that the route to the owner is not at fault. The manufacturers are normally extremely helpful when there are problems. Clinicians should make 100% certain that their controls (e.g. fridge temperature monitoring) are in place before blaming the owner.
2. The method of administration should be checked. Not only the route must be correct but also the actual technique, i.e. the vaccine must actually go into the animal.
3. We have discussed earlier the influence of maternal immunity. Vaccines given during the period of high maternal antibody circulation will not be effective and will have to be repeated.
4. Vaccination can be ineffective if disinfectants contaminate any of the equipment and needles. Equally vaccination will not be accomplished if there is bacterial contamination and abscessation.
5. Naturally the vaccine must be the correct vaccine for controlling the disease in question. There is always going to be doubt about the use of unlicensed vaccines.
6. The animals must be healthy when they receive the vaccine. Animals in very poor condition

or suffering from a deficiency will not be able to respond to the vaccine.

7. Animal owners should obtain advice when giving several injections at the same time. On the whole the less the animals are stressed by continual handling the better. However, giving anthelmintics, antibiotics and several vaccinations at the same time may be too much for the animal.

8. Vaccination is a numbers game. The majority of a group of animals may respond but certain individuals may not make an antibody response. They may actually be immune or of course they may not be immune.

When using more than one vaccine there are no hard and fast rules. However, following these guidelines constitutes a good code of practice:

1. If possible separate the two vaccines by at least 2 weeks.

2. If this is not possible it is better to inject them at the same time rather than separate them by only 2 or 3 days.

3. If two vaccines are going to be given it will take longer, so stress should be minimized by providing adequate food and water to waiting animals.

4. Always use separate vaccinators and needles.

5. Inject at different sites (e.g. left and right side of the animal).

Vaccines

Blackleg

There is a single component vaccine licensed for cattle and sheep against *Clostridium chauvoei* (blackleg), which can be given safely to SACs to provide good immunity. SACs require two doses separated by 6 weeks, boosted with a single dose annually. To obtain passive immunity in crias, female SACs should receive the second dose 3–4 weeks before parturition.

Blue tongue

SACs are definitely affected by this disease, which can be fatal. However, there are many strains. Clinicians should carry out a risk analysis and use the appropriate strains. Polyvalent vaccines do not seem to be effective and therefore single strain vaccines should be used. The vaccination regime recommended for cattle should be used, not that recommended for sheep.

Bovine respiratory disease

These cattle vaccines should be avoided in SACs until further research work has been carried out. The only exception is vaccination against parainfluenza 3 (PI3), which has been used to good effect in an outbreak of this virus in young llamas.

Bovine virus diarrhoea

Bovine virus diarrhoea (BVD) will affect SACs. However, there are no reports of the safe use of any cattle vaccines in SACs so practitioners will have to consider very carefully any use of vaccination with the owners of the SACs.

Brucella melitensis

There is a live vaccine available, which is not licensed in the UK but is available elsewhere. This organism has been isolated from SACs so in exceptional circumstances this vaccine could be recommended.

Cattle scour vaccines

These vaccines, which are injected into cows in their last 6 weeks of pregnancy, have been used in SACs. They offer protection against rotavirus, coronavirus and *Escherichia coli*. It would appear that the viral component is what is useful. Obviously immunity only occurs if the crias receive adequate levels of colostrum. There are passive immunity products that can be given to calves in their first 6 h after birth. These might be a safer option for use in SACs.

Chlamydophila species

If SACs are found to be suffering abortions from this organism, the sheep vaccine may be used *before* service for the next pregnancy. There appear to be no side effects.

Clostridial disease vaccination

This is the most important vaccination that needs to be carried out in SACs worldwide. SACs are very prone to getting tetanus. It is vital that they are fully vaccinated. If a practitioner is called to a SAC that has been cut or is going to perform a castration it is vital that the tetanus status is evaluated. If there is any doubt the practitioner should give not only a dose of a suitable tetanus vaccine but also a dose of tetanus antiserum (TAT). A dose for an adult SAC would be 3000 IU given either subcutaneously or intramuscularly. The dose for a cria is half of that, i.e. 1500 IU. It is a myth that TAT is toxic in SACs.

Other than *Clostridium tetani* the most important clostridia to affect SACs are *C. perfringens* type C and D. All SACs should be regularly vaccinated against these types by an initial course of two doses separated by 4–6 weeks then a booster every 6 months. The use of polyvalent vaccines including *C. novyi*, *C. septicum*, *C. chauvoei* and *C. sordellii* is worthwhile in most areas, particularly if there is any risk of liver fluke *Fasciola hepatica*, as this parasite damages the liver and makes the SAC more prone to succumbing to clostridial infections. There are vaccines containing 4, 7, 8 and 10 strains. Practitioners need to be familiar with the potential risks to the SACs in their area to advise their owners. The timing of vaccination for crias is open for debate. However, a safe regime would be to start vaccination at 10–12 weeks of age if the dams are fully vaccinated and have been given a booster injection in the last third of pregnancy. If the dams have not received an injection in the last third of pregnancy, crias should receive their first dose between 2 and 4 weeks of age with a second dose given 4–6 weeks later. All SACs should receive booster doses twice a year.

Eastern equine encephalitis

This disease has been reported to be a cause of death in the eastern part of the USA. No adverse effects from a killed multivalent equine vaccine have been reported in alpacas (Bedenice *et al.*, 2009).

Equine herpes type 1 vaccination (sometimes called *Equine Rhinopneumonitis*)

Equine herpes virus (EHV) type 1 has been isolated from SACs and has been shown to be the cause of death in SACs kept near to affected zebra. SACs could be vaccinated with an equine vaccine if the risk is thought to be high. Vaccination should be carried out quarterly.

Leptospirosis vaccination

In leptospirosis-endemic areas a biannual vaccination should be carried out in susceptible females using the cattle vaccine. This is prepared from formol-killed cultures of *Leptospira interrogans* serovar *harjo*. Initial vaccination requires two doses separated by 4–6 weeks.

Pasteurellosis

The *Pasteurella* vaccines prepared for sheep do not confer any immunity to SACs and therefore should not be used. However, if a specific vaccine is made for SACs it should be used according to the manufacturer's instructions to animals at risk.

Rabies vaccination

Rabies will occur in SACs. However, they are an end host so are unlikely to transmit the virus. Killed rabies vaccines can be used in endemic areas; however, their efficacy has not been proven.

Toxoplasmosis

If SACs are at risk the sheep vaccine may be used to help control this disease. It must be given *before* service.

West Nile virus

It has been shown that this virus may affect SACs causing death. If it is present in the area young and immune-compromised animals can be vaccinated. The suggested dose regime is three doses at three weekly intervals with the final dose given a month before the peak mosquito exposure. A single dose then should be given annually (Kutzler *et al.*, 2004).

8

Sedation, Anaesthesia, Surgical Conditions and Euthanasia

Pre-Operative Considerations

Legal aspects

This is a very difficult situation as the law is far from clear. There are no licensed medicines for use in camelids. Nor has it been decided whether they are pets or food-producing animals. There are certain medicines that are forbidden in food-producing animals. To get around this the practitioner should get assurance from the owner that the animal will not enter the food chain. Such an assurance is realistically impossible to enforce and the responsibility falls back on the veterinarian. Since Brexit the enforcing agency is the Veterinary Medicine Directorate (VMD).

General considerations

- Body weight. This is easy to overestimate in heavy-fleeced animals. It is prudent to actually weigh the animal, particularly crias.
- Trauma is a danger as camelids have long limbs and a long neck. They also have prominent eyes.
- The jugular groove is not easy to see because the skin is thick, and the fleece can be long and dense. Clipping is worthwhile as visualization of the jugular vein is very difficult. It should be remembered that the jugular

vein in the lower third of the neck is deep and lies just above the carotid artery.
- It should be remembered that camelids are herd animals and are often not halter trained. They will 'kush'. Chutes that crush and have a floor that drops are very helpful with wild animals.
- Male llamas will weigh between 140 and 175 kg. Female llamas will weigh between 100 and 150 kg.
- Male alpacas will weigh between 60 and 100 kg. Female alpacas will weigh between 50 and 80 kg.

Tetanus cover

SACs are very prone to getting tetanus. It is vital that every effort is made to cover all animals in the case of an urgent surgical procedure. In the case of an elective procedure it should be delayed until full vaccination has been carried out. Full vaccination involves a double dose of vaccine separated by 4 weeks. The boosters should be given at 6-monthly intervals.

If the procedure is urgent and the animal has had an initial course of two doses of vaccine some time ago a single booster dose will be sufficient. However, if this has not been carried out it is suggested that the patient should receive its primary dose of tetanus vaccine and 3000 IU of

© Graham R. Duncanson 2023. *Veterinary Treatment of Llamas and Alpacas*, 2nd Edition (G.R. Duncanson)
DOI: 10.1079/9781800623576.0008

tetanus antitoxin (TAT). This could be reduced to 1 500 IU in very young animals. Cover with antibiotics is also important. If tetanus is a consideration, the antibiotic of choice is penicillin.

Analgesia

This is very important. The drug of choice with both sedation and anaesthesia is butorphanol. This can be given post-operatively as well as pre-operatively at 0.1 mg/kg every 6 h either intramuscularly, subcutaneously or intravenously. Non-steroidal anti-inflammatory drugs (NSAIDs) can be given at the same time except it should be remembered that they are nephrotoxic, so they should be avoided if there is likely to be any kidney damage. The practitioner can use his judgement on which NSAID to use (see Chapter 6). Buprenophine can be used. The dose is 0.01–0.02 mg/kg. Other opiates can be given, e.g. morphine at 0.05–0.2 mg/kg intramuscularly every 6 hours. A single dose of fentanyl may be given intravenously at 0.002 mg/kg.

NSAIDs are very good pre-operative analgesics. However, it must be remembered that steroids are more potent anti-inflammatory drugs than non-steroidals. As inflammation causes pain there may be good reason to use steroids for some analgesia. The clinician has to consider the risks carefully. Steroids (e.g. dexamethasone) will delay wound healing. On the other hand wound healing is irrelevant if the animal has died from hyperlipaemia from inappetence caused by inflammation and pain.

Antibiosis

These should be given as soon as possible in urgent cases. In elective procedures they should be given before surgery is planned to allow for good tissue levels. Unless there are special considerations a combination of penicillin and streptomycin is the antibiotic of choice.

Gut fill

Ideally the gastroenteric organs should be as empty as possible. However, practitioners should

beware of withholding fluids from the young and from debilitated animals. Care should also be taken in hot climates. In some ways starving the patients is more important when heavy sedation or field anaesthesia is used as there is no cuffed endotracheal tube in place to prevent C1 contents being inhaled. A protocol suggested is to withhold concentrates for 24 h pre-op, forage for 12 h and water for 8 h. In young animals under 4 weeks of age, they should be treated as normal except they should not be allowed to suckle for 2 h before sedation or anaesthesia. It should be remembered that sedation decreases gut motility and increases urinary output.

Fly control

This is important in all animals, particularly fibre-producing animals. A cream containing acriflavin and benzene hexachloride should be applied to all wounds. The whole animal should be protected by synthetic pyrethrum compounds.

Sedation

Alpacas are gentle creatures and can readily be controlled so sedation is rarely required. They will often go into the 'kush' position or can easily be cast. This is not so with llamas, which can be difficult. The main thing is to get close into them so that any kick will not be as painful. Xylazine hydrochloride is very effective; an injection intramuscularly of 1 ml of a 2% solution will certainly sedate a llama, which may well then 'kush', whereas 0.75 ml of a 2% solution is quite sufficient for a large male alpaca. Guanacos and vicuna are more like wild animals and will require sedation for most procedures. Xylazine can be given as a gel either on the buccal mucosa or on the vaginal mucosa. Various other sedation combinations have been described, for example: for light sedation in a 50 kg animal, a combination of 1.5 ml of a 10 mg/ml solution of acetylpromazine and 0.35 ml of a 10 mg/ml solution of butorphanol given intramuscularly; and for heavy sedation in a 50 kg animal, a combination of 0.5 ml of a 20 mg/ml solution of xylazine and 1 ml of a 100 mg/ml of ketamine. Another sedation combination for which a wide dosage has been suggested is xylazine hydrochloride at 0.1 to 0.3 mg/kg given intravenously, intramuscularly or subcutaneously, butorphenol tartrate at 0.03 to 0.1 mg/kg given intravenously, intramuscularly or subcutaneously and metdetomidine at 10 to 30 μg/kg given intramuscularly.

Some authors (C. Gittel, personal communication) suggest that camelids are less sensitive to metomidine than to xylazine.

Azaperone has been suggested as a sedative in camelids. However, the author of this book has no experience of this drug other than in swine.

Morphine, a schedule 2 controlled drug, may be used in camelids. It is not licensed for food-producing animals. The dose is 0.05–0.2 mg/kg intramuscularly. The author has never used this drug except in conjunction with an alpha-2 agonist.

Yohimbine is not licensed for use in the UK. However, it is used elsewhere as a reversal agent for xylazine. It is obtained as a solution of 10 mg/ml. It should be given intravenously or intramuscularly at a rate of 0.25 ml/10 kg, although its usage is outside the author's experience. Many clinicians consider it to be a useful drug, equally others have found difficulties. There are anecdotal reports of acute cerebellar oedema causing fatalities. The author has never had any difficulties with recovery from xylazine sedation but considers monitoring very important. The short-term signs to be on the lookout for are: abnormal posture, reluctance to stand, reluctance to move, abnormal gait, reluctance to join the herd, bruxism (tooth grinding), raised temperature, pulse and respiration and marked pallor. If these problems persist then intravenous fluids are advised together with flunixin at 1.1 mg/kg.

Tolazoline is not licensed for use in the UK. However, it is used elsewhere as a reversal agent for xylazine. It should be given intravenously or intramuscularly at 1 to 2 mg/kg.

Atipamsole is not licensed for use in the UK. However, it is used elsewhere as a reversal agent for xylazine. It should only be given intravenously at 0.125 mg/kg.

As a rule of thumb alpacas on a weight for weight basis require between 10 and 20% higher doses of sedation to give the same effect as llamas. However, this may just be a factor of lower actual weights in the same way that ponies appear to require higher rates of sedation compared to horses.

Acepromazine is not a very useful sedative in SACs as it really only gives mild tranquillization at standard doses of 0.03 mg/kg intravenously or 0.05 mg/kg intramuscularly. It is useful in maiden females who are reluctant to allow crias to suckle. A single injection of 2.5 ml of a 10% solution and 2.5 ml of a 10 IU/ml of oxytocin given intramuscularly as soon as the problem is realized is helpful.

Detomidine and romifidine can be used in SACs. However, as xylazine is so reliable their use must be questioned and it is outside the author's experience.

Diazepam is a useful sedative for use in small crias. It can be given either intravenously or intramuscularly at 0.1 mg/kg. At this dosage it will give safe profound sedation. It is not nearly so effective in older and larger animals.

General Anaesthesia

General anaesthesia using gaseous anaesthesia is hazardous in SACs (Bradbury, 2008). There is a considerable danger of regurgitation. This is described as either passive or active. Passive regurgitation occurs under deep anaesthesia and manifests as a continual flow of stomach contents through the mouth. Active regurgitation occurs during light anaesthesia. It is projectile, as it is in fact antiperistalis. It is extremely dangerous and can lead to inhalation pneumonia particularly if it occurs during intubation. Adult SACs should be fasted for 12 h before surgery and water should be withheld for 8 h. Regurgitation is influenced by the anaesthetic agent used (Garcia Pereira et al., 2006). Ketamine causes less regurgitation than thiopentone, which should be avoided in SAC anaesthesia. Protocols using xylazine intravenously followed by ketamine intravenously may be used. This will allow intubation and gaseous anaesthesia with isoflurane. There are considerable difficulties with this protocol: (i) intravenous injections are not easy as the owners do not like the wool clipped – the skin is very thick so the jugular cannot be visualized. The carotid lies only just below the jugular particularly in the caudal third of the neck; (ii) intubation is very difficult unless you are skilled with a long laryngoscope; and (iii) there is a real danger of inhalation pneumonia on induction and recovery. There are various tips suggested to aid intubation. An adult alpaca will require an 8 mm endotracheal tube and an adult llama will require a 10 mm endotracheal tube. These sizes of tube are readily available for large dogs. However, the canine tubes are too short and so clinicians should try to obtain foal tubes or have longer canine tubes made specifically. A laryngoscope with a blade of 20 cm will be required. After premedication with atropine, which can be given intramuscularly at 0.04 mg/kg or intravenously at 0.02 mg/kg, the animal should be anaesthetized with one of the combinations of anaesthetics described below. With the animal in sternal recumbency the neck should be stretched vertically. The top and bottom jaws should be held open by an assistant with two loops of bandage. The tube can then be inserted into the trachea with the laryngoscope. This will be aided by an aluminium rod inside the tube to add rigidity. An ideal size of rod is the arm of an aluminium horse twitch with the string removed.

A preferred method is an intramuscular injection of a cocktail into the quadriceps muscle. The dose for a typical 18-month-old llama weighing 80 kg, which is a common time for castration, is 5 ml ketamine (10% solution), 2.5 ml xylazine (2% solution) and 0.5 ml butorphanol (1% solution). All these three medicines should be given in the same syringe. This will give 20 min of anaesthesia after an induction period of 5–10 min. The dose for a typical 18-month-old alpaca weighing 60 kg for castration is 3.3 ml ketamine (10% solution), 1.7 ml xylazine (2% solution) and 0.3 ml butorphanol (1% solution). Naturally larger or smaller animals can be anaesthetized with different dosages on a pro rata basis. As intramuscular injections may be sometimes less reliable than intravenous injections clinicians may prefer to inject a combined dose of 0.1 mg/kg of butorphanol, 3 mg/kg of ketamine and 0.3 mg/kg of xylazine intravenously. This method will only give approximately half the length of time of anaesthesia, i.e. 10 min.

This cocktail is prepared by many other clinicians in a slightly different manner; they prepare a solution of the three drugs, which they then give on a per kilogram basis.

The stock solution is:

- 10 ml of a 100 mg/ml solution of ketamine;
- 1 ml of a 100 mg/ml solution of xylazine; and
- 1 ml of a 10 mg/ml solution of butorphanol.

This solution can be given at 1 ml/34 kg intramuscularly to provide heavy sedation. If given at 1 ml/17 kg intramuscularly it will provide anaesthesia. This anaesthesia can be maintained by giving 1 ml/34 kg intravenously.

The following gives a very sensible anaesthetic protocol for a 68 kg animal:

- Inject 4 ml of the cocktail intramuscularly.
- Inject 4 ml of atropine sulfate in a 600 μg/ml solution intramuscularly.
- When anaesthetized, establish a drip line with a 14G over-the-top catheter pointing caudally (the skin will need to be incised after surgical preparation).
- Inject 2 ml of the cocktail every 30 min to maintain anaesthesia.

A combination of ketamine and diazepam has been recommended for anaesthesia following xylazine sedation for a 50kg animal:

- Inject 0.75 ml of a 2% xylazine (20 mg/ml) solution intramuscularly.
- After sedation, catheterize the animal (a bleb of local anaesthetic should be given under the skin).
- Inject 1 ml of a 100 mg/ml solution of ketamine intravenously.
- Inject 0.1 mg/kg diazepam intravenously.
- Inject 2 ml of atropine sulfate in a 600 μg/ml solution intravenously.
- Anaesthesia can be maintained by giving 0.5 ml of 2% xylazine, 0.5 ml of 10% ketamine and diazepam every 30 min.

One author recommends for general anaesthesia 4.7 to 6.0 mg/kg tiletamine/zolazepam followed by halothane isoflurane 1 to 5% by either orotracheal tube or nasotracheal tube (D. Anderson, personal communication). This author noted that an acute death had occurred after rapid intravenous administration of tolazoline at high doses.

The author of this book has no first-hand experience of the use of these drugs.

Thiopentone, guaifenesin and propofol have all been used for general anaesthesia in SACs; however, as ketamine is such a safe and reliable anaesthetic agent the author has never found a need to use them. Propofol can be given at 1–6 mg/kg intravenously to effect. It has a quick onset (E. Po, personal communication).

Taylor *et al.* (2017) published an evaluation of three intravenous injectable anaesthesia protocols in healthy adult male alpacas. The protocols given intravenously were: ketamine (4.0 mg/kg) and diazepam (0.1 mg/kg); propofol (4.0 mg/kg); and ketamine (2.0 mg/kg) and propofol (2.0 mg/kg). They found no significant difference in duration of anaesthesia. All animals recovered within 20 minutes after induction and with minimal ataxia.

Recovery from Gaseous Anaesthesia

SACs are obligate nasal breathers and gas exchange must be confirmed immediately after the endotracheal tube has been removed as the airway may be compromised during the transition from endotracheal tube breathing to nasal breathing. SACs tend to relax after the endotracheal tube is removed as the stimulus is also removed. The endotracheal tube should be left in place until the patient is able to swallow, chew, cough, and is actively trying to expel the tube. Sadly the tube is liable to damage, but at least the animal is not put at risk. If regurgitation has occurred, the endotracheal tube should be withdrawn with the cuff inflated until the cuff reaches the larynx. Any ingesta must be removed from the pharynx or buccal cavity. The animal's head should be kept elevated. Human assistance must always be present until a SAC is fully recovered. The author does not recommend the use of intra-nasal tubes to supply extra oxygen because if too wide a bore is used there may be severe haemorrhage or turbinate trauma leading to nasal oedema. The use of a very small tube will normally be counterproductive by restricting the airway.

Regional Anaesthesia

Local anaesthetics

- Procaine is licenced for use in cattle and therefore following the cascade it is the local anesthetic of choice. The maximum dose is 20 mg/kg.
- Lidocaine can be used unlicensed. The maximum dose is 8 mg/kg.

Epidural anaesthesia

The normal site used by practitioners is the sacrococcygeal space. A 1½ inch 20G needle should be used perpendicularly to the spine. The dose is 2 ml of 2% lignocaine for an adult llama. To give a longer action and some slight sedation 0.25 ml of 2% xylazine can be added to this. The dose of both lignocaine and xylazine should be reduced by 25% in alpacas.

Dental blocks

The only block used by the author is the maxillary block. A volume of 3 ml of procaine is injected above the infraorbital foramen. This lies 1.5 cm above the first molar.

Regional anaesthesia of the lower limb

Apply a tourniquet immediately above the carpal or tarsal joint. Two small rolls of bandage should be inserted either side of the Achilles tendon when applying the tourniquet to the hindleg. The mid area of the metacarpus or metatarsus should be clipped and surgically cleaned. A suitable superficial vein should be selected. A bleb of local anaesthetic should be put under the skin using a 25G needle. Using a 1 inch 23G needle, 2.5–10 ml (depending on the size of the animal) of 2% lignocaine should be injected extremely slowly into the vein. Within 5 min full regional anaesthesia will be achieved. This will last for over 1 h. Anaesthesia will cease as soon as the tourniquet is removed.

Common Surgical Conditions

Angular limb deformity

These deformities will be observed soon after birth. They should be monitored but no immediate action should be taken. Sometimes they will occur in crias with other congenital problems. Careful assessment will have to be carried out to decide if euthanasia is the most appropriate action. Assuming limb deformity is the only problem then the cria should be allowed to mature for 6 weeks. Radiographs should then be taken of the carpus and metacarpus, or in the case of the extremely rare hindlimb deformity, the tarsus and the metatarsus. If the carpus or tarsus is deformed euthanasia should be advised. Only if the metacarpus or metatarsus is bent should surgery be attempted. The author advises a periosteal strip as no specialized instruments, screws etc. are required, and the risk of a second operation is removed. There is also less risk of post-operative sepsis. Antibiotics and TAT should be given preoperatively. The cria should be masked down with halothane or isoflurane and the limbs prepared for surgery. Depending on whether it is varus or valgus the 2.5 cm long vertical incision should be made on the lateral or medial aspect of the metacarpus. The periosteum should be scratched off the metacarpus for a length of 12 mm and width of 6 mm. The skin should be closed with small interrupted skin sutures or staples. The wound should be covered by a protective bandage. The owners should be counselled that the cria has to grow more rapidly on the opposite side to straighten the leg. This growth cannot be accurately predicted.

Atresia ani

This congenital condition may be inherited but this has not been proven. However, it is prudent not to breed from these animals. Normally the condition is not seen until sometime after birth. The place where the anus should be located is bulging out full of meconium. This area should be clean and a skin bleb of local anaesthetic should be injected. A small cruciate incision should be made with a scalpel. No suturing is required. The tetanus status of the cria should be checked. The cria should be examined in 48 h to check that patency has been maintained.

Atresia recti

Unlike atresia ani this condition is often not readily seen and its correction surgically is extremely difficult. Euthanasia is likely to be the kindest and economic course of action.

Castration

There is a myth, strongly held by owners, that castration should be delayed until puberty, i.e. 18 months. They feel that if animals are castrated before sexual maturity the animals will get weak long legs. It is difficult to disprove this opinion as owners are reluctant to allow clinical audit.

Castration can be performed in two ways. Naturally the veterinary charge will reflect the manner of castration. This can be a proper sterile operation under general anaesthetic. The surgery is performed in a similar manner to castrating a dog. With the animal in dorsal recumbency the area around the penis and the scrotum is surgically prepared. One testicle is pushed cranially into a pre-scrotal position. A careful incision is made over it, and it is then drawn out within its tunics. Two pairs of artery forceps are then clamped above the testicle. The pair nearest to the testicle is removed and a tight ligature of absorbable material is placed in the groove. The testicle is then removed above the second pair of artery forceps. The forceps are then removed carefully allowing the stump to return to its normal position in the scrotum. This process is repeated with the second testicle through the same incision. The skin is then closed with a single continuous subcuticular suture of absorbable suture material and the area is covered with antibiotic spray. With skill and forethought there is time under intramuscular anaesthesia without a top-up to perform this surgical procedure provided the surgeon is assisted by a competent theatre nurse, who can prepare the patient and the instruments while the surgeon is scrubbing up.

The second method is to perform castration under local anaesthesia either standing or in the 'kush' position. Ideally the animal is well restrained behind a solid gate, e.g. in the front of a cattle trailer, with an inner partition. Access can be provided from behind, e.g. the 'jockey' door. The use of a trailer spares the surgeon from having to kneel down. Of course if there is no trailer the animal can be made to 'kush' or be 'chukkered' (see Chapter 1) on the ground. It is useful to lay a towel under the hindquarters to keep the surgery site as clean as possible. A total of 5 ml of anaesthetic is injected under the skin in the scrotum and up into the cord on each side. The area is thoroughly cleaned. The surgery is performed as for castration of an adult pig. The testicle is squeezed into the scrotum. An incision is made over the testicle and through the tunics. The testicle is then drawn from the scrotum and from the abdomen by pulling and twisting. There are two problems that may confront the clinician. The first is a prolapse of scrotal fat through the incision in a few hours, which will cause owners some concern. To avoid this either the fat can be removed at the time of surgery or the incision can be closed with a single horizontal mattress suture of absorbable suture material. The author prefers the former technique so the incision wounds can be left open for drainage. The second problem may be experienced when castrating small 18-month-old alpacas. The initial incision through the scrotum may be made too deep so that the testicular substance shells out and the tunics are hard to grasp. To avoid this, the clinician should make a careful incision through the scrotum so that the testicle is still inside the tunics as if a closed castration was being performed. A pair of artery forceps can be applied to the cord, and the testicle within its tunics can be drawn completely.

It is very important to remember to check the tetanus status. The animal should be given antibiotics and NSAIDs. The wound should be covered with antibiotic spray. If castration is carried out in the summer in the UK some sort of fly control should be considered.

Digital amputation

This procedure is not commonly carried out. However, it should be considered by clinicians if there is chronic septic arthritis in one intraphalangeal joint. The operation is welfare friendly. It is best to carry out the surgery under light sedation and a regional block. A tourniquet is required for both the regional block and for the operation. The animal is given pre-operative antibiotics and NSAIDs.

The foot is trimmed to remove any overgrown horn on the tip of the hoof. Then the whole leg below the middle of the metacarpus or metatarsus is clipped and surgically prepared. A length of embryotomy wire is positioned between the cleats. With an assistant holding the affected cleat with a pair of vulsellum forceps

the cleat is sawn off with the wire in a 45° upward angle. This cut will be made in the middle of the second phalange. The stump is then dressed with a suitable antibiotic cream and covered with a suitable dressing. The whole foot and leg to mid carpus/tarsus is bandaged with thin cotton wool and standard bandages. This is then covered by gaffer tape, taking care that the gaffer tape does not actually touch the skin. The animal is kept under antibiotic and NSAID cover for a minimum of 10 days. The dressing should be changed twice in this period. If a good healthy bed of granulation tissue has been formed a lighter protective bandage can then be applied.

Entropion

This is extremely rare in SACs. It is an inherited condition and causes severe welfare problems if it is not treated promptly. Every effort should be made to stop using sires that have the gene. Often if the condition is observed at birth the curled-in eyelid can be immediately uncurled and an entropion will not develop. However, if the condition is missed then treatment has to be initiated. Antibiotic eye ointment provided no steroid is included will help, but obviously will not influence the long-term disease. The curled-in eyelid needs to be turned out permanently. The best treatment is to treat the cria like a dog and carry out a 'cake slice op'. After putting in the local anaesthesia, the area around the eye needs to be clipped and prepared for surgery. A small slice of skin is then removed. The wound is then sutured with fine interrupted simple sutures. The eyelid is then permanently in the correct position. The sutures need to be removed in 10 days. Entropion has never been recorded in the top eyelid as well as the bottom eyelid although in theory it could occur. In this case two small slices of skin will need to be removed.

Enucleation of the eye

In all cases where there is no chance of the eye condition in any disease or traumatic problem recovering, enucleation should be considered on welfare grounds. It can be carried out under heavy sedation normally with xylazine.

Local anaesthetic should be instilled all around the orbit not only under the skin but into the deeper tissues with a single very deep injection of 5 ml behind the eye to block the optic nerve. The eyelids should then be sutured together and the whole area clipped and prepared aseptically. A careful incision is then made through the skin parallel to the upper eyelid margin but not entering the conjunctival sac. Using blunt dissection the eye muscles are sectioned around that half of the eye. The same procedure is then carried out to the lower half. Eventually a pair of curved scissors can be used to section the optic nerve and the eye can be removed. The remaining socket can then be obliterated with subcuticular suturing with absorbable material and the remaining eyelids can be sutured with non-absorbable material. The animal should receive antibiotics and NSAIDs for a minimum of 5 days. The sutures should be removed in 10 days.

Fracture of the mandible

These are quite common injuries from fighting and they appear horrendous. However, in fact they heal very well. The animal should have either heavy sedation or a general anaesthetic. Radiographs should be taken. The wound should be cleaned and debrided as necessary. The mandible should be stabilized with wire using the incisors, canines and rostral cheek teeth. Any loose teeth should be left *in situ* as they will often re-anchor. However, any actual fractured teeth should be removed as fractured enamel can not repair. The soft tissue should be sutured. The animal should be given antibiotics, NSAIDs and TAT. It should be fed on a sloppy diet or lush grass. The prognosis may well be good.

Limb amputation

This has been carried out in several species larger than llamas or alpacas. Practitioners must debate carefully the welfare aspects of limb amputation. On the plus side SACs 'kush' and so have an advantage over other Artiodactyla species of a similar size, in that they can rise up relatively easily. It has been performed on numerous occasions successfully in llamas and alpacas. The actual surgery is outside the author's experience.

Ovariohysterectomy

This surgery is outside of the author's experience. The rationale for such surgery can only be experimental and would be very difficult. Obtaining access to the ovaries would cause considerable problems. Hysterectomy alone would not be quite so difficult. However, the need to carry this out would be in the event of a uterine tear. If the tear was cranial then repair should be carried out from an abdominal incision. If the tear was caudal such a repair would be very difficult and euthanasia would be indicated.

It might be postulated that certain uterine conditions might require hysterectomy. However, treatment through the cervix would appear to be an easier and safer option.

Patella luxation

This is a deformity that is normally bilateral as a result of the patella grove being too shallow. Repair has been tried but was unsuccessful. Euthanasia must be advised.

Patent urachus

This condition is normally congenital. The urachus has failed to close at birth. Normally this can be ligated together with the vessels lying beside it, without need for anaesthesia. Prolonged antibiotic cover is vital as if sepsis develops further difficult surgery will be required. All the diseased infected tissue will need to be removed. This should be done under a general anaesthetic with the cria masked down with halothane or isoflurane. Once the diseased tissue has been removed the urachus and the vessels will need to be ligated inside the abdomen. Drainage will have to be established so that the healing can occur from within. Further broad-spectrum antibiotic cover will be required as well as wound flushing with dilute povidone-iodine.

Persistent hymen

If this condition is actually a persistent hymen it is relatively easily rectified. It also does not hold any ethical problems, unlike a similar but rarer condition of vagina aplasia. Vagina aplasia is genetic and so surgery should not be attempted.

The sign of both conditions in affected animals will be that of the male failing to fully penetrate the female. Normally the hymen containing uterine mucoid secretions can be perforated with a finger. The secretions are voided and the animal can be bred from in the normal manner. There is no need for further treatment. If this cannot be achieved the animal should be examined carefully with a small duck-billed speculum. If there is a persistent hymen it will be seen bulging towards the operator. It should be pieced with a stab incision with a small scalpel and widened with a finger. If there is aplasia of the vagina the animal should be left as a fibre producer and not be considered for breeding.

Repairing an inguinal hernia

Inguinal hernias are extremely rare in male SACs and are not seen in female animals. They are a genetic recessive disorder and therefore should only be repaired after castration. The left side is more commonly affected. If there is a strangulation of the intestine within the hernia, the animal will show colic-type pain. Because of the stoical nature of SACs these affected animals are often found dead. The animal should be given a general anaesthetic and placed in dorsal recumbency. The area is surgically cleansed in the normal manner. A careful scrotal incision is made over the testicle, taking care not to incise the tunics. The testicle is drawn through the skin incision milking any abdominal contents back into the abdomen. When the surgeon is 100% certain that this has been accomplished two large pairs of haemostats are placed over the cord. The proximal pair is removed and a trans-fixing ligature is tied in the grove left by the haemostats. The testicle is then removed distal to the remaining pair of haemostats. When the testicle has been removed the skin should be sutured with horizontal mattress sutures.

Similar surgery should be carried out on the other side even if there is no inguinal herniation. The animal should be given antibiotics, NSAIDs and TAT by injection.

Repairing an umbilical hernia

Umbilical hernias are extremely rare in SACs. They have a high heritability and so repair should not be carried out in males unless they are castrated. It is reasonable to repair an umbilical hernia in a female that is being kept for breeding on the understanding that her progeny will not be kept for breeding.

Repair of umbilical hernias should be delayed until the cria is at least 4 months of age. Often with age there is little reason to repair them as the abdominal opening is relatively small. If no more than three fingers can be inserted into the abdominal opening the hernia can be closed with an elastrator ring. The cria should be given antibiotic and NSAID cover with its tetanus status checked. It is then placed in dorsal recumbency. Raising the hernia sack to ensure there are no bowel contents, a rubber ring is placed as near to the abdominal wall as possible. Antibiotic cover and fly control should be maintained for a minimum of 10 days.

If the abdominal opening is larger than three fingers a full surgical operation will need to be carried out under general anaesthetic. The cria should be prepared as above under general anaesthetic and the area should be clipped and surgically prepared. An elliptical skin incision is made around the hernia sack. With blunt dissection the skin is removed. With great care, with blunt dissection, the hernia sac is undermined from the abdominal wall without entering the abdomen so that there is a rim of 1 cm around the orifice. Sterile nylon mesh is then sutured to the abdominal ring over the orifice with monofilament nylon continuous stitches. After closing the wound with a continuous layer of subcuticular sutures of absorbable material the skin is closed with single horizontal mattress sutures of monofilament nylon. The wound is covered with antibiotic spray. The cria should be confined for a minimum of 10 days and receive antibiotics and NSAID cover. Obviously fly control and tetanus cover are vital.

Repairing a ruptured bladder

This condition does not seem to occur in male alpacas or llamas at birth as it does in horses. It can occur in both males and females that are subjected to violent trauma from road traffic accidents or from falls from high places. It has been reported that a bladder has been ruptured during rectal examination. The author has large hands and so does not carry out rectal examinations in SACs. The more common cause is rupture as a result of urethral obstruction.

In the incidence of trauma the repair needs to be carried out as soon as possible and does not carry any welfare or ethical considerations. Diagnosis of bladder rupture is not easy. If it is suspected, the delay waiting for the blood urea to be raised will not be helpful. A peritoneal tap is required (see Chapter 4). Normal peritoneal fluid has a potassium concentration of below 5 mEq/l; urine has a potassium level ten times that figure.

Repair should be carried out under general anaesthetic with the animal in dorsal recumbency. In the male an incision will have to be made paramedian to get as much access to the bladder as possible. The bladder should be carefully examined and the patency of the urethra should be established by flushing before closure using a double layer of continuous inverting sutures. The abdomen should be flushed after closure of the bladder before closing with two layers of continuous sutures. The skin should be closed with single interrupted sutures of monofilament nylon.

The welfare and ethical dilemma arises when the bladder has ruptured because the urethra of a male has become blocked with calculi. If these calculi can be flushed out with flushing, the bladder can be repaired as described above. However, if the urethra cannot be cleared the clinician has a dilemma. Several surgical approaches have been described. These include ischial urethrostomy, urethrotomy and marsupialization. The problem is that invariably there is urine scalding, at best there is continual pyoderma. At worst there will be continual acute skin inflammation with fly strike in the summer. The author's own opinion is that euthanasia is required. This opinion is influenced by the author's poor surgical results in other species and therefore the author readily accepts that in better surgical hands the outcome may well be more favourable.

Replacing a prolapsed rectum

The causes of this very rare condition are obscure. It has been suggested that homosexual behaviour might be a cause. It does appear to be more prevalent in males. Severe coughing caused by lungworm or pneumonia has also been postulated as a cause in pigs but this is unlikely in SACs. The SAC should be given antibiotic and NSAID cover. The tetanus status should be checked and fly control implemented. With the SAC either in the standing position or in the 'kush' position an epidural regional anaesthetic should be given. The perineal area should be cleaned before a purse-string suture is put in place. It is important that this is placed before replacement of the rectum, otherwise the rectum will re-prolapse while the suture is being placed. After replacement of the rectum using plenty of obstetrical lubricant the purse-string should be drawn tight to only allow one finger in the orifice. The animal should be kept on a laxative diet and regularly checked. The suture should be removed in 10 days. In the majority of cases it will remain *in situ*. However, if it re-prolapses euthanasia is indicated. The wisdom of performing surgery on these animals is controversial. However, it is possible that with careful resection of the rectal mucosa the problem could be solved satisfactorily.

Rig operation

Retained testicles are very rare in SACs. A SAC that has only one descended testicle will definitely be fertile. In fact in the author's experience they have more libido and therefore cause more problems than normal males. There is every reason to suspect that retained testicles are more likely to become cancerous. Therefore these animals will need to be castrated. Such an operation should not be undertaken lightly as some retained testicles may be up near to the kidney. In these instances the best method is to carry out the removal laparoscopically. However, in most cases the testicle will lie just inside the inner inguinal ring. In these cases a straightforward surgical procedure can be carried out under general anaesthetic. The scrotum and the surrounding area should be clipped and surgically cleaned. An incision should be made over the external inguinal ring. The tunics covering the retained testicle will be found by blunt dissection over the inguinal ring. These should be grasped by a large pair of artery forceps and the testicle should be drawn, slowly and carefully, to the exterior. A transfixing ligature of absorbable suture material should be placed around the tunics dorsally to a second pair of artery forceps. The testicle should then be removed and the subcuticular tissues should be closed with a continuous row of sutures of absorbable material. The skin should then be closed with single horizontal mattress sutures of monofilament nylon. The animal should be given antibiotics and NSAIDs. The tetanus status should be checked.

Before deciding an animal is a rig, clinicians should examine the groin very carefully not only to see previous scars but also because often testicles have descended and do not lie in the scrotum but cranial to the scrotum lateral to the penis.

Tendon contraction

This is a rare condition when seen on its own. It will be seen in crias with other congenital defects. In these instances euthanasia may be indicated. If it appears to be the only defect then careful appraisal should be carried out. If the limb or limbs can be extended but the cria chooses not to, the author gives the cria an injection of 500 mg of oxytetracycline. There is considerable doubt on the effectiveness of this treatment. Its virtue is that it gives 48 h for further evaluation. It is not prudent to immediately splint or cast the limbs as many cases will self-cure. Splinting or casting is very hazardous as pressure sores are likely to be created with life-threatening results. If after 48 h the limbs can be extended then the owner should be instructed to house the cria and its mother. Then as many times as possible every day the limbs should be forcibly extended. In the author's experience this will have a 50% success rate. Should this fail or if the tendons are so contracted that the limb cannot be

extended then surgery should be attempted under general anaesthetic.

The cria should be masked down with halothane or isoflurane and the limbs prepared for surgery. The cria should be given antibiotics and TAT by injection. The author does not give NSAIDs as these may be toxic in very young crias. A 2.5-cm-long incision is made centrally in the palmar aspect of the metacarpus in the direction of the limb. The median artery and nerve will lie medially and the ulnar nerve will lie laterally. These should be reflected medially and laterally so that the two branches of the superficial digital flexor tendon can be severed. The skin should be sutured with small interrupted skin sutures or staples. The wound should be covered with a padded support bandage. The weight of the cria will hopefully stretch the deep digital flexor tendon.

Urethral obstruction

This is seen typically in young males fed on dry concentrate diets. Surgery as described for a ruptured bladder is possible but carries severe welfare implications.

Vasectomy

This operation is not required in normal circumstances. However, it may be required for reproduction studies. The scrotum is not pendulous and so the operation is best performed under general anaesthetic in dorsal recumbency.

The area of the scrotum and cranial to it is prepared for surgery. A 5 cm incision is made cranial to the scrotum over the spermatic cord but slightly medial to the cord. The spermatic cord is then exteriorized by blunt dissection. A pair of artery forceps is positioned between the skin and the cord. The shiny vas deferens will be seen on the medial aspect of the spermatic cord. It can be grasped with a pair of rat-toothed dressing forceps. A 5 cm length is removed having ligatured either end with absorbable suture material. The skin is closed with two horizontal mattress sutures of similar absorbable material. The process is repeated on the other side.

Euthanasia

Introduction

It must be stressed that veterinarians must at all times check that whatever method has been used has been successful. They must certify that death has occurred themselves and not rely on any helpers. In the normal circumstances euthanasia of any animal by a veterinarian using blunt trauma is *totally unacceptable*. However, every veterinary surgeon is an individual and is legally and morally in charge in euthanasia situations. The veterinary surgeon must use his judgement. For example, there is a fire in a shed and a very badly burned small cria. The off-duty veterinarian happens to be passing, and he has no firearm or lethal injection; is it better to administer one sharp blow with a hammer to the cria's head or to wait for another veterinarian to arrive?

Use of a firearm with a free bullet

This method is quite satisfactory in SACs provided the veterinary surgeon has a licence for the firearm. The point to aim for is the middle of a cross formed by two lines running from each eye to the opposite ear. This method should not be used in young crias. This method is not advised in normal circumstances in the UK.

Use of a captive bolt pistol

The same point of aim can be used for euthanasia of SACs with a captive bolt pistol as is used for euthanasia with a free bullet. Immediate bleeding out by cutting all the neck vessels is required. Captive bolt pistols should not be used in young crias. This method is not advised in normal circumstances in the UK.

Electrocution

In theory this method could be used commercially for euthanasia of SACs. Immediate bleeding out by cutting all the neck vessels is required. This method is not advised in normal circumstances in the UK.

Chemical euthanasia

This is the normal method of euthanasia for SACs. For skilled veterinarians who are used to giving intravenous injections in SACs there are few problems in injecting either a large volume (approximately 100 ml) of triple strength barbiturate solution or 25 ml of a solution containing 400 mg/ml quinalbarbitone and 25 mg/ml cinchocaine hydrochloride intravenously. However, normally the skin of SACs is too thick to allow the jugular vein to be visualized so inexperienced veterinarians will find this difficult particularly if the SAC is large and poorly handled. In these instances the SAC can be heavily sedated with 2% xylazine given intramuscularly (5 ml for a large male llama) or actually anaesthetized by a cocktail of agents given intramuscularly and then the triple-strength barbiturate or the solution containing 400 mg/ml quinalbarbitone and 25 mg/ml cinchocaine hydrochloride can be given intravenously when the animal is in lateral recumbency.

Small crias can be destroyed by injecting 15 ml of triple-strength barbiturate into the jugular vein. This in the authors experience may be difficult in a totally collapsed moribund cria. In these cases it is humane to inject the triple-strength barbiturate straight into the heart. To do this the cria should be held by the assistant either in lateral recumbency or with both arms across the assistant's chest.

9

Medicine and Surgery of the Gastroenteric System

Anatomy of the Teeth

SACs appear to have no upper incisors, only a dental pad. However, they do in fact have an upper incisor that has migrated caudally and resembles a canine tooth. Thus, in the upper jaw they appear to have two canines on each side. In the lower jaw they have a single canine tooth. These six 'canines' are called fighting teeth and can be very devastating structures.

Certain authorities maintain that the three pairs of deciduous incisors are present at birth. In reality this is rarely the case as the outside pair may not actually emerge for 3 months. These deciduous incisors are replaced sequentially starting with the centrals at just over 2 years of age. The middle incisors are replaced at approximately 3 years of age and the corners at approximately 4 years of age. These eruptions do not appear in such a standard manner as in horses but rough ageing of animals under 5 can be carried out. As practitioners are aware, most foals in a UK environment are born in the spring and technically have a birthday on 1 January. Therefore, teeth eruption and age can be linked fairly satisfactorily. However, although most owners aim to have SAC crias born in the spring in the UK this is often not accomplished and so crias are often born in the autumn. Therefore, accurate ageing is difficult as the time of the year of birth is not always known.

The migrated canine, which is actually an incisor in the upper jaw, may have a deciduous precursor. These are very rare in females but may be seen in the first 3 months of life in approximately 5% of males. The permanent migrated incisor teeth will erupt at approximately the same time as the real canines at 2 years of age.

SACs are anisomatic, i.e. their upper cheek teeth are wider than their lower cheek teeth. However, unlike equines, which tend to develop sharp enamel points on the buccal aspect of the upper cheek teeth rows from grinding, SACs maintain a normal occlusal table and do not develop sharp enamel points.

SACs have five cheek teeth in the four rows, two premolars and three molars in each row. The two premolars are present at birth but are not replaced rostrally from the front until 4 and 5 years of age. The three molar teeth erupt rostrally from the front before this time at approximately 9 months, 2 years and 3 years, respectively. Thus a SAC does not have a 'full mouth' until 5 years of age.

All the roots of the lower cheek teeth lie in the mandible, so if there is any apical abscessation it will start as a unilateral swelling on the mandible before it fistulates. The roots of the upper premolars lie in the maxillary bone so any apical abscessation starts as a swelling of the maxillary bone, which is likely to lead to a fistula. The roots of the upper molar teeth lie in the

© Graham R. Duncanson 2023. *Veterinary Treatment of Llamas and Alpacas,* 2nd Edition (G.R. Duncanson)
DOI: 10.1079/9781800623576.0009

maxillary sinus so an apical abscess will manifest as a malodorous unilateral nasal discharge.

Mouth and Dental Problems

Introduction

Obviously if several animals are affected with mouth and possible dental problems, the differential list is going to be different from a single animal being affected. However, in either case individual animals have to be examined. First the clinician needs to decide what signs are being shown. There is likely to be excess salivation. This may be coupled with cud spilling, which normally manifests as a green discolouration around the mouth. The whole head should be examined before the lips are peeled back to examine the incisors and to examine the mucosa. Then with the use of a gag and a good light source, preferably a head torch, the inside of the mouth and the teeth can be examined (Fig. 9.1). It is very important that clinicians examine the outside of the mouth carefully first. Squamous cell carcinomas will be found in the oropharynx of old animals. Tumours of the salivary glands will be seen but these seldom metastasize to the local lymph nodes. If there is

a fracture of one or both mandibles, the gag should not be used. If there is any doubt, a radiograph should be taken. This should be a lateral oblique with the plate against the side of the jaw most likely to be affected nearest to the plate. The x-ray machine should be placed lower than the head and point up at a 30° angle. The whole mandible should be radiographed, so a large plate will be required. If a fracture at the symphysis is suspected then a dorso-ventral view may be helpful. Once again a large plate will be required for the whole head. However, a small plate may be useful for an intra-oral radiograph of the symphysis and the incisors. This later projection is also useful for diagnosing the very rare dentigerous cysts usually found in the area surrounding the incisor roots.

Pytalism and pseudopytalism

Both these conditions occur in SACs. Owners will complain of cud staining or the appearance of digestive fluid on the ground overnight. It is important to establish whether feed material is present or not. Various behavioural vices or pathological lesions may provide an explanation for loss of saliva. Possible causes are: ulcerative stomatitis, lingual paresis, malposition of the

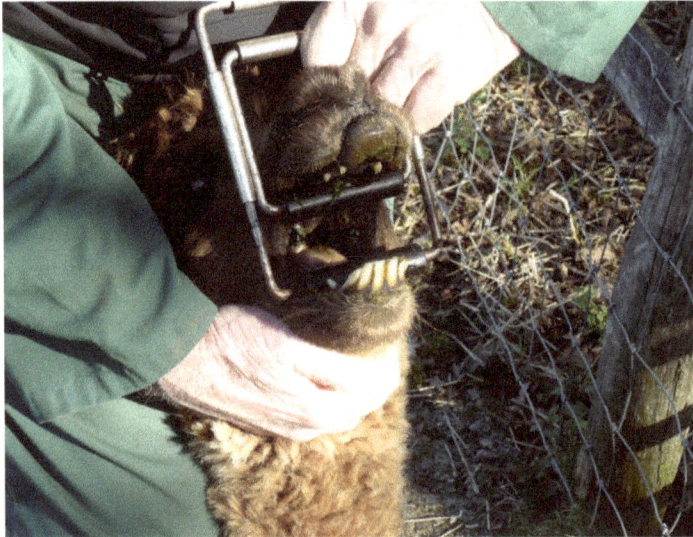

Fig. 9.1. Examination of the mouth.

parotid ducts, early mega-oesophagus, osteomyelis (often called lumpy jaw), soft tissue abscess (including *Corynebacterium pseudotuberculosis*), facial bone fracture, retained food bolus, malocclusion or choke.

Passive regurgitation during sleep is a relatively common problem in young SACs between 6 and 18 months. It tends to be self-limiting and stops after the age of 18 months. Parotid saliva in SACs is similar to ruminants. It is alkaline and copious. Its loss leads to acidaemia and hypokalaemia. Except in cases of choke, which are extremely rare, the saliva can be replaced orally.

Choke may be secondary to megaoesophagus. The normal cause of this is iatrogenic following jugular veni-puncture on the left side. It is very important that clinicians use the right-hand side for veni-puncture. Diagnosis can be confirmed by radiographs. In a normal SAC, plates exposed immediately after a barium swallow rarely show more than a trickle of contrast material, so any retained in the oesophagus is diagnostic. Treatment should include long-term antibiotics and non-steroidal anti-inflammatory drugs (NSAIDs) and the animal should be fed on pelleted lucerne or grass nuts.

Incisor and canine problems in SACs

Introduction

This whole area related to the incisors and the dental pad is very contentious. The author has fairly radical views. However, he will endeavour to put forward a balanced argument. First of all there is the problem of the over-extension of the mandible, prognathia, and under-extension, brachygnathia (Fig. 9.2). Both these conditions are inherited and therefore such individuals should not be bred from. Contrary to popular opinion neither of these conditions affects the animal concerned. There have been no welfare problems recorded related to either prognathia or brachygnathia. Animals with these conditions do not suffer from any degree of dysprehension and therefore suffer no problems with loss of weight. Brachygnathia is rare; however, prognathia is common and is a fault recognized by show judges and buyers. Therefore routine grinding of these incisors is carried out (Fig. 9.3). Not only is this practice inhumane but also it is being used to

mask an inherited conformation fault for monetary gain. Clinicians should consider carefully whether they can condone such a practice.

Incisor removal

This is a relatively straightforward procedure if an incisor tooth is loose. However, even then it is quite easy to fracture the root so elevation is worthwhile. Local anaesthetic should be instilled under the mucosa rostral and caudal to the tooth. An amount of 1 ml either side is sufficient. A dental syringe makes this task easier. The clinician must use judgement on whether removal is a help to the animal or not. Normally incisors should be left unless they are very loose or much displaced.

In rare cases the deciduous incisor teeth may fail to fall out and in other cases animals will appear to grow an extra row of incisors (Fig. 9.4). The clinicians are advised to radiograph these teeth and think long and hard before attempting to remove them. Obviously if they are loose they should be removed. They should also be removed if they are causing problems and it is easy to see which are the permanent teeth. Otherwise monitoring the problem must be the best advice.

Canines

There is the problem of fighting teeth in adult uncastrated males. These are very vicious weapons and can inflict severe wounds on other animals,

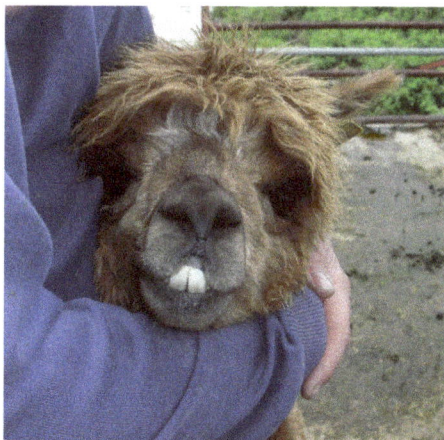

Fig. 9.2. Prognathia.

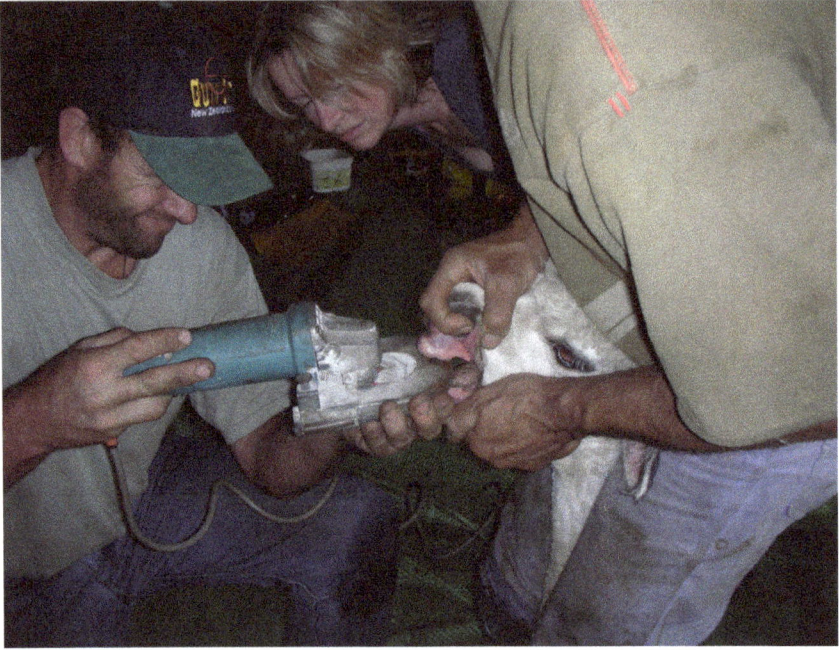

Fig. 9.3. Grinding incisors.

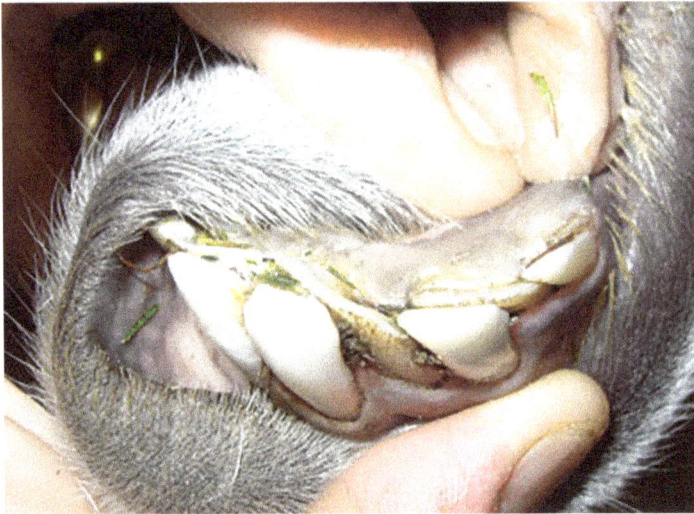

Fig. 9.4. An extra row of incisors.

particularly other mature uncastrated males. The general opinion of eminent veterinarians in the UK and elsewhere is that the erupted crown of these teeth should be removed at the age of 2 to 3 years. This procedure will have to be repeated at regular intervals of roughly 2 years. I question the wisdom and the ethics of this procedure. First of all it will only be a problem if stud males run together or if inadvertently two stud males get in the same compound as one another. Should such males be kept together? Certainly no farmer would consider running mature bulls or mature male goats together except in a very extensive area. The author is aware that rams, outside of the breeding season, are run in groups. However, shepherds are very careful to pen such animals tightly together for 24 h before letting them loose to help to control fighting. Outside the breeding season rams are less aggressive.

Whichever stance practitioners adopt one thing is for certain, that removal of 'fighting teeth' needs to be carried out in a humane manner. La Rue W. Johnson, DVM, PhD of Colorado State University (personal communication), an extremely experienced SAC veterinarian, considers the procedure should be carried out under a short-acting anaesthetic (see Chapter 8), using embryotomy wire that is continuously bathed in cold water to prevent excess heat. This must be considered best practice. Any other method is likely to be unethical, particularly the use of 'canine nippers', which are liable to cause the tooth to fracture possibly in a vertical plane. This will result in apical abscessation.

Cheek teeth problems

These are common. The normal referring sign is a facial swelling. Swellings of the soft tissue that enlarge rapidly are unlikely to be tooth related and are normally abscesses, although they could be insect or reptile bites. The fibre should be trimmed away and the area cleaned before an 18G needle is inserted. Pus will be seen in the needle and then the abscess may be lanced. Digital exploration should be carried out into the abscess to make sure there is no foreign body, e.g. a slither of wood or an air-gun pellet. Antibiotics should be given and the tetanus status checked. If the swelling is unrelated to the underlying bone and not rapidly enlarging it is likely to be an *Actinobacillus ligneriesii* infection, which can also involve the mandible and is often termed lumpy jaw. Lancing will be unrewarding. Treatment with daily injections of streptomycin for a minimum of 7 days should be carried out. Lymphomas will cause soft tissue swellings as will cud retention. The latter might be tooth related, e.g. a loose tooth or a displaced tooth. Careful

cheek teeth examination should be carried out. Normally a tooth problem manifests as a slowly progressive hard swelling related to the mandible or less commonly to the maxilla (Fig. 9.5). Mandibular thickness measurements in alpacas can aid early detection of animals in need of specialized dental care. Most animals with an increased mandibular thickness suffer from advanced dental disease. However, routine dental examinations remain necessary to allow the early detection of dental disorders in alpacas (Proost *et al.*, 2022). While osseous remodelling is taking place there will be changes to the swelling. On the other hand, often these swellings will remain unchanged for months. There may be some weight loss but other signs of food spilling or anorexia are rare.

A novel treatment was described by Po *et al.* (2022). Diagnosis was confirmed by computerized tomography, and near-complete restoration of bone architecture and no evidence of active bone destruction was observed on CT 14 months later.

An overview of tooth root infection

This is a relatively common problem in camelids. Owner and veterinarian awareness is probably responsible for the increasing frequency of diagnosis of these lesions. Dental surgery in camelids can be rewarding, but proper facilities and equipment should be available for optimal treatment and outcome (D. Anderson, DVM, MS, Diplomate, American College of Veterinary Medicine, Ohio State University Columbus, Ohio, USA, personal communication).

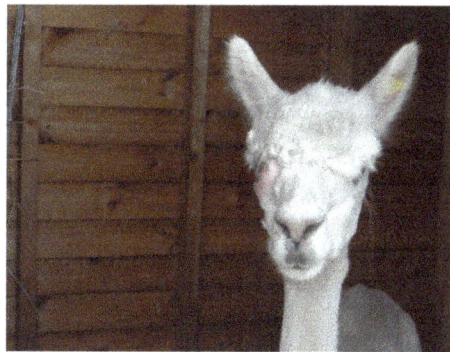

Fig. 9.5. A hard swelling on the maxilla.

Extremely rarely there will be a malodorous unilateral nasal discharge. Owners normally seek veterinary attention in these cases and in cases where the swelling fistulates. However, on occasion the abscess will drain into the mouth and the owner will only notice the malodorous breath.

Radiographs, particularly with metal probes in the fistula, will be helpful to diagnose which tooth has an apical abscess. Radiolucency will be observed surrounding the affected tooth and bone proliferation may be noted. Long-term antibiotics may be tried but the result is rarely satisfactory. At least a month of daily injections of penicillin or ceftiofur has been tried or a ten-shot series of florfenicol at the higher dose given every fourth day is claimed to have a success rate of 50%. The fistula may appear to close but will re-open when the antibiotic cover ceases. Tooth removal is the only option. These lesions are most commonly seen along the horizontal ramus of the mandible (>90%), and, less commonly, the maxilla (<10%) and affect both the premolars and the molars. However, if the SAC is pregnant such a stressful operation is best left until after parturition.

Some authorities advise a buccostomy approach. This requires very careful surgery under general anaesthetic and is not advisable for practitioners in the field. Removal by repulsion is not an option on account of the fragile mandible or maxilla. The author's preference is removal per os with the SAC in the 'kush' position under very light sedation with xylazine. Radiographs should be taken to accurately pinpoint the diseased tooth. This is easier if there is external abscessation as a radiopaque probe can be inserted into the fistula. However, if the roots of the upper molars, i.e. the caudal three cheek teeth, are involved there will be no external fistula as the roots lie in the maxillary sinus. In these cases there will be a unilateral malodorous nasal discharge. The clinician will have to study the roots very carefully on oblique radiographs to decide which tooth is diseased. If in doubt, referring the radiographs to a more experienced practitioner or to a human dentist is advisable. As stated earlier, unless the tooth is loose removal is extremely difficult. Before surgery, antibiotic cover should be given, normally a mixture of penicillin and streptomycin. NSAIDs should also be given and the tetanus state of the animal checked. The animal should be allowed to 'kush' with a holder astride the SAC holding the head in a normal position. If the animal is fractious a very small dose of xylazine (0.05 mg/kg: 0.125 ml of a 2% solution/50 kg) may be given intramuscularly. A second holder using both hands should keep the gag open and in the correct plane. With a head torch the tooth to be removed should be examined and then with a very small equine dental pick the gingival mucosa should be elevated on both the lateral and medial aspects of the tooth. The dental pick should be forced between the tooth and the alveolar socket. A pair of small molar separators should be placed rostral and caudal to the tooth to try to obtain some tooth movement. Then the tooth should be grasped with a pair of small right-angle molar extraction forceps. Careful, persistent medial/lateral rocking motion should be commenced. When the tooth is loose it should be elevated using a long pair of artery forceps as a fulcrum. Antibiotic cover and pain relief should be maintained for several days.

The alveolar socket does not require packing but flushing through the fistula daily is helpful. The socket rapidly granulates.

Congenital and Hereditary Conditions Affecting the Gastrointestinal Tract

Atresia ani

It is reasonable to treat these cases but the owners should be warned of the genetic implications. The diagnosis is normally straightforward as a young cria will be presented with a swelling below the tail and an absence of an anus. A small bleb of 1 ml of local anaesthetic should be injected over the swelling where there should be an anus. A small stab incision is made with a very small scalpel blade into the swelling and faeces will be extruded. Sutures are not required and normally the anus will remain open if the owner cleans the area for a couple of days.

Atresia coli

In the authors opinion euthanasia is the correct option in these cases. However, in theory a skilled surgeon could draw the colon back to the anal area and create a rectum and anus.

Mega-oesophagus

This is an extremely rare condition but it does occur in SACs. It appears to occur in llamas more commonly than alpacas. The main sign is repeated regurgitation. However, animals will show multiple non-specific signs such as weight loss, ptyalism, choke and halitosis. The cause is mainly unknown although a persistent right aortic arch has been shown to be the cause in one case. Trauma to the vagus from jugular vein puncture is the most likely cause but this is difficult to prove and clinicians are unlikely to raise this hypothesis. Diagnosis is normally possible on radiographs without contrast material. There is no worthwhile treatment but cases can normally be managed by only feeding the animal from an elevated position with regular small feeds of highly digestible well-soaked feed at a lower level. Affected animals can live for several years if owners are prepared to persevere with this feeding regime and construct a suitable ramp for the animal to stand on.

Viral Diseases Affecting the Gastroenteric Tract

Blue tongue virus

Blue tongue virus (BTV) is arthropod borne. It is therefore infectious but not contagious. It is found in many parts of the world where it affects wild and domesticated ruminants. It used to be thought to be primarily a disease of wool sheep. However, that is no longer the case. There are 24 serotypes of this Orbivirus. The serotypes tend to be restricted to certain areas and vary in virulence and in which species they affect. The vectors are various species of *Culicoides*. One of the most important found in Africa and in the southern Mediterranean area is *Culicoides imicola*. *C. pulicaris* and *C. obsoletus* are found in the UK. These midges can live up to 3 months. The virus is maintained in the *Culicoides* spp. and in the infected ruminants or SACs. The climate has to be not only warm enough for the *Culicoides* spp. to breed but also warm enough for the virus to replicate in the *Culicoides*. All stages of *Culicoides* are influenced by moisture and require a semi-aquatic breeding habitat. They are strong fliers and also can be passively dispersed by wind. This has been shown to occur in the Mediterranean area for over 300 km. Therefore the disease is restricted to warmer temperate areas and the tropics. The disease is found all through the USA and Europe. The disease has been controlled in the UK, having first been detected from an infected plume of *Culicoides* from Belgium on 4 August 2007. Of the 24 serotypes worldwide, there are only five serotypes in the USA and four serotypes in northern Europe. There are more than 1400 species of *Culicoides* worldwide, but only 20 or so are possible vectors of blue tongue virus. Only female *Culicoides* are involved in disease transmission.

BTV first replicates in the local lymph nodes. The viraemia seeds other lymph nodes, spleen, lung and vascular endothelium and replicates. The viraemia normally lasts for 3–5 days but can last up to 60 days. Endothelial damage and disseminated intravascular coagulopathy (DIC) cause the clinical signs. The incubation period is 6–9 days. Antibodies can be detected from 6 days post-infection. The clinical signs are associated with virus replication in endothelial cells, which results in haemorrhage, ischaemia, inflammation and oedema. The lesions are common in areas subject to mechanical trauma and abrasion, e.g. the feet, mouth and eyes. There is fever up to 42°C. There are respiratory signs and abortion. BTV causes not only gross abnormalities to the central nervous system of the fetus, but also generalized growth retardation and fetal lymphoreticular hyperplasia (Richardson *et al.*, 1985). There is conjunctivitis, mucosal inflammation and oedema. Petechiae, ecchymoses and cracked lips will be seen, leading to excess salivation. There is coronitis causing lameness.

The diagnosis is confirmed by polymerase chain reaction (PCR) for viral RNA. It can detect all 24 serotypes. Virus can be sequenced and isolated. If serology is required there is an enzyme-linked immunosorbent assay (ELISA), a serum neutralization test (SNT) and a virus neutralization test (VNT).

When treating affected animals all handling should be gentle with as little movement as possible.

The differential diagnosis in SACs must include foot-and-mouth disease (FMD) and vesicular stomatitis. On the whole, in FMD there is a much lower mortality than in BTV. Facial swelling is much more marked in BVT compared with FMD. On the other hand vesicles and ulcers are characteristic of FMD but are less common in BTV. Clinicians should remember that FMD is highly infectious but BTV requires a vector.

There is no specific treatment for BTV. Antibiotics and NSAIDs are helpful. Nursing is vital. This should include offering water and mushy food, and providing deep bedding out of the sun and heat. Affected animals will never return to full health. There is an increase in the incidence of mastitis. There is an increased incidence of lameness. There will be long-term fertility problems including abortions, stillbirths, weak crias and early embryonic deaths. In alpacas there will be wool loss and staple breaks. There is an increase in pneumonia cases and long-term 'poor doers'.

Since 1998 there have been 12 different invasions of BTV into Europe with 12 different vaccines required to help control them. The vaccines available are inactivated (dead) vaccines against specific serotypes. The most up to date are highly purified by liquid chromatography (see Chapter 7).

Bovine viral diarrhoea

Bovine viral diarrhoea (BVD) virus will affect SACs. It can spread in a herd of SACs as well as to other species, e.g. cattle, sheep and goats. Crias will show weight loss and diarrhoea. Some crias will be stillborn or show congenital neurological signs. Ill-thrift and weight loss will be shown in adults. Diarrhoea is rare. The virus will cause abortion. Persistent infection (PI) has been demonstrated. SACs that are infected in early pregnancy, i.e. between 32 and 133 days, are 82% likely to be PIs. Most of these will be light at birth, i.e. 6 kg rather than the normal alpaca cria weight of 8 kg. They will grow slowly and will die before they reach 30 months of age. The disease is spread by mixing animals. Both type 1 and type 2 virus have been isolated in Chile but only type 1 has been found in the UK. The recommended test for detecting the virus in SACs is a PCR. Seroconversion can be diagnosed by the use of SNT. The standard serological antigen and antibody tests used in cattle are not validated and may give false results.

Coronavirus

This is a relatively common finding in SAC crias. It is often brought into the herd by animals returning from a show. The main sign will be diarrhoea. With careful hygiene and the use of electrolytes it is fairly easily controlled. However, both hands and any equipment should be carefully cleaned between animals. It appears that crias will self-cure. There is rarely a need for antibiotic support or NSAIDs.

Foot-and-mouth disease

SACs definitely contract FMD as do camels. They may only be carriers for a few days but they definitely do spread the disease. This is contrary to the popular belief of SAC owners and many veterinary surgeons working with SACs. The severity of FMD will vary markedly with the strain of virus, the breed of animal and the type of husbandry. The disease spectrum will range from inapparent infection detected only by subsequent herd sero-surveillance through to high morbidity outbreaks with very noticeable diseased animals.

The main signs are lameness and reluctance to move. Excess salivation is invariably seen at some stage of the disease in SACs. A thorough examination of the whole herd will reveal the typical erosions and ulcers on the mouths and feet of a considerable number of animals. Crias suckling their mothers will be crying and hungry as a result not only of the disease but also as a result of the milk drop experienced by their mothers. Several animals will be acutely ill with pyrexia. With some strains recovery is quick with the disease passing through the herd in a few days. Recovery is not quite so quick with some strains and may take a considerable time. The earliest signs are vesicles, fluid-filled sacs within the epithelium. The fluid is clear, slightly yellow and slightly viscous. The vesicles are thin walled and therefore very transitory. Often the whole infection will only last 2 days in an animal. Over 90% of the herd will have foot lesions and sudden severe lameness will be very evident. This is the most common clinical sign associated with FMD in SACs. Whole groups will frequently lie down and be very unwilling to rise. Serum will need to be tested for antibodies to confirm FMD. It is possible that FMD may be confused with BTV but careful assessment of clinical signs will clarify the diagnosis.

The spread of FMD virus can occur in a number of ways. The most important is by direct contact between infected and susceptible livestock. However, it can also occur with feeding infected milk, using infected semen or infected embryos. The virus can be airborne or carried by people or species of animal not susceptible. The virus can be carried by vehicles and any other fomites.

Virus production in infected animals remains high until antibodies develop at approximately 4–5 days post-infection. Some animals will remain as carriers for a considerable length of time but most owners and their practitioners are in denial about this. In the UK the disease is notifiable and the animals will be slaughtered as soon as possible.

Malignant catarrhal fever

Malignant catarrhal fever (MCF) is a disease of cattle caused by a group of herpes viruses. These include Alcelaphine herpes virus 1, Ovine herpes virus 2 and Caprine herpes virus 2. The most important is Alcelaphine herpes virus 1. The normal host of this virus is the wildebeest (gnu) in which it is asymptomatic. The disease in cattle appears in the Masai cattle in Kenya and northern Tanzania at the time of the wildebeest calving season from the end of January to the beginning of March. Goats are not affected but occasionally Masai sheep will show symptoms. These are lethargy and pyrexia. There is inflammation of the mucosal surfaces, mainly mouth necrosis and keratitis with conjunctivitis. The sheep are likely to recover unless they are suffering from malnutrition or some other disease. However, in the UK the sheep is normally an asymptomatic carrier like the wildebeest in Africa. Cattle are the main host. In cattle there is a grave prognosis. Diagnosis is either with an ELISA or a PCR. There is no treatment or vaccine available. SACs are not kept in Africa and therefore are not likely to be infected. However, they can contract the disease in the UK by close contact with infected cattle or sheep. It is a very

serious disease in SACs with a high mortality but an extremely low morbidity. Bovine herpes virus 3 has been found in pigs in the UK and these animals could be infective to SACs.

Nairobi sheep disease

Nairobi sheep disease (NSD), which occurs in sheep and goats, is caused by a nairovirus. It is spread by ticks, mainly the brown ear tick, *Rhipicephalus appendiculatus*. It is mainly seen in areas in Eastern Africa where this tick occurs. SACs are not kept in these areas, which is probably why it has not been reported in SACs, but it is likely that it would cause deaths.

Diagnosis can be confirmed by blood samples for an ELISA test. There is no treatment. Prevention can be carried out by very strict twice-weekly dipping in a suitable acaricide or regular use of pour-on cypermethrin products. It is hoped that there will be a vaccine prepared in the near future.

Peste des petits ruminants

Peste des petits ruminants (PPR) is caused by a morbillivirus and is related to rinderpest. However, unlike rinderpest it is not contagious to cattle. On the other hand rinderpest can affect goats but appears to be less virulent as the mortality rate may be as low as 50%, whereas the disease in cattle in the author's experience causes 100% mortality. It is hoped that rinderpest has been totally eradicated. PPR is often termed goat plague. It is a disease with a high morbidity and mortality in goats, sheep and camels. It is seen in Africa, the Middle East, central Asia and the Indian subcontinent. The Food and Agriculture Organization (FAO) were concerned at the end of 2010 about an outbreak in Tanzania, which was threatening over 13.5 million goats and 3.5 million sheep in the country. FAO advised an emergency vaccination around the disease outbreak with further vaccination campaigns in the bordering areas of Malawi, Mozambique and Zambia. Sheep and goats are critical to food and income security for pastoral communities in sub-Saharan Africa. An Asian lineage strain of virus has been isolated in Sudan and has spread to

Morocco (Kwiatek *et al.*, 2011). It is therefore now very close to Europe. SACs would be very susceptible but clinicians should not be concerned that they will miss this disease as the signs are very obvious. There is high fever with erosions on the mucous membranes of the mouth and eyes. There is acute bloody diarrhoea and also signs of pneumonia. Whole herds will quickly become infected and the majority will die. There is no specific treatment. However, oxytetracycline injections seem to reduce the number of deaths. NSAIDs may be useful. There is a vaccine available for use in sheep and goats. This might be effective in SACs. It is likely that there would be immediate slaughter of affected animals within the EU.

Rotavirus

Rotaviruses have been found in most farm animals in many countries. There are seven serotypes recognized. However, their pathogenicity in crias is not clear cut. They will definitely cause diarrhoea but often there is another pathogen isolated at the same time. This may be a bacteria, e.g. *Escherichia coli*, or a protozoan, e.g. coccidia. Clinicians cannot treat the virus so attention should be drawn to the other pathogen.

Bacterial Diseases Affecting the Gastroenteric Tract

Introduction

Physiological diarrhoea is seen in crias, particularly in bottle-fed animals. The signs are normally self-limiting. Unformed pasty faeces are commonly seen in bright neonatal crias and are related to dietary change in the immature gut. The eating of solid food before the stomach has sufficient microorganisms may be the cause. The crias continue to suck and thrive. If owners and clinicians are concerned, samples should be taken. However, it is wise not to rush in with antibiotic treatment as this may well make the situation worse. Careful monitoring of the crias should be carried out. Normally the condition is transient. If the faeces become profuse and watery much more aggressive treatment will be

required while the clinician is waiting for diagnostics to be carried out. Electrolytes are very useful but should be given at half dilution as prescribed for calves as crias do not need as much glucose or sodium. *E. coli* infections will occur in crias but they are not common. There have been no K99 hypersecretory types isolated. Oral and injectable antibiotics and injectable NSAIDs will help support the cria. The isolation of either *E. coli* or *Salmonella* spp. as a septicaemia is very serious but will occur even if the bacteria are not isolated in the faeces.

Clostridial disease

Clostridial diseases are important in SACs. There are some differences from other species.

Bacillary haemoglobinuria

This has not been reported in SACs. It is primarily a disease of cattle in central Ireland and is sometimes called bacterial redwater. It is caused by *Clostridium haemolyticum*. It might well occur in SACs in the future if they are kept in large numbers in Ireland. It is likely to cause sudden death. The disease might occur in other areas of high rainfall, particularly when summers are wet. The signs likely to be shown would include abdominal pain, jaundice, dysentery and as the name suggests haemoglobinuria. The latter is likely to be the main sign. Aggressive treatment with penicillin, fluid therapy and particularly whole blood may be successful (see Chapter 10). On postmortem, anaemic liver infarcts are pathognomic for the condition.

Blackleg

This is primarily a disease of cattle and is not known in SACs. It is caused by *Clostridium chauvoei*. The disease is meant to follow shearing wounds and dog bites. However, it could occur in SACs as a result of dirty injection technique. The organism is common in the soil. The first sign shown would be lameness. On careful examination the animal will show a very swollen painful area over a wound. Treatment with high doses of penicillin and NSAIDs is unlikely to be successful.

Black's disease

The correct name for this condition is infectious necrotic hepatitis. It is caused by *Clostridium novyi* type B. It has not been recorded in SACs. The trigger factor is acute fluke activity, i.e. the migration of immature flukes through the liver. Acute fluke activity will occur in SACs but they tend to get the chronic form. Control can easily be carried out by vaccinating all animals against *C. novyi* type B. Fluke control is vital not only to prevent Black's disease but also to prevent the damage caused by the flukes in the liver.

Botulism

Unlike the previous two conditions, the organism *Clostridium botulinum* multiplies in the soil, or in silage and not in the animal. The organism produces toxin outside the body. Therefore the severity of the disease will be related to the amount of toxin ingested. It has not been recorded in SACs. It could occur as it has been reported in camels in Chad. The author has seen a flock of sheep affected with botulism in Western Australia. There was a mortality of over 50%. The animals had been in drought conditions and there was no association with silage feeding. Diagnosis is not difficult if the pathognomic sign of a flaccid anus is seen when the rectal temperature is taken. There is no specific treatment. However, animals will recover if they can be kept alive with oral fluids.

Braxy

This is a disease that only occurs in sheep. It is caused by *Clostridium septicum*. It appears to be a 'British disease', as the author has discussed it with European colleagues and they are unfamiliar with the condition. Australian, New Zealand and South African veterinarians also have not recorded the disease. The trigger factor is thought to be eating frosted root crops. These are fed classically in Norfolk in the UK throughout the winter. They include stubble-turnips and sugar-beet tops. When they are consumed in a frosted condition they cause an abomasitis, which is thought to allow entry of *C. septicum*. *C. septicum* is included in several polyvalent vaccines. This disease has not been recorded in SACs. It could easily occur following the feeding of frozen root crops.

Enterotoxaemia

Enterotoxaemia is more commonly called pulpy kidney and is caused by *Clostridium perfringens* type D. It is a sheep disease, but it is also a very common disease in SACs. It is the most common clostridial disease in the UK not only in sheep but also in SACs. It is found in growing crias and adults that have not been vaccinated adequately. The toxoid is included in *all* the vaccines and so there is little excuse for vaccination failure.

The disease normally manifests as sudden death although observant keepers will see sick lifeless cold moribund animals. There is no treatment. Diagnosis will not pose a problem on post-mortem. The abdomen, pleural cavity and pericardium will be filled with fluid, usually bloody. The kidneys will be friable as the common name suggests.

Lamb dysentery

This is a rare condition in commercial flocks because of vaccination. It does not seem to occur in hobby flocks. It is caused by *C. perfringens* type B and is a disease of young lambs. Often they die before they develop dysentery. It is not seen in SACs.

Malignant oedema

This disease, which is found in SACs, is caused by several clostridial organisms, namely *C. septicum*, *C. chauvoei*, *C. perfringens* and *C. novyi*. Animals can be found dead or *in extremis*. They show swellings, which are often gaseous. The disease may follow wounds obtained by male SACs fighting. The organism may gain entrance at parturition and cause massive swelling of the hindquarters. Aggressive treatment with penicillin and NSAIDs may be successful if started promptly.

Sordellii abomasitis

C. sordellii causes this disease in SACs in compartment three of the stomach (C3). It produces two toxins, one is haemolytic and the other is lethal. It attacks C3 and has different manifestations in the various age groups. In young crias over 3 weeks of age it will cause acute inflammation of C3. In older crias it will cause sudden death from damage to C3. In adults it will cause sudden death or damage to C3, which leads to death often from ulceration and peritonitis. It is one of the main clostridial diseases of SACs. There is now a vaccine available, which is highly recommended in SACs. As the same vaccine is prepared for cattle it should be pointed out that there are two different dosages. It is a 2 ml dose for cattle and a 1 ml does for sheep. SACs should receive the sheep dose.

Struck

This disease in sheep is common in Kent but very rare elsewhere in the UK. It is caused by *C. perfringens* type C. As the name suggests it causes sudden death. There is no standard trigger factor. However, the author believes the very heavily fertilized grass under fruit trees is likely to be the culprit. *C. perfringens* type C has been recorded in SACs in similar conditions.

Tetanus

The causative organism *Clostridium tetani* is well known as is its pathogenesis. In the author's experience it is now very rare in sheep, mainly owing to vaccination. The disease is also seen in SACs. Vaccination is advisable. The condition can be diagnosed by observing the clinical signs. Adult animals will appear stiff and reluctant to feed. They often appear slightly blown. Movement in C3 will be absent. The neck will be straight out and there may well be saliva coming from the mouth. The jaws may eventually become clamped together. Initial treatment should be large doses of tetanus antitoxin (TAT) and also large doses of penicillin. Animals may recover if they are given adequate nursing. Acetylpromazine given twice daily by intramuscular injection at 0.1 mg/kg may help to control the tetanic spasms.

Escherichia coli 0157

This is not a pathogen in SACs. However, it is carried by them and therefore they are a danger to humans. The commensal bacterium of concern is VTEC 0157:H7. It causes no clinical signs in alpacas or llamas but precautions must be taken by owners, particularly those with farms open to the general public. In the UK it is found by routine testing to be present in approximately 3% of alpaca faeces samples (see Chapter 17).

Escherichia coli pathogenic to crias

This disease is rare in crias because of their extensive husbandry and the extremely rare birth of twins. Basically *E. coli* infection is largely about poor management rather than virulent pathogens. *E. coli* are the normal inhabitants of a cria's intestine. In the second day of life a healthy cria will have 10^{10} *E. coli* bacteria/g of its faeces.

Crias will harbour the *E. coli* bacteria with the K99 antigen but these enterotoxigenic *E. coli* are extremely rare. However, they may be found in 2% of herds. With this disease there is nearly always a septicaemia. The condition may be peracute so that death may occur before the cria is seen to scour. Isolation of the organism from heart blood is diagnostic. Often colostrum will be seen in the stomach but will be unclotted. Of these strains of *E. coli*, 40% are resistant to ampicillin. Amoxicillin with clavulanic acid is likely to be the antibiotic of choice. In the author's experience oral combinations of neomycin and streptomycin are not effective. There is no licensed *E. coli* vaccine available in the UK.

To sum up, *E. coli* is not a major pathogen in crias but its importance should not be discounted. Good management is vital. Antibiotics should not be used to supplement bad management.

Johne's disease

Johne's disease is found in SACs throughout the world. Johne's disease is primarily a pathogen of cattle but the strains affecting SACs tend to be fairly species specific. However, clinicians should not be complacent and should always beware of the dangers, e.g. milk or colostrum from infected cows should not be fed to crias, nor should colostrum from goats be fed to crias without checking on the health status of the goats. In cattle the main sign is diarrhoea. This is not the case in alpacas and llamas, which tend to suffer ill-thrift. In all animals once clinical signs develop the disease is always fatal. On very rare occasions certain animals will show signs of remission. However, remission will be short-lived and deterioration will soon set in. Euthanasia is the only option.

It should be remembered that there is thought to be a link-up between Johne's disease and Crohn's disease in humans and therefore the disease may be a zoonosis. Normally the infected alpaca or llama will slowly suffer weight loss, which will eventually lead to emaciation.

The normal method of transmission is from dam to offspring soon after birth through colostrum, milk and faeces. Transplacental infection can also occur particularly in animals showing advanced signs of ill-thrift.

Johne's disease can be diagnosed by an ELISA blood test, which is fairly sensitive once the animal shows signs of the disease. However, it is too insensitive to be used as a screening test in clinically normal animals. Faecal smears stained with Ziehl-Neelson (ZN) have a high specificity but a sensitivity of only 30% as the shedding of the organism is very intermittent in SACs. The strains found in alpacas and llamas are very difficult to grow on culture. They are particularly slow growing and can take over 3 months to grow. The use of liquid cultures may speed up a positive diagnosis but 3 months is required as a minimum for a negative result, which may not be that sensitive.

Clinicians might think that a post-mortem examination is definitive. However, gross pathology is not very reliable. There may be granulomatous lesions in the intestines and local lymph nodes but these may not be obvious. Histology from multiple sites is vital. The key point about this disease in SACs is that it is difficult to diagnose and does *not* manifest as diarrhoea as in cattle. However, like in cattle, the disease is likely to be present in many more situations than would be imagined and it may not be clinically apparent until the animal is not only an adult but has had several offspring.

Figures for the incidence of Johne's disease in SACs are unreliable in the UK as the disease is not notifiable. There was a useful questionnaire sent to owners in 2004. There was only one case reported in a population of 38 llamas, 18 alpacas and 8 guanacos surveyed in the UK. In Australia there are much more reliable figures as the disease is notifiable. However, there was only one case in the whole country in 4 years 2005–2008.

Diagnosis in SACs is notoriously difficult. The gold standard is culture but this may take several months. Sheep strains are notoriously difficult to culture. It is presumed that if SACs are infected with cattle strains culture is easier. There is faecal shedding of bacteria earlier in the disease; only later is there a cell-mediated response, which will show up on serology, and so serology is much more reliable later in the course of the disease. Smear testing of faecal samples with ZN stain is very unreliable as the animals are intermittent shedders. On post-mortem a piece of large bowel is more reliable than bowel contents. In sheep and goats the agar gel immunodiffusion test (AGIDT) has been used to screen suspect cases for antibodies. This test does not require species-specific reagents and so could be used in SACs, but the specificity and sensitivity of the test is unknown. Workers (Kawaji *et al.*, 2011) have found that a faecal quantitative PCR assay was a sensitive and specific ante-mortem diagnostic test for *Mycobacterium avium* ssp. *paratuberculosis* (MAP) in sheep. They concluded that quantification of MAP DNA in faeces by PCR could provide immediate information to estimate the stage of infection, as well as the risk of transmission from infected animals. It is possible that a similar test might be developed in SACs.

The disease spread in SACs is not known. Feeding of infected colostrum either from cattle or goats is thought to be a danger but this has never actually been proven.

Control of Johne's disease in SACs is possible using the Weybridge vaccine. Crias should be given half the cattle dose into the brisket at less than 4 weeks of age. Owners should be warned of the unsightly lumps that may occur at the site of injection. Snatching crias at birth to ensure adequate colostral intake from known negative dams and rearing them artificially away from the dam's environment might be worthwhile but is extremely difficult. It is vital to maintain clean rearing environments for crias. The infection may be spread congenitally as well as via infected milk and colostrum; family line culling may be worth considering. All floor feeding should be stopped and all the water troughs should be raised.

Protozoal Diseases Affecting the Gastroenteric Tract

Coccidiosis in SACs

Coccidiosis is one of the most frequently diagnosed diseases of British SACs, with affected animals usually showing clinical signs of weight loss and diarrhoea (Twomey *et al.*, 2010a). There are five species involved: *Eimeria alpacae*, *E. lamae*, *E. macusaniensis*, *E. ivitaensis* and *E. punoensis*. Perhaps the most pathogenic are the two larger species *E. macusaniensis* and *E. ivitaensis*. They both originate from Peru, probably over 1000 years ago. *E. macusaniensis* has been a problem in the UK for several years. *E. ivitaensis* has only been isolated recently. *E. ivitaensis* also occurs in Germany, the USA and Argentina. *E. macusaniensis* is one of the most important pathogenic parasites in SACs in North and South America and in Australia.

The coccidia life cycle includes several stages of multiplication; consequently a low dose can result in a high level of infection. The average life cycle takes approximately 3 weeks and as the initial stage is confined to the small intestine, symptoms consist of weight loss and hypoproteinaemia with little diarrhoea until the infection spreads to involve the spiral colon and large intestine. Thus, there may be extensive damage to the small intestine before it is possible to diagnose the infection via faecal samples. It is very important that the laboratories give the practitioner an estimate of the numbers of the large and the small species.

Although immunity does develop with age, it is species specific, so such individuals remain susceptible to new species and any immunity will wane in geriatric animals. Even immune animals may continue to shed, leading to huge environmental contamination, which can be exacerbated by overcrowding. Animals can maintain infectivity for many years. Pastures can also maintain infectivity for several months when not grazed. The animals most at risk are those lowest in the pecking order, that are likely to eat leavings that fall out of feeders.

Diagnosis is straightforward with chronically infected animals by floatation techniques on faeces samples. Rapid diagnosis can be made from dead animals by impression smears taken from the gastrointestinal (GI) mucosa. The problem diagnosis is within the pre-patent period when the animals can be very sick and yet are not shedding oocysts. ELISA and PCR tests have been developed to aid diagnosis in the pre-patent period.

There are several lines of treatment. There are old-fashioned treatments using amprolium as a drench at 10 mg/kg for 3 weeks or sulfonamides

at 160 mg/kg of sulfamethoxine twice daily for 5 days followed by 80 mg/kg for 10 days as a drench or decoquinate at 0.5 mg/kg for 28 days mixed in the feed. Sulfonamides have been proven to be effective in crias but there is poor absorption of sulfonamides from the GI tract in adults and therefore this treatment is not recommended for adults. Also oral sulfonamides upset the flora in compartment one of the stomach (C1). The old-fashioned ionophores should be avoided in SACs as there is a very low safety margin. On the whole clinicians are likely to advise modern treatments licensed for sheep and cattle of diclazuril at 1 mg/kg as a drench repeated in 3 weeks or toltrazuril at 5 mg/kg also as a drench. Both these treatments affect all intracellular stages, and hence will not only cure the infection but also reduce oocyst shedding.

Cryptosporidiosis

The incidence of this disease in crias is rising in the UK. Cryptosporidiosis is the result of an infection caused by a protozoan of the genus *Cryptosporidium*. There are as many as 16 species. However, few of them are pathogenic to domestic animals and SACs in particular. The most important species is *Cryptosporidium parvum*. This will cause diarrhoea in crias and will also affect humans, although the most important species in humans is *C. hominis* (see Chapter 17). *C. parvum* has a direct life cycle with infection occurring by the faecal-oral route. Normally the infection in SACs is not a monoinfection but more commonly a mixed infection with other pathogens. The highest mortality rates occur in crias under 21 days of age. Obviously it is impossible to ascertain whether the deaths are due to the *Cryptosporidium* or another pathogen. The oocysts are fully sporulated and infective when they are excreted in the faeces. Very large numbers are excreted during the pre-patent period resulting in heavy environmental contamination. Transmission can occur directly from cria to cria or indirectly via a fomite, which may be a human. Infection in crias can result from faecal contamination of food or water. For bottle-fed llamas or alpacas infection can be via contaminated milk. For suckling crias infection can occur from dirty contaminated teats. Female llamas and alpacas can contaminate the environment, as if they are harbouring *C. parvum* they will show a periparturient rise in oocyst excretement. Oocysts are resistant to most disinfectants and can survive for several months in cool and moist conditions. Their infectivity can be destroyed by ammonia, formalin, freeze-drying and exposure to temperatures below freezing or above 65°C. The contamination of the environment rises sharply as the numbers of crias increase. The crias born later in the season are at more of a risk, particularly if colostrum intake is low. Age-related resistance, unrelated to prior exposure is observed in lambs. This does not occur in crias. Case fatality rates in cryptosporidiosis are generally really low unless another pathogen, e.g. a rotavirus, is also involved. The possibility of auto-infection should not be ruled out in crias, nor should an infection from calves either nearby or when they have been housed in the shed earlier in the year. The infectious dose of *C. parvum* oocysts for a neonate is very low.

In clinical cases in crias the faeces tend to be pale and liquid. Fresh blood may be seen but tenesmus is not a feature. In severe cases the animal will be depressed and dehydrated. Abdominal pain is common. The condition is easy to diagnose as large numbers of oocysts will be seen in the infected faeces. Ziehl-Neelsen is a useful stain as the oocysts are small and relatively non-refractile.

Control of the condition requires attention to detail in all aspects of hygiene to lessen cross-contamination and auto-infection. Halofuginone lactate can be used for prophylaxis and treatment. It is licensed for use in cattle in the UK and is available as an oral solution containing 0.5 mg/ml of halofuginone lactate. The dose is 2 ml/kg daily for 7 days.

At the end of the breeding season it is vital to steam clean the houses used for birthing SACs.

Cryptosporidiosis does not seem to be a problem in adult SACs, only in young animals.

In conclusion it should be stressed that cryptosporidiosis is a zoonotic disease. Naturally, keepers of SACs must be warned. However, what is more important is that members of the public, particularly children, must adopt strict hygiene measures. These must be prepared in writing on farms that are opened to the public commercially.

Giardia

This is a zoonotic pathogenic protozoan, which is transmitted by the faeco-oral route. It can affect SACs but only young animals where it is associated with diarrhoea. It does not affect adults. However, it can affect adult humans as well as children (see Chapter 17). It has a long maturation period of 2 or more weeks so it is not found in crias under 4 weeks of age. In animals it rarely actually causes disease unless there is a massive environmental contamination. This usually occurs when wildlife contaminate the drinking pond. The organism has a predilection for the small intestine. Treatment should be either with fenbendazole at 10 mg/kg orally for 3 days or metronidizole at 25 mg/kg given either orally or as an enema for 3 days.

Sarcocystis

This parasite is seen all over the USA and in South America. It has only been seen in imported animals in the UK. It is spread by dogs and wild carnivores and so safe carcass disposal is vital to prevent the spread of the organism. The SAC is the intermediate host. They may exhibit a variety of signs, e.g. anaemia, fever, vasculitis, myositis, abortion, chronic wasting and sudden death. However, these signs are so diverse that the disease is rarely diagnosed in life.

Parasitic Diseases of the Gastroenteric Tract

Intestinal cestodes

Adult tapeworms (e.g. *Moniezia expansa*) occur in SACs if they are running with sheep in the UK. This species is found throughout the world. *Moniezia benedeni* and *Thysaniesia giardi* are found in Peru. The secondary host for all intestinal cestodes found in SACs is an oribatid mite found on the pasture. The pre-patent period is 40 days. Some authorities suggest that they are of no clinical significance. However, in large numbers they may cause ill-thrift and intussusceptions have been reported on post-mortem.

They are well controlled with albendazole. Care should be taken in pregnant animals as it is thought by owners to cause abortion. This has not been substantiated. A further tapeworm *Thysanosoma actinioides* can be considered here. It does not actually live in the intestines but in the bile ducts and the pancreatic ducts. They are considerably smaller and their presence often goes unnoticed. It is also found in the Rocky Mountains in North America. Control is not easy, weekly dosing with double strength albendazole for three treatments is recommended. This species causes clinical signs that vary from mild diarrhoea to violent diarrhoea and liver failure signs. Liver enzymes will be raised in serum samples.

It should be remembered that the metacestode stages of *Taenia multiceps* referred to as *Coenurus cerebralis* cause 'gid' in sheep and goats. It has been suggested that it occurs in SACs in the UK but this has never been substantiated. They are also found in the muscles and subcutaneous tissues as well as the brain. The metacestode stages of *Taenia hydatigena* referred to as *Cysticercus tenuicollis* occur in sheep and rarely in SACs. In very rare cases these may result in acute manifestation and death. Hydatid disease or echinococcosis, due to *Echinococcus granulosus*, occurs frequently in sheep in the UK but only rarely in SACs. This is not the pattern elsewhere in the world where *E. granulosus* is quite common in llamas and alpacas.

Cysticercosis was seen in 7% of 9000 lambs reared in Somerset on a single holding in 2009 (Eichenberger *et al.*, 2011). The infection was linked to footpath contamination by dogs. In such a situation SACs would become infected. Metacestodes possibly found in llamas and alpacas are shown in Table 9.1.

Intestinal nematodes

Practitioners, like the owners of alpacas and llamas, need to radically change their thinking on the control of intestinal nematodes. The old instructions of regular use of anthelmintics should be totally discarded. Animals should only be treated if they need to be treated. The difficulty for practitioners and owners is the problem of knowing when they need to be treated. The overuse of anthelmintics has brought on universal resistance to the standard three types of anthelmintic. It is vital that the new class, which has recently been released, is not rendered useless by overuse and the build-up of resistance. One of the main new instructions is that no animal must be under-dosed. So if animals are in a group it is important that the dose is worked out for the largest animal in the group and that is the dose which is used for the whole group. Now certain anthelmintics have a narrow safety range in SACs, e.g. levamisole, so it is important that accurate weighing and dosing is carried out. This will not be a problem in small herds where each animal can be treated as an individual. However, in larger herds it is important if there is a marked difference in size that the dosing groups can be small enough to

Table 9.1. Metacestodes found in sheep and SACs.

Cestode species	Primary host	Metacestode species name	Where found in the secondary host	Comment
Echinococcus granulosus	Small carnivores	Hydatid	Abdomen and pleural cavity	Very common worldwide with a high zoonotic risk. Found in SACs.
Taenia hydatigena	Small carnivores	*Cysticercus tenuicollis*	Travel through the liver to end in the mesentery	Deaths have been reported in SACs from the damage caused by migration through the liver.
Taenia multiceps	Small carnivores	*Coenurus cerebralis*	Brain, muscles and subcutaneous tissue	Will possibly cause the neurological condition of 'gid' in SACs.
Taenia ovis	Small carnivores	*Cysticercus ovis*	Heart and skeletal muscles	Asymptomatic, not reported in SACs.

accommodate the variations. When dosing animals with anthelmintics it is important that if there is mixed grazing of different species that the species are separated and the correct weights for the two groups are estimated accurately. When decisions have to be made regarding the need for worming, the two species groups should be treated separately. Equally it must be remembered that there is a close crossover of helminth species between sheep, goats and SACs. Therefore there will be a crossover of resistant species of worms between species.

If llamas and alpacas are running together they can be treated as one group as regarding the need to dose is concerned. However, it is vital that the weights of the two subspecies are considered accurately for dosing.

It is vital to separate animals into age groups as the need for dosing will be different for most situations. However, clinicians should remember that where *Haemonchus contortus* is involved it is likely that all the animals regardless of age are treated. To complicate the situation further the hormonal state of the females must be considered. Historically it was thought that there was a rise in faecal egg output by animals in the spring. This was called the 'spring rise'. It is now known that spring was not the trigger but parturition was. Llamas and alpacas both have a post-parturient rise, which is not related to the season of the year, the coming of the rains, nor the hemisphere where the animals are kept.

In SACs it is important to remember that helminths should not be considered in isolation. The clinician has a goal of maintaining the status quo, i.e. each animal has a relatively small worm burden so that it maintains some immunity to a large worm burden but does not suffer disease or subclinical disease. This balance is much easier to attain if nutritional status of the grazing is adequate, particularly if the amount of protein available to the animal is adequate. The provision of sufficient minerals and trace elements will also help to maintain the status quo.

The aim of the practitioner and the owner must be to minimize the use of anthelmintic treatment. Anthelmintics should *only* be used when it is necessary to prevent clinical disease. In this way the rate of selection for resistance will be reduced. The drug efficacy will therefore be preserved for as long as possible. To do this it is important that the number of worms in *refugia* is

increased. Worms that are not selected by anthelmintic treatment are said to be in *refugia*. This includes worms whose larvae are on the pasture. It also includes worms in untreated animals or whose larvae are at stages in animals that are not affected by treatment. The larger the population of worms that are in *refugia*, compared to the population of worms that are exposed to treatment, the slower resistance will develop. After treatment there are always some worms that survive in the host. These are resistant worms. If the offspring of these worms are in the majority, resistance to the anthelmintic will develop rapidly. To prevent resistance developing, a substantial number of worms needs to be left untreated each time anthelmintics are used so that these non-resistant worms essentially provide the subsequent generations of worms. It is now considered that where SACs are continually exposed to worms it is a good idea to have a few worms inside the animal to not only help develop a form of immunity but also to prolong the effectiveness of the available anthelmintics. The selective treatment of animals significantly increases the percentage of the worms in *refugia*.

Every holding and every group of animals must be considered separately. There should be no blanket treatments. In fact effective worm control prevents unnecessary dosing, which is also good economically. However, it is vital to prevent resistant worms being brought on to a holding. Therefore in a closed or semi-closed situation the aim with any new animals is total deworming. This may involve a combination of the 'old' three wormers given at the correct dosage or the 'new' wormer recently available. Drugs may be given at the same time but should not be actually mixed. After drenching, the animals should be housed or at least kept off the pasture for 48 h to allow any still viable eggs to be shed. The new animals can then be introduced on to the originally grazed pasture to pick up the 'non-resistant' worms and thus dilute any resistant worms.

Controlled grazing methods will help to avoid infection. Any method of allowing pastures to rest will be beneficial as soil organisms (e.g. earthworms, dung beetles and nematophagus fungi) will reduce pasture burdens. Mixed species (e.g. rabbits and horses) will also be helpful. However, owners must realize that sheep, goats and SACs are infected by the same helminths. There are some species-specific worms (e.g.

Lamenana spp.) in SACs that will be killed by sheep and goats. Cattle grazing will also help but there are some species of helminths that cross between cattle and sheep or cattle and goats or indeed between cattle and SACs, so practitioners should not give blanket advice but continue to monitor the situation. Preventing close cropping of grass is good as rarely do worms climb more than 3 cm up the stems. The ideal control of pastures is to plough and have a break crop (e.g. lucerne or kale). Making hay also considerably helps pasture contamination as does resting a pasture for a year, but neither is totally effective. Only resting a pasture for 3 years can be considered totally effective. Of course zero grazing is the ultimate method of control and may be considered in large herds of SACs. Young llamas and alpacas are most at risk, so it is important to protect them from contaminated pastures and also to remember that their mothers will be contaminating the pasture on account of the 'post-parturient rise phenomenon'. Each herd has different problems. However, there are various ideas that can be put forward to the owner. The time of parturition can be altered. This is easier with sheep and goats with their 5-month gestation period but harder for SACs with their 11-month gestation period. Parturition can be carried out indoors and turn out delayed until the mothers faecal egg output is lower and the overwintered larvae have died on the pasture.

The minimum frequency of dosing should be used and as stated earlier the correct dose must be used to avoid under-dosing. The dose of the anthelmintic has been tested in sheep so that is not a problem provided the sheep are weighed. It should be stressed that *only anthelmintics licensed for sheep should be used* (not products licensed for cattle or horses). The problem lies with SACs, which have no licensed products. General advice would be to use twice the sheep dose with benzimidazoles and avermectins, which have a wide safety margin, in SACs. As stated earlier levamisole does not have a wide safety margin and so the dose can be increased to one and a half times the sheep dose but no higher than this. When to change anthelmintics is problematic. The most up-to-date advice must be only to rotate drugs when resistance is suspected, not on an annual basis. Faecal egg outputs should be monitored. It is important to sample individuals and not a bulked-up sample or the egg count will be diluted.

The number of samples is difficult to decide upon. In very small herds each animal can be treated as an individual. In larger herds 10% can be used as a yardstick. In very large groups a compromise has to be reached. Testing before treatment will provide information about the worm status of the group and whether anthelmintic use is necessary. Testing after treatment will show the efficacy or otherwise of treatment. It takes 3 days for all the eggs in the gastrointestinal tract to pass out, so if treatment is 100% effective there will be virtually no eggs present at that time. However, there is a shock effect of the anthelmintic, where it will stop egg production but not actually kill the mature worms. It is therefore prudent to wait for 2 weeks after treatment before sampling. Worms acquired after treatment will not normally produce eggs for 3 weeks. The practitioner can therefore advise the owner on the likelihood of anthelmintic resistance to the drug being used and the advisability of a change of drug. Practitioners must stress that if there is resistance to one drug in that group of drugs then there will be resistance to all the other members of that group of drugs. Owners can easily get confused by the different packaging of the products.

As yet there are no natural anthelmintics available in plants, e.g. garlic, which are effective at controlling worms, although many owners are totally convinced of their efficacy.

Although SACs are affected by the same nematodes as sheep (Table 9.2), it is thought that llamas are more susceptible because they are principally browsing animals and their resistance to these endoparasites is less highly evolved. However, alpacas that are grazing animals should therefore follow more closely to the sheep model. This may be unlikely as alpacas tend to dung on certain areas of the pasture forming dung hills. This may affect their resistance to intestinal helminths. Alpacas may be more sensitive than sheep to endoparasites when kept on lush pastures with poor parasitic control. They may carry heavier nematode burdens, which will be reflected in higher faecal egg counts. These may persist for longer periods, especially in alpacas with crias at foot. The post-parturient rise may last for the whole summer. An indication of clinical disease would be 2000 eggs/g. However, it may be that above 500/g will also indicate clinical disease.

Table 9.2. Intestinal nematodes found in SACs.

Where found in the SAC (Where found in the sheep)	Helminth species	Where found	Comment
C3 (Abomasum)	Bunostumum trigonocephalum	Americas and UK	Uncommon but will cause serious disease
C3 (Not found in sheep)	Camelostrongylus mentulatus	Americas and Australia, not found in UK	Found in camels as well as in SACs. Very similar to Ostertagia spp.
Small intestine (Small intestine)	Capillaria longipes	Rare in UK	Clinically significant in SACs but not in sheep
Large intestine (Large intestine)	Chabertia ovis	UK	Uncommon, of very doubtful clinical significance
Small intestine (Small intestine)	Cooperia curticei	UK	Common
Small intestine (Not found in sheep)	Cooperia mcmasteri	Americas and Australia	Found in SACs and cattle, will cause serious disease
Small intestine (Found in cattle)	Cooperia onocophora	Americas and Australia	Caught from cattle and may cause clinical signs
C3 (SAC specific)	Graphininema aucheniae	South America, not found in UK, Australia or New Zealand	Only found in SACs
C3 (Abomasum)	Haemonchus contortus	Worldwide	Will cause very serious anaemia
Small intestine (SAC specific)	Lamanema chavezi	Only in South America	Passes through the liver causing damage
Small intestine (Small intestine)	Nematodirus battus	Worldwide	Life-threatening disease
Small intestine (Small intestine)	Nematodirus filicollis	Australia and South America	Common and may well cause clinical disease
Small intestine (SAC specific)	Nematodirus lamae	South America, not found in UK, USA, Australia or New Zealand	Found in SACs
Small intestine (Small intestine)	Nematodirus spathiger	Australia	Common and may well cause clinical disease
Large intestine (Large intestine)	Oesophagostomum venulosum	Australia	Common but causes little disease
C3 (Abomasum)	Ostertagia circumcinta	Australia and Americas	Common cause of clinical disease of diarrhoea and weight loss
C3 (Abomasum)	Ostertagia leptospicularis	Europe	Infections caught from deer
C3 and duodenum (Duodenum)	Ostertagia marshalli	USA	Will cause problems in SACs
C3 (Abomasum)	Ostertagia ostertagi	Worldwide	Will cause problems in ruminants and SACs when encysted in the mucosa
C3 (Abomasum)	Ostertagia trifurcata	USA	Common cause of clinical disease of diarrhoea and weight loss
C3 (Abomasum)	Skrjabinagia kolchida	South America	Infections caught from deer
Large intestine (Large intestine)	Skrjabinema ovis	South America	Very common oxyurid parasite
C3 (SAC specific)	Spiculopteragia peruvianus	South America, not found in UK, Australia or New Zealand	Found near Lake Titicaca in Peru and Bolivia in SACs

Continued

Table 9.2. Continued.

Where found in the SAC (Where found in the sheep)	Helminth species	Where found	Comment
C3 (Found in kids not in sheep)	*Strongyloides papillous*	South America	Will cause clinical disease in young crias
C3 (Abomasum)	*Teladorsagia davtiani*	South America	Common cause of clinical disease
C3 (Abomasum)	*Trichostrongylus axei*	Worldwide	Very common in cattle seen also in equids
Small intestine (Small intestine)	*Trichostrongylus colubriformis*	Australia, USA and UK	Common cause of disease
Small intestine (Small intestine)	*Trichostrongylus vitrinus*	Worldwide	Common cause of disease
Large intestine (Large intestine)	*Trichuris ovis*	Worldwide	Common but of no clinical significance

It must be remembered that the problems caused by nematodes will be very different in SACs kept in the semi-arid areas of the altiplano to those kept on lush pastures in the UK or well-kept fields in the USA, Australia or New Zealand.

Infection with just a single worm species is uncommon in all animal hosts grazing under natural conditions (Carmichael *et al.*, 1998). The clinical signs of infection with worms are a mix of those caused by the various worm species contributing to the infection. There will be host factors, e.g. immune status, nutrition and age. Animals under two years of age are usually more affected both clinically and subclinically. Interestingly geriatric animals also seem to be more affected. This may be because the nutritional state of these animals is not so good because of poor teeth, poor locomotion and bullying by younger stronger adults. Animals kept on massive acreages on the altiplano will have very different worm burdens to animals kept in small lush paddocks. However in the Andes the animals are often brought together to give birth and so the risks of severe parasitism are increased. This particularly occurs as the females are stressed by giving birth, lactating and becoming pregnant again in a very short space of time. Other factors in the Andes also will bring animals together, e.g. shearing. There will also be factors relating to the worm, e.g. numbers and species.

If alpacas are grazed with sheep they are certainly more likely to have high worm burdens. The author assumes this would happen with alpacas grazing with cattle but that is beyond his experience. If other species are grazed with alpacas the benefits of their discrete common latrines are negated.

Practitioners are hampered by the fact there is no magical figure for worm egg counts in faeces that are dangerous or should trigger dosing. Figures in excess of 1000 eggs per gram might not be alarming during the dry season in the altiplano but such figures would be very alarming in other parts of the world. Therefore practitioners should err on the safe side and suggest that all intestinal nematodes in SACs will cause various signs and symptoms depending on the species of nematode, which determines the place where the adults are found. The author considers statements like 'even one nematode egg is too many' are in error but equally it is difficult to give a definite figure. Probably the most serious is *Haemonchus contortus*, which is a blood sucking parasite in C3. It will cause severe life-threatening anaemia in all ages of SAC. Diagnosis by faecal worm egg output is normally too late. Clinical diagnosis by assessing the pallor of the mucous membranes is vital so that prompt anthelmintic treatment can limit the number of deaths. Ocular membranes can be examined and categorized as: 1 = deep red (non-anaemic), 2 = red-pink (non-anaemic), 3 = pink (mild anaemia), 4 = white-pink (anaemic), and 5 = white (severely anaemic). Both eyes should be examined in direct sunlight. If any animals are 3 but there are no 4 or 5s, these animals alone should be treated. If any animals are 4 then all the animals should be treated. If any animals are 5 then all the animals should be treated with at least two different groups of anthelmintics.

'Ostertagian nematodes' cause the gastric glands in C3 to become hyperplastic and cause an increase in pH. This leads to a leakage of pepsinogen into the plasma. This can be measured in a serum sample to aid diagnosis. On post-mortem following heavy infections the mucosa of C3 in SACs will show necrosis and sloughing. The sign in the living animal is violent blackish diarrhoea.

Intestinal nematodes produce villous atrophy and crypt hyperplasia. Diarrhoea is then of a more chronic nature. There is a protein-losing enteropathy. This will cause setbacks in growth rates of young animals and weight loss in older animals. Diagnosis will be made by raised individual faecal worm egg counts. Individual counts are important to avoid dilution effects, which may give misleading results.

Many of the intestinal nematode species encountered in SACs are encountered in sheep but there are also other species which are found in SACs but are not found in sheep. All these species are shown in Table 9.2.

Nematodirus battus is a very serious nematode, which causes scouring in lambs and crias. It may well be associated with viral, bacterial or coccidial infection. A heavy infection will cause profuse watery yellowy green diarrhoea, leading to severe dehydration and death even before eggs are seen in the faeces. The eggs are roughly twice the size of other intestinal nematodes found in SACs and are easily recognized. Lower levels will cause 'ill-thrift'. The classically described condition is changing in the UK. Historically *N. battus* affected 4–8-week-old lambs that had been grazing on pastures grazed by young lambs in the previous summer. The eggs required a frost before they could become infective. Now the pattern in the UK is changing with infections occurring in older lambs. A similar clinical syndrome is seen in older crias. Owners should be urged not to graze either young or older crias on the same pasture in consecutive years. This is difficult on most smaller holdings. Pastures that have been grazed by young cattle or ewes are no longer safe. *N. battus* has now been found to be resistant to benzimidazole anthelmintics in the UK (Mitchell *et al.*, 2011). However, at the present time the benzimidazole anthelmintics are still recommended for treatment of *N. battus* as resistance at the time of writing was not widespread. Many of the other species of nematode worms are becoming resistant to the three standard wormer types. Treatment is difficult. It has been suggested that worms should receive a therapeutic dose of all three wormer types at 3-weekly intervals if multiple resistance is encountered. The use of monepantel should be very carefully controlled.

Trematodes

Introduction

In the UK there has been a massive increase in prevalence of fascioliasis. It is no longer just found in the wetter, western areas of the UK and Ireland. The distribution is dependent on the presence of the snail intermediate host, *Lymnaea truncatula*. This aquatic snail is now fairly ubiquitous. The levels of infection and incidence of disease are linked to the rainfall from May to October. The adult flukes in the bile ducts of ruminants and SACs lay eggs in the faeces on the pasture. The eggs hatch in the warmer months (>10°C) in water, releasing motile miracidia. These infect the snails in which the development continues through sporocyst and redia stages releasing cercariae. In wetter summers there is a massive shedding of cercariae on the pasture during August to October. These encyst into metacercariae on the herbage and are ingested by the ruminant or SAC. The immature flukes migrate through the liver to the bile ducts. In cattle and to a large extent in llamas and alpacas this is not a dangerous stage, but in sheep there is often massive damage to the liver resulting in death from acute fascioliasis. Practitioners should be aware that acute fascioliasis can occur in llamas and alpacas but it is not a common manifestation. In the UK deaths will occur from September to December. A useful description of the clinical disease is described in an alpaca in Eire (Hayes *et al.*, 2021). It showed colic signs and moderate anaemia. Eggs were found in the faeces. Neither albendazole nor triclabendazole were effective. The animal had a blood transfusion and other supportive treatment but was eventually destroyed. The diagnosis was confirmed on post-mortem. More chronic infections are seen in llamas and alpacas with adult flukes in the bile ducts and will occur in February and

March (see Fig. 9.6). Llamas and alpacas with chronic fascioliasis will be weak and anaemic. The classic sign is oedema in the mandibular space 'bottle jaw'. Mild winters increase the numbers of hibernating snails, which shed more cercariae in the following spring.

SACs seem to be particularly susceptible to *Fasciola hepatica* infection. This may be because of a deficiency of their immune response. SACs have a relatively small liver so they may more readily be severely affected by the infection. SACs, particularly alpacas, are like sheep and graze very close to the ground and therefore are very much at risk. Liver fluke infection is becoming more common not only in the UK but also in the USA.

The most common clinical sign is weight loss. However, some will show pain and recumbency. Diarrhoea is not a feature. Generally the infection follows the more chronic cattle-type model rather than the acute or even peracute sheep model. Fluke eggs may be seen in the faeces using a sedimentation test. However, the eggs will only be present in the chronic cases after the long pre-patent period. In the live animal, diagnosis may not be easy as the ELISA test used in cattle has not been validated in SACs. The disease is fairly straightforward to diagnose on post-mortem examination. The signs seen will include ascites, hydrothorax and subcutaneous oedema. The liver will be increased in size. Experienced operators will be able to evaluate this on ultrasonographic examination. Naturally this could be confirmed on liver biopsy. However, raised live enzymes will help diagnosis in the live animal. Examining the faeces for fluke eggs is not very rewarding. In one study (Kutzler *et al.*, 2009) only seven animals were shown to have fluke eggs in the faeces out of 25 animals that had adult flukes in their livers on post-mortem. At post-mortem in the acute case the liver will show the pathognomic signs of the immature fluke tracts through the liver. In the more typical chronic case there will be hepatic fibrosis, fibrinous perihepatitis, thickened bile ducts and the presence of adult flukes. Mural endocarditis has been described in a series of fascioliasis cases in North America (Firshman *et al.*, 2008). This has also been seen in the UK by the author in 2009.

Control programmes must take into account topography, geographic location and prevailing weather conditions. Draining endemic areas will help to eliminate snail habitats. Fencing off wet areas in the autumn prevents access to these snail habitats. In average rainfall years all SACs likely to have become infected should be dosed twice in October and January with a drug that is effective against immature stages, e.g. triclabendazole. They will need to be dosed again in May.

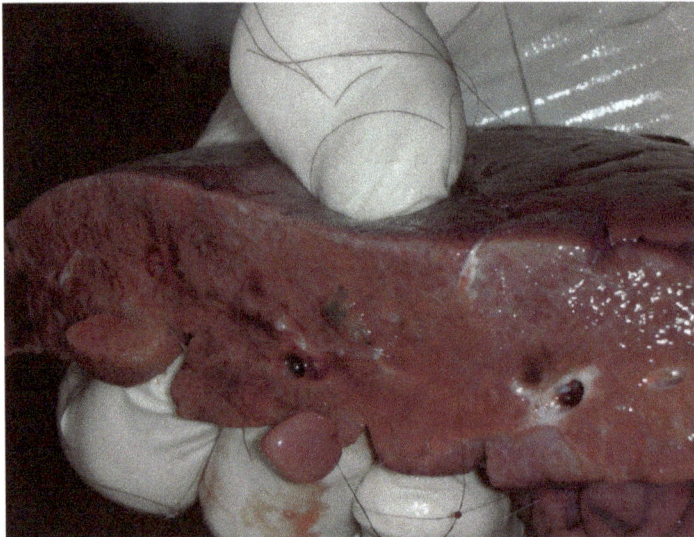

Fig. 9.6. Adult flukes in the bile ducts.

This can be with a combination roundworm and fluke drench at this time only (see Chapter 6). In high rainfall years SACs may require additional dosing in both the winter and the summer season.

There is strong evidence (Sargison and Scott, 2011) that there is resistance of *F. hepatica* to triclabendazole. This has serious economic consequences. The population genetics of *F. hepatica* will inevitably prove to differ from those for parasitic nematodes, and therefore refugia-based strategies that have been developed to slow the emergence of resistance in parasitic nematodes cannot be extrapolated to *F. hepatica*. Owners should attempt to develop evasive strategies, such as: fencing off snail habitats; managing snail habitats and areas that are conductive to the survival of free-living stages of *F. hepatica*; and the strategic use of fasciolacidal anthelminitic treatments with the aim of reducing *F. hepatica* egg shedding and miracidial infection of snails. The diagnostic signs of fascioliasis in llamas and alpacas are shown in Table 9.3.

Conditions of the Stomachs and Intestines

Anatomy

The stomachs

SACs have a long oesophagus, which leads to their stomachs. Examination of the viscera in the abdomen of a camelid from the left-hand side reveals instead of a reticulum, rumen, omasum and abomasum as a ruminant, three compartments, called compartments 1, 2 and 3 (C1, C2 and C3). There are no papillae and there is glandular tissue in all three compartments. C1 occupies the entire left-hand side, except for the triangular spleen lying caudally. It has cranial and caudal sacs, which are separated by a horizontal pillar. The oesophagus enters the C1 midline from a cranio-dorsal aspect. There is only a single lipped oesophageal groove. Looking from the right-hand side directly behind the diaphragm a small part of C2 and C3 can be seen but the rest will be hidden behind the liver, which lies entirely on the right and has a fimbriated caudal border. Camelids are like horses and do not have a gall bladder. Behind the liver will be seen part of C1. Both C1 and C2 have glandular saccules (see Fig. 9.7), which contain mucus-producing glands. C2 lies on the cranio-dorsal aspect of C1 with C3 lying as a long slipper-like organ on the cranio-mesial aspect of C2. Only the final fifth of C3 contains true gastric glands and is the true acid-forming stomach. C3 has five longitudinal ridges of mucosa-like pleats. The lesser omentum has no sling. The greater omentum is attached along the greater and lesser curvature of C2 and C3 and along the right surface of C1.

The small intestine

The duodenum is dorsal to the right side of C1 running into the jejunum, which is folded around the root of the mesentery in the right caudal abdomen. The jejunum joins with the ileum, which begins ventrally and courses medially and dorsally to enter the large intestine at the caeco-colic junction.

Table 9.3. The diagnostic signs of fascioliasis in llamas and alpacas.

Disease type	Peak incidence in northern hemisphere	Clinical signs	Fluke numbers	Eggs per gram of faeces
Acute	October–January	Sudden death or dullness, anaemia, dyspnoea, ascites and abdominal pain	1000+ mainly immatures	0
Subacute	October–January	Rapid weight loss, anaemia, submandibular oedema and ascites in some cases	500–1000 adults and immatures	<100
Chronic	January–April	Progressive weight loss, anaemia, submandibular oedema and ascites	200+ adults	100+

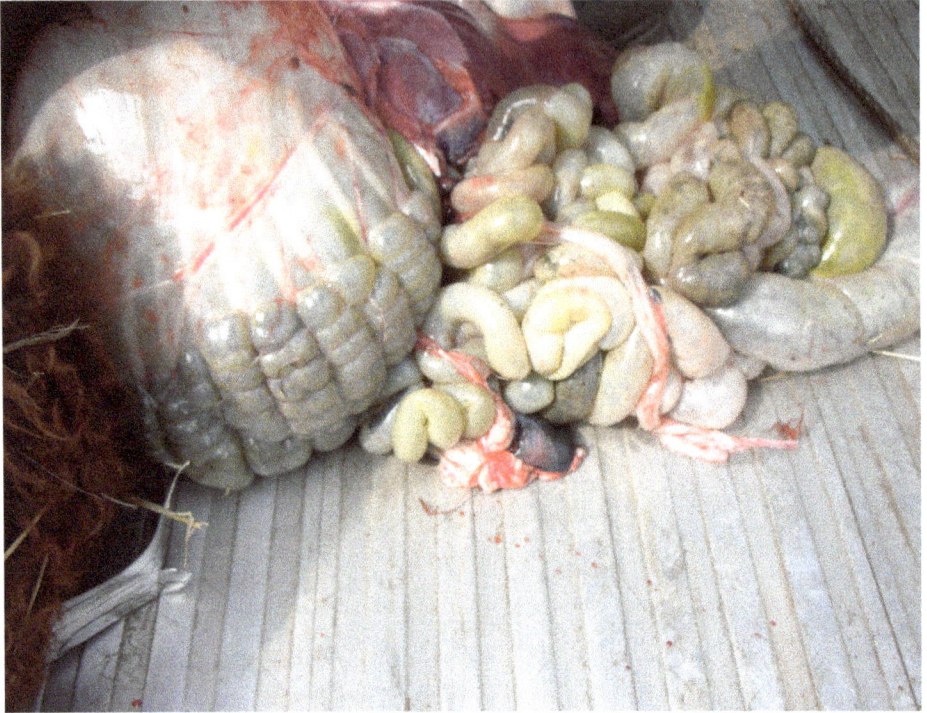

Fig. 9.7. Glandular saccules on C1.

The large intestine

The caecum lies midline and runs towards the pelvis. The colon is roughly similar to that of the ruminant in that it runs cranially and ventrally before entering a spiral loop. However, there are five coils in the spiral colon contrasting with three in the sheep. The colon narrows from a diameter of 5 cm to 2 cm in the spiral colon but widens again as it becomes the transverse colon, which runs caudally to the rectum.

Physiology of digestion

SACs are adapted to survive in a harsh, nutrient-poor environment. Their gastric fermentation of fibre is more efficient than ruminants. It is likely that the non-keratinized epithelium of their gastric saccules contributes to this efficiency by providing a large surface area for rapid absorption of volatile fatty acids from the gut lumen. The pH in C1 in a camelid eating a natural high-fibre, low-energy diet is 6.5, which encourages the loss of a hydrogen molecule from volatile fatty acids, thus slowing absorption. However, once in the gastric saccules, the volatile fatty acids can become reionized by claiming a hydrogen molecule from the carbonic acid that is a by-product of fermentation, thus increasing speed of absorption and leaving behind bicarbonate.

High-energy diets

On a high-energy diet the pH is much lower (i.e. 4.5), the volatile fatty acids retain their hydrogen molecule and are rapidly absorbed, leaving carbonic acid rather than bicarbonate, thus reducing the buffering effect so the bicarbonate is generated when fatty acids are absorbed under low-energy conditions. This has led to the myth that camelids are more resistant to grain overload. This is not the case as bicarbonate is not generated under high-energy conditions. Camelids are very susceptible to grain overload.

A second myth is that camelids are discriminate feeders and thus not prone to engorgement. High-density confinement increases competition between animals and alters feeding behaviour. Camelids with access to highly fermentable feedstuffs will certainly gorge themselves. Naturally, engorging can be prevented by dividing grain feeding over the day, making feed changes slowly and providing adequate roughage. Feeding of grain should not be encouraged. If really necessary whole grain rather than crushed or cracked grains should be fed. Oats are preferable to barley and wheat should definitely be avoided. Owners should make sure that the feed-room door is locked.

Other than a break-in there are two other likely chances of grain overload. First in the debilitated, or old, animal, which requires feeding up to increase its body weight. Such animals will develop acidosis with the addition of very little grain to their diet. Second, in the housed camelid group where an aggressive animal will consume more than its fair share of the grain ration. In either case the signs will be similar and include acute depression, gastric atony, subnormal temperature and neurological signs including pain.

Confirmation of a diagnosis of acidosis can be made by taking a sample from C1 with a long 16G needle through the flank. This avoids salivary contamination. The normal pH of the contents of C1 is 6.4–6.8. This will rise with anorexia or salivary contamination. Camelids suffering from acute acidosis will have pH values lower than 4.5. In reality anything under 6 is suspicious. Some camelids on grain-based diets have subclinical acidosis with pH values of 5.5. However, unlike ruminants, camelids cannot adapt to low gastric pH and will suffer from bouts of low-grade pain, diarrhoea and weight loss. Such animals may well suffer from gastric ulcers. This is a relatively common condition and is usually associated with stress, e.g. movement, mixing or parasitism. All three stomach compartments can be affected, although lesions are most common in C3. They can perforate the stomach wall and cause peritonitis. The condition can be seen in crias as well as in adults.

Gastric ulceration is a common problem

Neubert *et al.* (2022) state that gastric ulcers are a common finding in post-mortem examinations of SACs, but diagnosis in living animals is often difficult. Their study was to provide an overview of the incidence of gastric ulcers in alpacas, common concomitant diseases, and clinical as well as laboratory findings to facilitate diagnosis for veterinarians. For this purpose, a total of 187 necropsy reports of alpacas were evaluated, including clinical and laboratory findings on the living animal. A total of 23 of the 44 animals (55%) were found to have gastric ulcers, nine were perforated. C3 was most frequently affected by gastric ulcers. No sex predilection could be detected, but animals 1 year of age and older were more frequently affected by gastric ulcers than animals under 1 year of age. Alpacas with gastric ulcers were presented to the clinic due to different non-specific symptoms. In alpacas with gastric ulcers, significantly more organs or organ systems beside the stomach revealed clinical findings than in animals without gastric ulcers. Of the 44 animals, a total of 21 alpacas (47.7%) had a poor nutritional status, but cachexia was not significantly more frequent in animals with gastric ulcers than in other dissected animals without ulcers. Haematological investigations revealed a significant lower white blood count and significantly lower segmented neutrophils than in deceased animals without ulcers. Compared to animals discharged after treatment, alpacas that died with gastric ulcers had significantly higher levels of band neutrophils and fewer eosinophils and basophils. Occult blood in faeces was found in 3 of 12 animals with gastric ulcers examined for occult blood. In summary, gastric ulcers are a common problem in SACs, which are difficult to diagnose clinically or by laboratory investigations. As there are often chronic processes involving other organ systems, regular monitoring of the animals' nutritional status and early detection of disease symptoms may help to prevent gastric ulcers.

It is important to treat the acidosis before gastric ulcers develop as they are a very serious sequel, which may cause the death of the animal if an ulcer should perforate. Treatment for acidosis if ulcers are not suspected should be prompt and aim to correct dehydration and systemic acidosis. Intravenous fluids containing magnesium bicarbonate or magnesium hydroxide are ideal. If intravenous fluids are not practical then oral fluids containing magnesium oxide should be given. Antibiotics such as penicillin or ceftiofur should be given by injection together with B vitamins to prevent secondary complications. Cover with NSAIDs by injection is useful together with activated charcoal by mouth. Most affected animals will survive with immediate diagnosis and this treatment. A few may become chronic poor doers with intermittent fever, depression, hypoproteinaemia and weight loss. These animals will be likely to have gastric ulcers.

Ulcers typically form at the point where C3 abruptly turns dorsal and cranial. The mucosa at this point is 0.7–1.0 cm thick, where the rest of the mucosa in the rest of the organ is only 0.3–0.5 cm thick. There is a small region in this area that secretes hydrochloric acid at a constant rate. It is likely that gastric emptying function is very important in ulcer development. Ulcers are seen in 6% of camelids on postmortem. In a normal camelid, the acid secretion would be rapidly propelled against gravity by peristalsis and the onward push of digesta, out of C3 into the intestine for neutralization. Stress factors tend to decrease appetite and peristalsis. Under conditions of poor gastric emptying, such as anorexia, intermittent feeding, dehydration and electrolyte imbalance, the acid contents would remain unneutralized and damage the mucosa. This would be exacerbated by a low gastric pH in cases of grain overload. Bile reflux is seen in half of camelids with ulcers. It is not known if this is a cause or an effect but is a useful sign to look out for when performing a postmortem. Ulcers are often seen in the mouths of these cases. They are secondary to uraemia due to renal failure from acute nephritis, which is seen in the end stages of these cases.

Diagnosis of ulcers

A definitive diagnosis is difficult to make. The history will be helpful. Ulcers take some time to form so the animal will have been off colour for some time. It is only when they become acute that the clinician is normally called. Practitioners might consider testing the faeces of affected animals for occult blood. Sadly this is unreliable. C3 may be full of blood and yet the test is negative. Equally if the soil is high in iron the test will show positive in normal animals. There is no evidence that *Helicobacter* spp. are involved in camelid ulcers. There is debate that copper deficiency is linked with ulcers in cattle but this has never been confirmed. Gastric ulcers are so widespread in camelids that such a sole cause is unlikely in this species. Clinicians are well aware of the large number of foreign bodies found in the reticulum of cattle, occasionally with disastrous effects. This phenomenon is not seen in camelids as they are selective feeders. Erosive hairballs may lead to gastritis in youngsters at weaning when they tend to suck each other's coats and ingest large amounts of hair. These are not seen in adults. However, adult camelids do suffer from gastroliths.

The non-keratized epithelium of the gastric saccules is protected from the abrasive action of ingested fibre by muscular sphincters coated with keratinized squamous epithelium. If large particles pass this sphincter, they are trapped in the saccular lumen. Large grains may do this. Once in the lumen, mineral is laid down around them forming stones. The minerals occur out of solution by minor shifts of pH. However, these stones are very common in adult camelids that appear fit and well. They can be seen on radiographs. There is no reason to believe that they cause any ulceration.

Clostridium perfringens and other *Clostridium* spp. are known to cause disease in camelids. It is possible that these organisms that cause haemorrhage in the bowel wall might cause ulceration. However, these organisms are normally associated with acute or peracute disease. Gastric ulcers are normally chronic in nature and only cause acute disease on perforation. Therefore the cause of gastric ulcers remains an enigma as they also occur in the Andes on the altiplano but certainly not as frequently as in camelids fed a high-energy low-fibre diet.

Treatment of ulcers

All treatment in camelids is difficult as there are no licensed medicines in the UK. Although clinicians are allowed to use medicines on the cascade principle they are well advised to discuss all treatments with the owners and obtain written consent to their use.

Treatment of ulcers is not going to be easy. Obviously prevention is to be encouraged. Measures would include: feeding high-fibre and low-energy diets, avoiding stress and treating all underlying disease particularly intestinal parasites. On being faced with a possible acute ulcer liable to perforate a human drug sodium pantoprazole (marketed as PROTIUM i.v.™ Nycomed GmbH Konstanz Germany) should be injected intravenously after dissolving the 40 mg powder in the vial with water for injection. This should be followed with further injections of sodium pantoprazole on a daily basis. Ideally the sodium pantoprazole should be given intravenously at 1 mg/kg but it can be given subcutaneously at double the dose, i.e. 2 mg/kg. Pain can be controlled with NSAIDs, but these should be discontinued as soon as appetite is re-established.

There is another proton-pump inhibitor related to sodium pantoprazole named Omeprazol, which has been extensively used commercially in the last three years in horses to treat gastric ulcers. There is every reason to think that it will be a useful treatment for ulcers in SACs. The dose is 4 mg/kg injected intramuscularly for four doses at weekly intervals. The author has no experience in its use in SACs but there has been favourable news from the USA in recent months. A second generation of Omeprazol called Esomeprazol has recently been used experimentally in horses. It has yet to be used in SACs but this may be even more efficacious.

Left displacement of the third gastric compartment.

This is an extremely rare condition and has only been reported once by Song *et al.* (2022).

Case presentation: A 2-year-old brown female alpaca (*Vicugna pacos*) was presented to evaluate a 3-day history of abdominal distention causing loss of both appetite and thirst, along with oliguria and low to no defecation. Clinical examination, X-ray examination, surgical exploration and determination of gastric pH (pH ~2.35) confirmed that left displacement of C3 resulted in abdominal distention. The gastric wall of the displaced third gastric compartment was incised for the expulsion of pneumatosis, and a medical-grade silicone tube was inserted into the incision to remove the effusion by siphoning. Surgical treatment proved to effectively alleviate the abdominal distention caused by left displacement of C3 without apparent side effects.

Spitting/vomiting

SACs have a largely unfair reputation for spitting, since they will rarely spit at people unless they have become over-familiarized. The activity is part of the animal's natural defensive mechanism and is usually a response to the invasion of personal space. An unwary person can be caught in the crossfire of two spitting animals. An animal that commonly spits at people is extremely rare. The actual contents of the spit can take three forms – food, saliva or stomach contents. The latter is the so-called green spit. Adults and more commonly crias will spit food and/or saliva when they are eating to warn other animals to back off and give them space. The green spit, which is much more unpleasant both to humans or other SACs, is used in more severe confrontations. It is used by SACs to establish dominance. Most animals will pre-warn the challenger by pinning their ears back very tightly and tilting their head back so that the nose is pointing up in the air. If this warning is ignored then the animal will spit.

Vomiting is extremely rare. It is indicative of gastritis, normally from ingestion of poisonous plants, e.g. rhododendron. It may be associated with mega-oesophagus, which, although recorded in camelids, is very rare.

Colic

Because camelids are foregut fermenters, tympanic colic as occurs in horses is extremely rare. However, SACs, like horses with colic, pose a diagnostic challenge to the practitioner. They need to be divided into surgical and medical cases.

Recognition of colic in camelids has two major difficulties. Many clinicians expect colic to be an active violent process as in equine practice. This is extremely rare. Equally inexperienced owners may mislead clinicians by over-interpreting non-specific signs such as sternal recumbency, anorexia and lack of faeces and so many animals that do not have colic will be included.

At first animals will appear bright and alert when handled but will lie down when left alone. They may appear restless getting up and down. Then they may go from sternal recumbency to lateral recumbency (see Fig. 9.8). They may keep

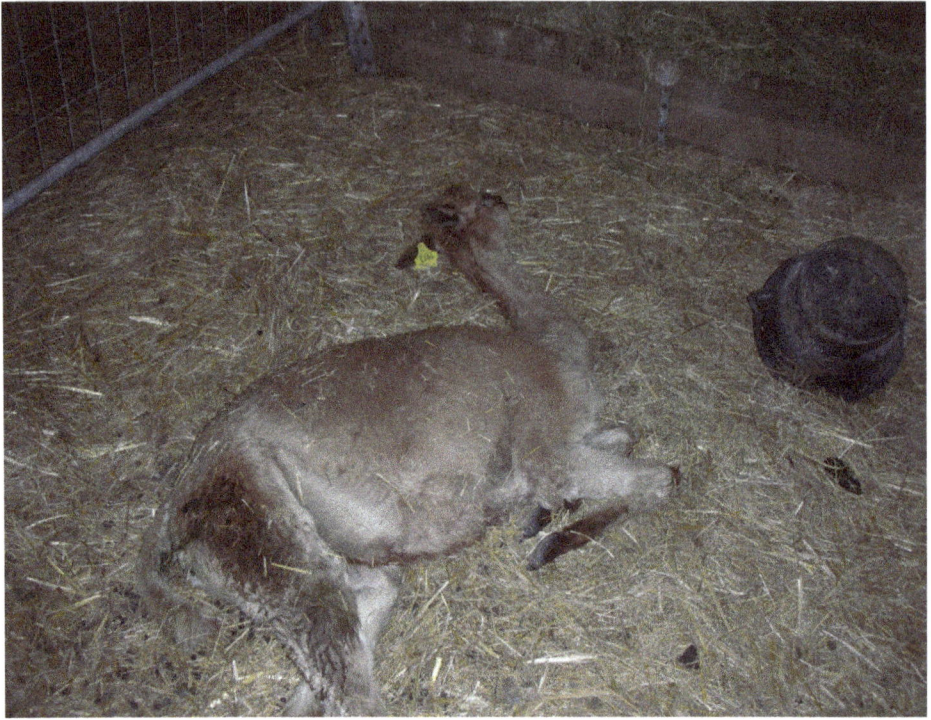

Fig. 9.8. Lateral recumbency in a colic case.

stretching out their legs. Signs may become more violent or may lessen if shock sets in. Clinicians will have to examine their patients carefully. The mucous membranes will be helpful as will the tightness of the skin. Naturally pulse strength and heart rate will be extremely helpful. Respiratory rate will be raised in severe cases. Mouth breathing will occur in animals that are just on the edge of extremis. Rectal temperature will be raised with peritonitis, pancreatitis, nephritis or hepatitis but otherwise will be subnormal in most cases of colic where shock is setting in. Gastric atony will occur. A tense painful abdomen is a more serious sign.

Most gastrointestinal colic is due to ischaemia, inflammation or fluid-distended gut tugging on mesentery. Large-diameter gastric compartments, full of fibrous material, empty into the small intestine, which is not only narrow but tortuous. Intraluminal obstruction can occur in the duodenum or the first two-thirds of the jejunum. The last third of the jejunum to the transverse colon and the spiral colon have long mesenteric attachments. These pendulous parts of the bowel are very susceptible to torsion, entrapment or strangulation. These are surgical cases (see Fig. 9.9).

Abdominal distension due to the accumulation of fluid within the gastric compartments is commonly seen with phyto/trichobezoars or other obstructions between the pylorus and the cranial jejunum. Obviously grain overload and gastric acidosis will need to be ruled out. Only mild colic signs will be seen with cranial intraluminal obstruction. Faeces distal to the obstruction will continue to be passed for 24 h. With enteritis or pancreatitis, diarrhoea as well as colic signs will be seen. Small amounts of raspberry jam faeces will occur in cases of intussusceptions. Tenesmus without diarrhoea is often seen with faecoliths, other obstructions or impactions in the large intestine. It will also be seen in colitis, peritonitis and peri-rectal abscesses. Tenesmus with diarrhoea is indicative of internal parasites.

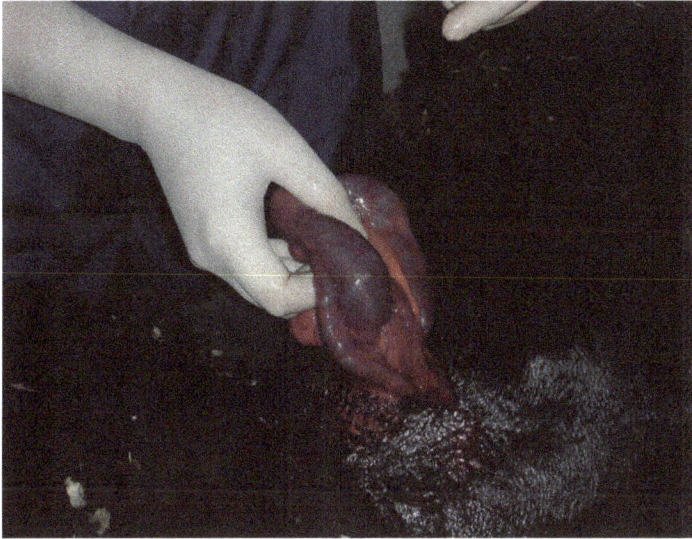

Fig. 9.9. Torsion of the intestine.

The diameter of the spiral colon decreases rapidly. It has short mesenteric attachments between loops. In the lumen the faeces are dehydrated. Whether the cause is due to impaired motility, too rapid dehydration of faeces or abnormal material in the faeces is unknown and probably varies from case to case, but this part of the gut is very susceptible to impaction or faecolith obstruction. These are normally medical cases in adults but will require surgery in crias (see below).

Torsion of the spiral colon may well be linked with coccidiosis as nearly all cases have a significant coccidian burden. Intussusceptions are extremely rare in the jejunum but are not that uncommon at either the ileocaecal junction or at the caeco-colon junction. In theory visualization should be possible with ultrasound, however it is not easy. All that can be seen is an excess of fluid. As these cases are likely to be surgical the clinician has little choice but to perform an exploratory laparotomy.

Differentiation between a surgical and medical case in gastroenteric disease in camelids is difficult for even experienced clinicians. Restlessness is a key sign. Constant shifting indicates pain, and trembling more severe pain. If clinicians are in any doubt a laparotomy must be performed even if the case turns out not to be a surgical case.

Spiral colon impaction

This is a relatively common condition in crias under 4 months of age. There are known trigger factors, e.g. recent diet change, recent diarrhoea, parasitism, pneumonia and hospitalization. They do not normally show colic but have a reduced appetite with reduced gastrointestinal sounds and faecal output. Ultrasonographic examination is useful. The small intestine will appear to have a thinner wall with an increase in fluid showing as black rather than grey loops. The blood picture will show a raised total protein and an increase in polymorphs. Diagnosis is straightforward on laparotomy. Enterotomy should be avoided as such surgery lowers survival rates. The obstruction should be milked through giving a possible survival rate of 33.3%.

Computed tomography of the abdomen

This is a useful diagnostic tool used with, but not to replace, other imaging modalities, particularly ultrasonography which gives a moving picture. The tissues show up in a similar way to radiographs, i.e. mineralized tissues and bone appear radiopaque, soft tissue appears as shades of grey, and air appears black. Fat can be differentiated from fluid. Fasting and a contrast agent are required. The animal will require heavy sedation. The small intestine, spiral colon, C1, C2, C3, spleen, pancreas and kidneys can be seen. The caecum can be seen in most animals.

Tumours affecting the stomach

Tumours affecting the gastric compartments of the SAC stomach are extremely rarely recorded and are only seen on post-mortem. The most common are lymphosarcomas. Practitioners must always be alert for tuberculosis if such masses are seen on ultrasound.

Tumours of the intestines

Squamous cell carcinoma is the most common primary tumour affecting the intestines of SACs. However, the most common tumour to actually affect the intestines is multicentric lymphoma but these are seen as secondaries in the intestines. Obviously the primary site will be in the lymphatics with secondaries not only in the intestines but also in the lungs, heart, liver, kidney and spine. The main presenting sign will be diarrhoea. The course of lymphoma in young animals (i.e. 2 year olds) is really quick and so diarrhoea signs should be taken very seriously. Squamous cell carcinomas and adenocarcinomas tend to occur in older animals. The early signs are often missed and so they will appear to owners to have a rapid onset. Surgery is not justified and euthanasia should be carried out.

Ultrasonographic imaging of the gastrointestinal tract

Transabdominal ultrasonographic imaging of the abdomen is useful to aid diagnosis of sick SACs (see Fig. 9.10). Starting on the right flank the liver will be seen ventral to the diaphragmatic lobe of the right lung. C2, C3, the intestines and the right kidney can be seen. If time is taken compartmental contractions and fluid movement will be seen. On the left side C1 can be seen. With careful observation the sacculated

and non-sacculated regions can be seen together with their motility patterns. The left kidney is superficial to C1 and immediately caudal to the spleen. Ventral to the kidney will be seen the small intestine and the spiral colon. The larger diameter loops of the colon compared to the small intestine will contain more echo-dense fluid. Visceral oedema will possibly be seen ventrally between C1 and C3 in the right paralumbar fossa. Visceral oedema may also be seen in the left paralumbar fossa near the left kidney, spleen and C1.

Radiographic imaging of the abdomen

Ideally this is best performed with the animal standing. However, this may not be possible in severe colics and therefore radiographs in these cases should be taken in lateral recumbency. If there is distension of C1 there will be cranial distension of the diaphragm and compression of the thorax. There may be displacement of the intestine into the pelvis. Small gas pockets or fluid lines in C1 are abnormal. Gas-filled intestines indicate intestinal obstruction. Bezoars may be seen.

Diseases of the Liver

Introduction

Practitioners should be aware that the liver of the SAC is very different in gross appearance from the liver of a ruminant. It is multilobulated with a fringed pattern (see Fig. 9.11). SACs do not have a gall bladder.

Abscesses

These may form in the livers either by haematological spread or by local invasion from C1.

They may be caused by a variety of organisms. The most common is *Escherichia coli*. Clinically the animals will be ill with pyrexia. Jaundice may be a feature. There does not seem to be a chronic condition as seen in cattle. Diagnosis may be helped by raised liver enzymes, liver biopsy and transabdominal

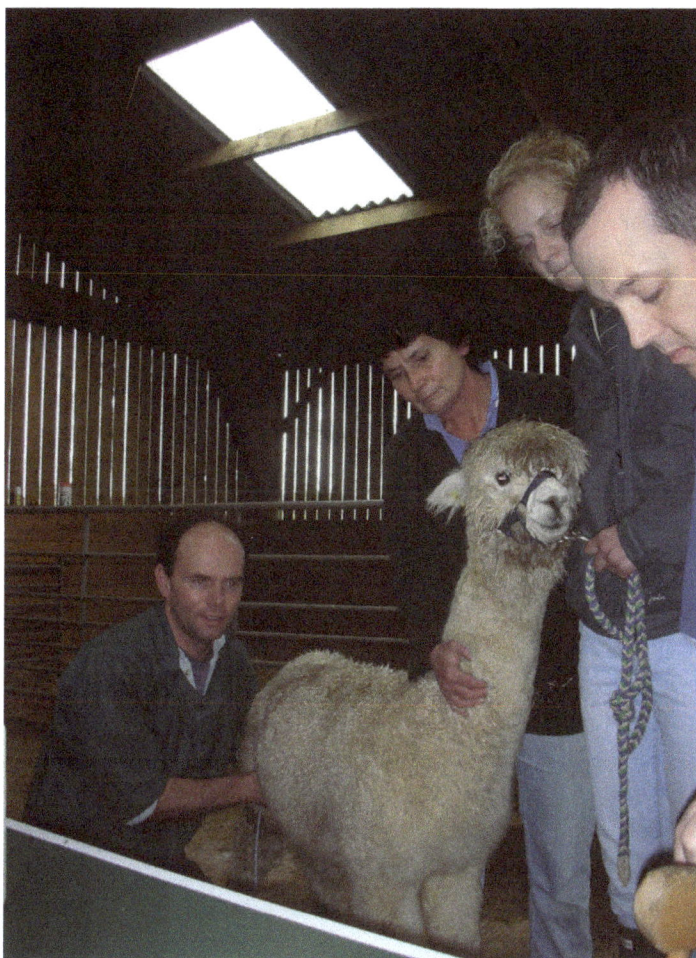

Fig. 9.10. Transabdominal ultrasonography.

ultrasonography. Obviously, aggressive anti-biotic treatment is required.

Black disease

This is caused by *Clostridium novyi*. It is mainly a sheep disease but the author suspects that it may also occur in SACs.

Dicroceliasis

This condition, mainly seen in the eastern USA, is becoming more common. It is caused by the 'lancet fluke' *Dicrocoelium dendriticum*. It has been recorded in the UK. The first intermediate host is the terrestrial snail, *Cionella lubrica*. The second intermediate host is the ant *Formica fusca*. Ants are eaten on the herbage by the SAC. The young flukes do not migrate through the liver tissue but reach the bile ducts from the intestine and begin to lay eggs 10–12 weeks after infection. There appears to be no immunity so there may be heavy infections causing cirrhosis. Clinical signs are only seen in heavy infections. Diagnosis can be made on seeing the eggs, which are quite small, 25 × 40 microns, and yellowish brown, in the faeces. There will be raised liver enzymes. Treatment is with albendazole at 7.5 mg/kg on

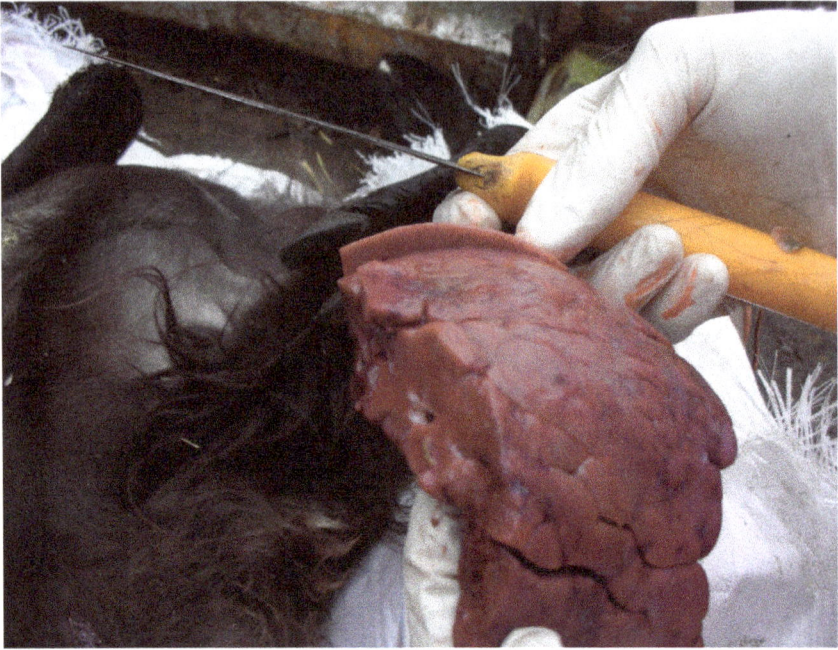

Fig. 9.11. Liver of a llama.

successive days. If the patient is pregnant it is advisable to spread the dosage further and give 3 mg/kg of albendazole for 5 days.

Fascioliasis

This is the most important liver disease in SACs.

Hyperlipaemia

This is an important condition of SACs (see Chapter 2). It is widely thought that insulin is a useful treatment. This has not been the author's experience.

Plant toxicity

This can occur in SACs (see Chapter 16). As there are very few toxic plants on the altiplano SACs are likely to ingest toxic plants with which they are not familiar.

Rift Valley fever and Nairobi sheep disease

Rift Valley fever (RVF) is a viral disease occurring primarily in sheep and goats. It will occur in camels and so potentially could occur in SACs. However, hopefully it will not be exported to areas where SACs are found and so it will not be a problem. It does affect humans and so technically it is a zoonosis. However, it is normally spread by insect vectors. The disease is caused by a bunyavirus.

Another bunyavirus is Nairobi sheep disease (NSD), which also in theory could affect SACs. Both diseases are spread by mosquitoes and maybe by other insects. It is also possible that there is direct spread from viraemic sheep and goats. It is only likely to be a problem in SACs kept in Kenya, Uganda and Tanzania.

Sheep blood taken from a live animal and heart blood taken from a newly dead animal can be tested with an ELISA for confirmation of the diagnosis. The liver shows grey-yellow necrotic foci distributed throughout its parenchyma. Virus isolation will give a definitive diagnosis.

There is no specific treatment. Administration of 30 ml of serum collected from convalescent animals given intravenously or intraperitoneally may reduce mortality rates.

Tumours of the liver

Tumours of the liver are found. They are nearly always formed from liver tissue except for very rare melanomas that have normally started in the lungs and spread through the diaphragm. Primary liver tumours are rarely malignant and do not cause emaciation. This is only seen in malignant tumours that rapidly grow large and invade the lymph nodes. Polycystic lesions are commonly seen in the liver of healthy animals and are not cancerous. In theory liver tumours could be seen on ultrasound or by luck picked up on liver biopsy.

Diseases of the Pancreas

Pancreatitis as a clinical entity on its own is not recorded in SACs. However, it may become an entity as a secondary complication to peritonitis or liver disease. The pancreas may also be infested with cysticerci from *Taenia* spp, whose primary host is a small carnivore.

10

Medicine and Surgery of the Respiratory and Circulatory Systems

Non-Infectious Conditions of the Upper Respiratory Tract

Hyperplasia of the soft palate

This condition of unknown aetiology is rare. The main clinical sign is a rattling noise on inspiration. The animals do not appear to be ill or to suffer from respiratory distress. Neither antibiotics nor anti-inflammatory drugs seem to alleviate the signs. The author has seen the condition on post-mortem when the adult gelding had died from a twist of the spiral colon. The conditions appeared to be unrelated.

Rhinitis

This condition is extremely rare and is thought to be allergic. The main sign is an intermittent clear nasal discharge from both nostrils. Sneezing is not seen but there is an eosinophilia on blood test. Antibiotics and non-steroidal anti-inflammatory drugs (NSAIDs) do not seem to be helpful, nor do antihistamines. In the UK the condition seems to get better in the autumn. Owners think nasal nets are helpful but the author is not convinced.

Infectious Conditions of the Upper Respiratory Tract

Nasal myiasis

Oestrus ovis is found in SACs in the UK and Europe but it is extremely rare. The adult fly of *O. ovis* deposits larvae around the nostrils. These invade the nasal cavity and develop into second stage instars, which invade the sinuses in the head. The mature larvae are sneezed out up to 1 year later.

The signs of sneezing can be controlled by eliminating the larvae with ivermectin treatment at 0.2 mg/kg by subcutaneous injection.

Cephenemyia spp. are nasophyngeal bots found in the USA. The primary host is the deer. SACs are very rarely affected. The infection can also be controlled with ivermectin. However, as the SAC is not the primary host there may be a granulomatous reaction in the nasopharynx. This will be manifest as severe dyspnoea, i.e. mouth breathing. Diagnosis can be made with radiography of the skull. Treatment has to be aggressive with prolonged antibiotics, NSAIDs and double dose ivermectin, i.e. 0.4 mg/kg injected subcutaneously.

DOI: 10.1079/9781800623576.0010

Non-Infectious Conditions of the Lower Respiratory Tract

Aspiration pneumonia

So called 'inhalation pneumonia' is a real danger in SACs undergoing a general anaesthetic, particularly if a gaseous anaesthetic is used. The occurrence can be lessened by careful monitoring of the animal on recovery. Aspiration pneumonia can also occur after faulty drenching technique in adults. This is particularly common in SACs that have not been handled regularly. It is also seen in lactating females that have hypocalcaemia and have been treated *per os* by the owner.

Diaphragmatic paralysis

This is a condition of the young SAC between the age of 2 months and 3 years. It tends to occur in the winter in the northern hemisphere. The cause is unknown but might be damage to the phrenic nerve, which has a motor component, which supplies the diaphragm. This nerve comes from the lower cervical region. It could be damaged by trauma. The main clinical signs are tachypnoea and dyspnoea. There is an abdominal effort and paradoxic breathing, i.e. the chest goes out as the flank goes in. Often the animal will adapt a dog-sitting posture.

Diagnosis is on clinical signs, having ruled out upper airway obstruction. Diaphragmatic hernia and pneumothorax can be ruled out by radiography. Diaphragmatic paralysis is better seen on fluoroscopy. Treatment is non-specific and supportive. Survival rates are 75%.

Drowning

SACs can swim well. However, in winter in the UK they become exhausted if they are not able to get out of the water on account of the heavy fleece. If artificial respiration is attempted, expiration may be aided by pressing the ribs firmly behind the shoulder with the animal in lateral recumbency. Blowing into the nostrils does not seem to inflate the lungs and so inspiration can be aided by lifting the ribcage behind the last rib. This procedure can be used very carefully in newborn crias.

Pleural effusion

This will occur with infectious pneumonia and with tuberculosis. However, it will occur idiopathically. The animal will be in respiratory distress and will be mouth breathing. There will be dullness on percussion of the ventral thorax and a fluid line may be seen on ultrasound. Clear straw-coloured fluid may be drawn off by aspiration below this line. This will bring about some clinical improvement. Sadly this is not sustainable and euthanasia is then warranted. A full post-mortem (see Chapter 15) should be carried out to eliminate infectious pneumonia and tuberculosis.

Trauma

This can have a variety of causes. The most important cause in adults is road traffic accidents causing rib fracture. Trauma can also occur when there is fighting between males causing thoracic penetration by bite wounds. Radiographs are useful in the former. Aggressive antibiotic treatment is required in the latter. NSAIDs are useful in both incidences.

Trauma of the ribcage can occur in crias from problems at parturition. Owners should be urged to take care when assisting birth and when trying to revive crias.

Infectious Conditions of the Lower Respiratory Tract

Introduction

Infectious pneumonia is extremely rare in SACs. Bovine respiratory viruses could affect SACs if cattle and SACs are housed closely together. Equally SACs could develop pasteurellosis if they are housed closely with sheep and goats. Finally, equine herpes virus was isolated from SACs in close proximity to infected zebra and *Rhodococcus equi* has been found in SACs in close contact with infected foals.

Actinomycosis

Actinomyces lamae has been isolated from lung abscesses. It is not clear whether this was an opportunist pathogen or a primary cause as it was isolated at post-mortem. The animal had shown signs of semi-acute pneumonia. Antibiotic treatment with tetracyclines had been given and was not effective. Large prolonged doses of streptomycin might have been effective. However, tuberculosis should always be considered as a differential diagnosis and therefore any treatment was unwise.

Anthrax

This may cause sudden death (see Chapter 15). The pulmonary form has been described in the USA and in South America. The animal will show marked dyspnoea and have an extremely high rectal temperature, as high as 44°C. Treatment is possible with large doses of crystalline penicillin every 6 h intravenously. The diagnosis can be confirmed on a blood smear stained with 'McFadyeans stain' (see Chapter 4). The zoonotic problems with the disease need to be addressed not only with the owners but also with the disease control authorities.

Colibacillosis

Escherichia coli will cause neonatal septicaemia and will often be isolated from the lungs of dying crias. It is unlikely to be a primary respiratory pathogen.

Coronavirus

There are early reports of a coronavirus causing respiratory disease in SACs. There is no concrete evidence at the time of writing. However, the author has included this comment for completeness.

Melioidosis

This disease is caused by *Burkholderia pseudomallei*. It is often called 'pseudo glanders'. It causes disease in many species, including humans (see Chapter 17). The organism lives in warm swamps in tropical and semitropical areas. In llamas and alpacas it is mainly a respiratory disease with abscesses in the lungs and associated lymph nodes. The organism may be cultured from the purulent nasal discharge and confirmed with a polymerase chain reaction (PCR). Treatment with broad-spectrum antibiotics is rarely successful and so euthanasia must be advised.

Pasteurellosis

The causative organism is *Mannheimia haemolytica*, so 'pasteurellosis' is actually nowadays a misnomer. However, the organism historically was called *Pasteurella haemolytica*. This organism will cause pneumonia in alpacas and llamas, which can be serious if not treated promptly with broad-spectrum antibiotics and NSAIDs. It is particularly prevalent in 1–2-year-old animals that have been stressed by travelling or have been in the same airspace as infected lambs or calves. Diagnosis can be confirmed by culture of nasal swabs or paired serum samples. Clinicians should note that the 'pasteurella vaccines' prepared for cattle or sheep do not seem to provide immunity in SACs.

Rhodococcosis

This is an equine disease and is caught by SACs kept in close proximity with infected foals. It causes chronic pneumonia and so clinicians must have tuberculosis as a differential. Both conditions will show infected lungs on radiography. As the treatment with rifampicin and erythromycin used orally in foals cannot be used in SACs, euthanasia should be carried out and a proper diagnosis should be obtained by a post-mortem and culture of the abscesses.

Streptococcosis

Streptococcus equi causes the mainly upper respiratory disease of strangles in equines. SACs will become infected but it is rare in the UK. However, it is relatively common in Peru and is known as 'alpaca fever'. It is a very serious disease in crias and young adults, causing a high fever and pneumonia. The normal manifestation of abscesses in the parotid and mandibular lymph nodes as seen in equines is not commonly seen in alpacas. Diagnosis on culture of the purulent nasal discharge is relatively straightforward. As in horses the fear is that a carrier state may be established. However, this does not seem to be a problem in SACs, perhaps because they lack a guttural pouch. Therefore the author considers antibiotic therapy with high doses of penicillin to be very worthwhile. Resistance of a *Streptococcus* to penicillin is unlikely. Clinicians should remember that *S. equi* can live for a considerable time outside the animal. Therefore biosecurity is important to prevent the spread of the disease.

Tuberculosis

This disease is increasing in the UK in SACs, which is a worrying phenomenon. It does in some way mirror the increase in bovine tuberculosis (TB). However, the disease in camelids should not be considered to be just a spill-over disease from cattle. The capacity of camelids to function as an amplification host and a reservoir means that camelids may have a very active role in the epidemiology of the disease, which had not been considered earlier. The zoonotic potential has been highlighted, with vets and owners becoming increasing targets. This is mainly on account of the close contact between camelids and humans, not least because of the presence of camelids in petting zoos, open farms, trekking and even therapeutic animals visiting hospitals. The author even experienced the attendance of a camelid at a formal dinner in Oregon (Fig. 10.1).

The disease in camelids is a legal nightmare. The UK government Department for Environment, Food and Rural Affairs (DEFRA), and owners who are represented to some extent by the breed societies, namely The British Alpaca Society (BAS) and The British Llama Society (BLS), cannot decide whether a camelid is a pet

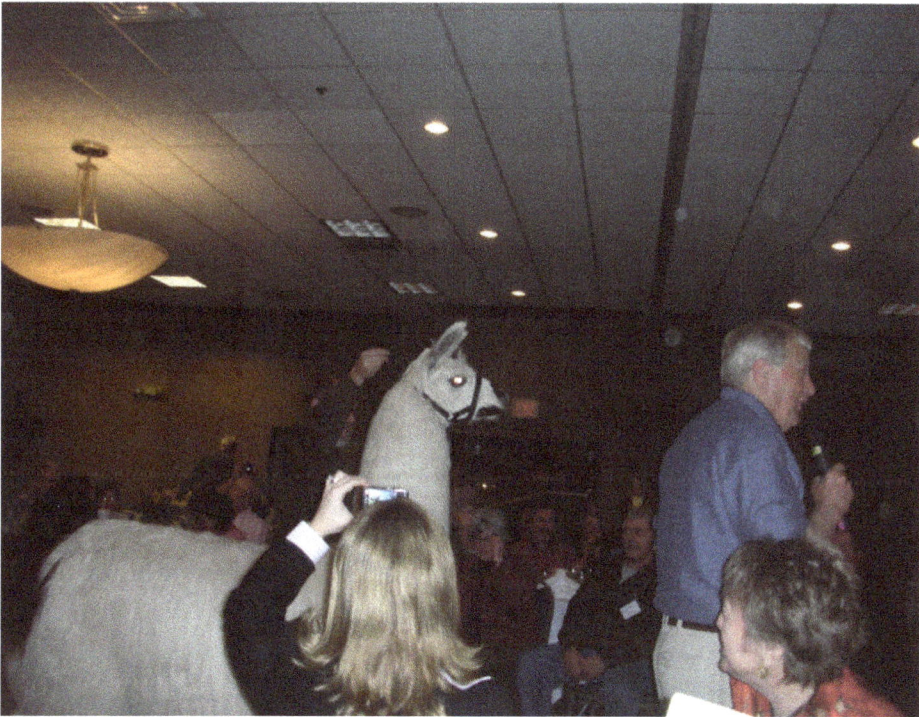

Fig. 10.1. Formal dinner.

Table 10.1. Data from the Animal and Plant Health Agency on the total number of camelids destroyed due to confirmed or suspected/direct contact with bovine TB in the UK from 2002 to 2017.

Year	Number of reactors removed	Number removed due to suspicion/direct contact
2002	0	Data not available
2003	3	Data not available
2004	1	Data not available
2005	1	Data not available
2006	9	Data not available
2007	20	Data not available
2008	22	Data not available
2009	68	Data not available
2010	43	Data not available
2011	79	3
2012	401	191
2013	97	95
2014	78	39
2015	237	104
2016	51	10
2017	288	12

or a farm animal, nor whether a camelid is a food-producing animal. Identification is not compulsory. Many owners do not like ear tags but prefer microchips. The latter are not encouraged in food-producing animals. Passports are not compulsory. As the disease is particularly difficult to diagnose in live SACs, because the skin test is unreliable, it leaves the industry and the government regulatory body, DEFRA, in a difficult position. See Table 10.1 and Table 10.2.

There are blood tests available, which have been validated at the Central Veterinary Laboratory, for example the Enferplex test. See Table 10.3.

The main pathogen is *Mycobacterium bovis*. This was isolated from 68 submissions to the Veterinary Laboratory Agency from 14 alpaca herds in 2009. However, there were also two submissions of *Mycobacterium microti* and a single isolation of *Mycobacterium avium* in the same year. Other mycobacteria have been isolated from camelids.

The clinical signs are very confusing as individuals vary enormously. There may be ill-thrift and loss of weight. Coughing may be a feature but it does not occur in all lung cases and certainly does not occur if another organ (e.g. the liver) is infected. Occasionally a peripheral lymph node will be swollen.

Even the post-mortem signs are confusing. The most marked signs are in the lungs, trachea and liver. There is extensive caseous necrosis and

little mineralization. It is often difficult to link the post-mortem findings with the clinical picture. Sometimes the animal is in explainable poor condition but in other cases with extensive post-mortem lesions the animal is in good or even fat condition. Sometimes there are cavities in the lung lesions, which are likely to be very infectious if the human model is followed. Lymph nodes in normal camelids are small and difficult to find. However, in tuberculous cases they may be much enlarged. They may contain a large amount of caseous material or they may contain multiple small foci. The lesions in the liver are usually not as marked as in the lungs. They may be multifocal. Clinicians must be careful not to confuse mineralized lesions in the liver, caused by parasitic migrations, with multifocal tuberculous lesions. Cutaneous lesions are often linked with a discharging superficial lymph node. There may be other granulomatous lesions in the body. These should not be mistaken for lymphosarcomas.

Clinical signs reported in camelids with tuberculosis

Associated with lung pathology

1. Exercise intolerance.
2. Chonic persistent coughing and other respiratory signs.

Table 10.2. Different mycobacteria isolated from camelids.

Mycobacterium strain	Complex	Natural host	Endemic in the UK	Zoonotic potential	Infects camelids
Mycobacterium tuberculosis	TB complex	Humans	Yes, but most cases are carriers entering the UK from endemic countries	Yes, the number of cases is very low (less than 10 per year)	Possibly, but very rare
Mycobacterium bovis	TB complex	Bovines, amplication in badgers, deer, goats and camelids	Yes, most common cause of bovine TB in wild and domestic animals	Yes	Yes
Mycobacterium microti	TB complex	Rodents	Yes (this may be under-reported as the organism takes longer to grow than M. bovis and cultures are destroyed too early)	No	Yes
Mycobacterium ulcerans	TB complex	Ubiquitous	Reported in Australia	Yes, causes Buruli ulcer	Yes
Mycobacterium caprae	TB complex	Goats	Prolific in Spain, reported in Germany	Yes	Yes
Mycobacterium kanasii	Atypical non-TB complex	Ubiquitous	Yes	Yes	Possible, but very rare, the author is only aware of a single case
Mycobacterium avium subspecies avium	Avium (non-lung intracellulare complex	Birds	Yes	Yes	Possible, but very rare, can clinically mimic Johne's disease
Mycobacterium avium subspecies paratuberculosis	Avium (non-lung intracellulare complex	Ruminants	Yes	Disputed, possible link with Crohn's disease	Yes, causes Johne's disease, mimicking clinical TB

Non-specific symptoms

1. Sudden death.
2. Bruxism.
3. Anorexia.
4. Weight loss and emaciation.
5. Weakness and lethargy.
6. Agitation.
7. Discharging skin lesions.
8. Superficial lymph node swelling.

Practitioners should be aware that there can be severe side effects following the skin test. These side effects appear to be linked to actual infection. Clinicians should warn the owners accordingly.

What has not been validated is the use of tuberculin as a primer to increase the sensitivity (extrapolated from cattle) with a corresponding decrease in specificity. The author is at a loss as to why DEFRA has refused to do this despite funding being offered by the industry.

Nematodes which Affect the Lungs

In general in SACs, lungworms are of no real significance. However, there is one exception to that rule. When there is mixed grazing with cattle, *Dictyocaulus filaria* can cause real problems in younger animals, i.e. first-season crias. There is a vaccine available in cattle using live irradiated larvae. This has not been used in SACs and therefore cannot be recommended. Treatment with injectable ivermectins is very effective. *Dictyocaulus filaria* has a direct life cycle in SACs so that cattle are not required to continue an infection. The signs that occur in late summer are pathognomic. They are a rasping cough in animals at grass. Although ivermectins by injection will eliminate the adults in the lungs, supportive therapy with antibiotics and NSAIDs is useful. A second dose of ivermectin should be given at an interval of 3 weeks. The pasture will be contaminated the following year so it is advisable for it to be used as a hay or silage field until later in the season.

Protostrongylus rufescens, *Muellerius capillaris*, *Neostrongylus linearis* and *Cystocaulus* spp. have all been found on post-mortem in the lungs of SACs but they have not been associated with clinical disease.

Parelaphostrongylus tenuis, the 'meningeal worm', will cause transitory respiratory signs, e.g. coughing, as it passes through the lungs (see Chapter 12).

Table 10.3. Different available tests in camelids.

Test name	Works by	Sensitivity (SN)/specificity (SP)	Notes
Single intradermal comparative cervical tuberculin	Evoked cell-mediated response causing a delayed type hypersensitivity reaction	Varies greatly between authors but is generally presumed to be low	Purified protein derivative or mixed complex antigens used for the test
Gamma interferon	Cellular-mediated response	Unclear, in the past SP has been likely compromised by microti strains in camelids	
IDEXX Elisa	Serological response	SN 69.2% SP 96.7%	Antigen: MPB83/MPB70 (mix)
DPPVetTB lateral flow	Serological response	SN 57.7% SP 96.7%	Antigen: MPB83/CFP10/ ESAT 6 (mix)
IDEXX+DPPVetTB	Serological response	SN 81.3% SP 95.8% SN 55.8% SP 99.7%	Parallel/breakdown testing Serial/voluntary testing
Enferplex	Serological response	Two spot: SN 66.7% SP 96.9% Four spot: SN 55.1% SP 99.8	Antigen: MPB 70 MPB 83 MPB 70 ESAT 6 ESAT 10 Alfa-crystalline-2 Rv36180

Diseases of the Cardiovascular System

Heart attacks

Heart attacks as described in humans are very unlikely to occur in SACs. Therefore, sudden death cannot be attributed to this cause. However, muscular dystrophy, 'white muscle disease', affects crias (see Chapter 2). It can occur in neonates and also in older animals. The animal will normally be found dead.

Iliac arterial thrombosis

This condition can occur in SACs. However, the author has only diagnosed the condition once in a large old male llama with right hindleg lameness. This animal showed pain on movement and the right hind was noticeably colder than the left hind. The condition was confirmed on rectal ultrasound examination. The animal was given daily doses of a combination of penicillin/streptomycin for 10 days. The lameness after 2 days made a steady improvement.

Poisonous plants

There are very few poisonous plants that actually stop the heart. Foxgloves and oleander (see Chapter 16) are the most common plants in the UK to actually cause cardiac signs.

Schistosomiasis

These trematode parasites live in blood vessels and as such they cause a variety of different signs and symptoms. They occur throughout the tropics but are also found in central Asia, the Middle East and the Mediterranean. They are elongated trematodes that have separate sexes unlike liver flukes. The male lives in a groove in the female. They are found in SACs as well as a variety of other species including humans. They mainly live in the mesenteric and portal veins and so they cause diarrhoea, dysentery, anaemia, emaciation and death. The pulmonary form causes respiratory signs. Oral praziquantel at 25 mg/kg is an effective treatment if repeated at weekly intervals for a minimum of 5 weeks.

Vegetative endocarditis

This condition occurs in SACs (Fig. 10.2). If the tricuspid valve is affected it is called right-sided heart failure. There will be ascites and peripheral oedema. There will be a marked jugular pulse. A jugular pulse is difficult to feel and impossible to see in SACs as their skin is relatively thick. If the bicuspid valve is affected it is called left-sided heart failure. There will be oedema of the lungs. This may show as a dull area in the ventral thorax. The animal may well have a cough when it is exerted. The resting pulse rate may well be raised. Clinicians should remember that dropped beats are normal in SACs. It is possible to have vegetative lesions on both sides of the heart. The combination of signs will be confusing.

Diagnosis can be confirmed with a 5.0 MHz scanner. There are a variety of bacteria that can cause the condition. *Erysipelas rhusiopathiae* is a common cause. Animals should be treated for at least 2 weeks with antibiotics. The author normally uses a penicillin/streptomycin combination. However, clinicians may prefer to use a longer-acting antibiotic if the owners are unable to inject the animals themselves. The condition may be incurable. However, if the signs diminish that is excellent, but if the animal is pregnant the owner should be advised to give a 2-week course of antibiotics immediately after parturition in case the condition flares up.

Ventricular septal defects

Ventricular septal defects are relatively common in crias. Clinicians are advised to check the hearts of young crias.

Viral myocarditis

This condition is seen in SACs. It is associated with foot-and-mouth disease infection and results in sudden death.

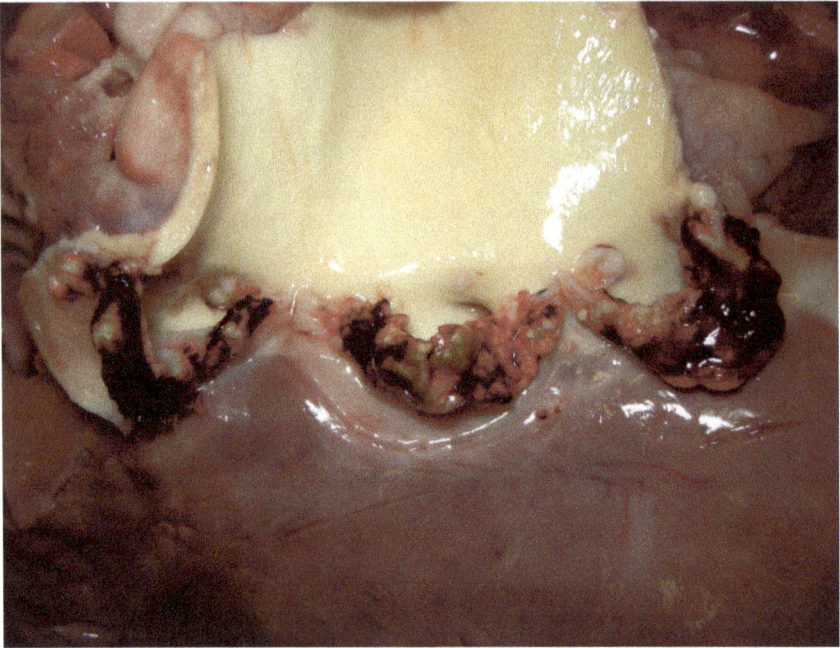

Fig. 10.2. Vegetative endocarditis.

Diseases Affecting the Haemopoietic and Lymphatic System

Anaplasmosis

This is an arthropod-borne, bacterial disease of ruminants. There is confusion as the main organism *Anaplasma phagocytophilum* used to be classified as a rickettsia. The disease is normally called 'tick-borne fever'. It is an obligate intracellular bacterium. The predominant vector in the UK is the tick *Ixodes ricinus*. In the north-eastern USA it is *Ixodes scapularis*. Ixodid ticks feed on most terrestrial vertebrates. There is a potential for cross-species transmission within such a large reservoir of different species, e.g. sheep, goats, cattle, deer, rodents, humans and SACs.

The clinical signs are very variable but include fever, lethargy and anorexia. Some animals may show neurological signs, mainly ataxia. These are thought to be caused by focal central nervous system lesions secondary to localized vasculitis. The blood picture will show lymphopaenia, anaemia and thrombocytopaenia. Intracytoplasmic inclusions are commonly seen in the neutrophils and are diagnostic. The diagnosis can be confirmed by a PCR test on anticoagulated blood. Paired serology showing rising titres is also diagnostic. Splenomegaly will be seen on post-mortem.

Mixed infections with *Mycoplasma haemolamae* may be seen. Treatment is the same for both infections, which is 20 mg/kg of tetracyclines on alternate days for a minimum of 10 days.

Babesiosis

Babesia spp. are tick-transmitted protozoan parasites of the red blood cells. In the UK SACs can be infected with *B. motasi* caught from sheep and *B. capreoli* caught from red deer.

Ticks become infected when they ingest a blood meal from a parasitaemic host. Within the tick, the *Babesia* spp. probably reproduces sexually, and is transmitted between larval, nymph and adult stages, and transovarially by infection of the eggs by a vermicule stage of the parasite. *Babesia* spp. enter the salivary glands of the ticks and are transmitted to the SAC. Rapid, asexual division of the parasite occurs within the host's red blood cells; this leads to haemolysis. The severity of the disease depends on the pathogenicity of the *Babesia* spp., host immunity and the level of challenge. The diagnosis of babesiosis is based on knowledge of *Babesia* spp.-infected tick activity and can be confirmed by identification of the parasite in Giemsa-stained red blood smears. It is an extremely rare condition. Treatment is with imidocarb, which is supplied in a multidose vial as a 12% solution. An amount of 1 ml/100 kg should be given intramuscularly. Abscess formation is possible, so owners should be warned.

Mycoplasma haemolamae

This used to be called *Eperythrozoon* spp. It will affect SACs worldwide and it has been isolated in the UK. Affected animals are not necessarily anaemic but normally will show an acute onset of weakness, fever, depression and recumbency. They will have pale mucous membranes and often are anorexic. They often show respiratory distress. It can affect all ages. Show animals may be symptomless carriers. On careful questioning the owners may have noticed weight loss. The pathogen is believed to be an opportunistic invader. It may be seen on thin blood smears stained with Giemsa and examined under the oil emersion power of a microscope. Care has to be taken as *Mycoplasma haemolamae* attaches to the surface of the red blood cells, causing damage without penetration. The blood film should be examined immediately after collection to avoid missing the organism. It can be positively diagnosed by a PCR test on a blood sample collected in EDTA (purple top). The organism has been seen in healthy animals, which may then become ill if stressed or immunosuppressed.

The normal mode of transmission is thought to be by biting insects but this has never been proven. Clinicians should take care as the organism can be transmitted on contaminated needles. Transmission may also be transplacental. Workers in Oregon have investigated crias born to infected dams. They found that crias may be PCR-negative both before and after suckling from an affected dam. Equally, other crias born to infected dams are positive before and

after ingestion of colostrum, and remain positive for up to 6.5 months (Tornquist *et al.*, 2011). Large doses of tetracyclines (i.e. 20 mg/kg every other day for 10 days) should be used for treatment. This may not totally eliminate the organism, so a carrier state may occur and there may be recrudescence if the animal is subsequently immunosuppressed. Florfenicol and enrofloxacin do not seem effective.

Theileriosis

Theileria ovis and *Theileria recondite* cause this disease. They are tick-borne protozoa similar to *Babesia* spp. They initially infect the lymphocytes followed by the erythrocytes of the SAC. They have been isolated from SACs, but have not been associated with disease.

Trypanosomiasis

Trypanosomes are, except for a very few exceptions, spread by tsetse flies (*Glossina* spp.). These flies are found in Africa south of the Sahara and north of the Limpopo river. Trypanosomiasis is therefore mainly restricted to this very large belt of Africa. The tsetse cannot withstand low temperatures and so it is not found at altitudes of over 1500 m. As SACs are not kept in these areas of Africa, they are not affected by trypanosomiasis caused by the three main species *Trypanosoma brucei*, *T. vivax* and *T. congolense*. Camels can be infected with these three species as well as with a fourth specific trypanosome, *T. evansi*, which is spread by biting flies. In theory SACs could be infected by this trypanosome but such an infection has never been recorded. *T. evansi* has been recorded in North Africa, the Middle East and India. If ever SACs are imported into these areas they are likely to become infected. Diminazene aceturate would be the drug of choice for treatment. It is supplied in 1.05 g sachets for reconstitution in 12.5 ml of water to make a 12.5% solution. This is the normal dose for an adult cow weighing 500 kg. The author has only had experience using it on a pro rata dosage for camels. It would be reasonable to use it on a pro rata basis by weight for treating *T. evansi* in SACs.

Investigating and Treating Anaemia in SACs

SACs have a different basic haematology from ruminants with respect to red cells. They have small ellipsoid erythrocytes with higher haemoglobin content. Therefore, their normal packed cell volumes (PCVs) are lower (25–45%) and they have a higher mean corpuscular haemoglobin concentration (MCHC). It is thought that these attributes have been helpful to SACs living at altitude with reduced oxygen. Any condition that causes a reduction in the number of erythrocytes, a reduction in haemoglobin concentration or a lower PCV will cause anaemia. The signs are normally weight loss, dyspnoea, lethargy and pale mucous membranes. However, the anaemia will have to be severe for the colour of the mucous membranes to be a reliable indicator. Blood samples should be taken into EDTA for a full haematological profile together with blood smears stained with Giemsa. A serum sample should be taken for biochemistry. Practitioners who are used to anaemia in other species will be very alarmed by the low PCVs shown by SACs.

Parasitic gastroenteritis, particularly *Haemonchus contortus*, will cause severe anaemia and death. The mucous membranes will be as white as a sheet. The faecal egg count (FEC) may be very high or zero if the clinical signs manifest before completion of the pre-patent period. The vast number of worms will be found in compartment three of the stomach (C3). Acute fascioliasis will also cause anaemia and death. There will be raised liver enzymes and low albumen. Eggs are not likely to be found in the faeces unless the condition has become chronic. However, chronic fascioliasis is more common than the acute disease. In the acute disease the migrating immature fluke tracts in the liver are easily seen. Although gastric ulcers are quoted as causing anaemia in SACs, such a cause is rare. Death will be caused by a ruptured ulcer, which will be obvious on post-mortem. *Mycoplasma haemolamae* has been isolated in the USA, in the UK and in South America. It will cause anaemia and can be diagnosed from an EDTA blood sample with a PCR. TB and Johne's disease are always said to cause anaemia. However, signs of anaemia will only occur very late on in these diseases. The lack of iron, copper, zinc and phosphorus all has been associated with anaemia. The diagnosis can be confirmed with blood samples taken: serum for iron, heparin for copper, serum in a non-rubber tube for zinc, and oxalate for phosphorus.

In old SACs neoplasia is common. Tumours, usually lymphosarcomas, will be seen on post-mortem.

Apart from haemorrhage the only other likely causes of anaemia are the ingestion of mouldy sweet clover or anticoagulant rodenticides.

Treatment of the primary cause of the anaemia is vitally important. Then the clinician has to decide if a transfusion is appropriate. Increased heart rate, mucous membrane pallor, acute lethargy and recumbency are all signs for consideration. The ultimate deciding factor will be the PCV. In cases of acute blood loss, if it falls below 15% a transfusion is warranted. In chronic anaemia cases a PCV of 12% would be an indicator for a transfusion.

In large herds, donor selection is relatively straightforward. Large males, usually geldings, with high PCVs are the animals of choice. Ideally their PCV should be greater than 30%. Cross matching is not required for a first-time single transfusion.

SAC blood volume can be estimated at about 8% of the body weight in kilograms. It is safe to remove up to 20% of the donor's blood volume. This equates to approximately 2 l from a 100 kg animal. The blood should be collected aseptically into specially prepared bags.

With the administration of the blood it is prudent to start slowly for the first 10 min at a rate of 1 ml/10 kg. If there is no evidence of anaphylaxis the rate can be radically increased. Up to 40% of the blood loss can be replaced.

In small herds when there is no suitable donor or if the clinician feels collection is not possible, SACs can be given polymerized ultra-purified bovine haemoglobin (PUBH). This is available in 125 ml bags but is naturally very expensive.

Tumours of the Cardiovascular System

By far the most common tumours are haemangiomas. These may be found in the spleen, the liver, the intestine and the subcutis. They are normally benign but will haemorrhage and cause anaemia. The clinical signs will resemble haemonchosis. Extremely rarely fibromas are seen in the heart muscle. These do not normally show clinically, only on post-mortem.

Malignant Round Cell Tumours

The malignant round cell tumours (MRCT) group includes lymphoma, neuroblastoma, rhabdomyosarcoma and MRCT. They are extremely rare in SACs but will occur. Using immune-histochemistry they can be further classified as B cell lymphoma, T cell lymphoma and MRCT. Diagnosis is normally at post-mortem as they rarely show lymphadenopathy and therefore biopsies are not carried out in the live animal. The signs are all non-specific and include anorexia, weight loss, respiratory distress and weakness leading to recumbency. The disease is normally insidious but they can die suddenly. The blood picture is also non-specific with hypoalbuminaemia, anaemia and raised liver enzymes. The main differential is TB.

11

Medicine and Surgery of the Urino-Genital System

Congenital and Hereditary Conditions of the Urinary System

Renal agenesis

This condition may be hereditary. However, it is normally seen as a terminal condition and so euthanasia is advised. It is often linked to gonadal agenesis. If it is unilateral both renal agenesis and gonadal agenesis may well go unnoticed in females. In males there may be a misdiagnosis, considering them to be rigs. Hopefully surgery will not be attempted. In the author's experience ultrasonography is not helpful, but perhaps with more sophisticated equipment and a more skilled operator, that may be the way forward. Equally laparoscopy could make diagnosis clearer.

Persistent patent urachus

This is usually a congenital condition as the urachus fails to close at birth. However, if it occurs a few days after birth it is likely to be as a result of a septic omphalophlebitis. Differentiation is important as treatment is likely to be different. If the urachus remains patent at birth, it can be ligated immediately. The animal should receive antibiotics for 10 days. Its tetanus status should be ascertained. A careful check by the

clinician should be carried out in 10 days. Fly control is important.

In the event of the urachus not closing with this treatment or if it has become patent some days after birth as a result of infection, more aggressive surgery needs to be carried out. The cria should be anaesthetized by masking down with halothane or isoflurane and surgically prepared. The practitioner should perform a laparotomy so that the urachus can be traced back to the bladder. It should be sectioned and the bladder closed with a double layer of continuous Lembert sutures of an absorbable material. The umbilical vessels should be ligated proximally to any infected and diseased tissue. This tissue should then be totally removed. The abdomen should be closed with interrupted sutures of monofilament nylon. These all should be laid individually before any are tightened in a 'vest over pants' configuration. When the practitioner is satisfied that there are enough sutures to close the abdomen and that no small intestine is trapped the sutures can be tightened. It is very important that no extra sutures are added after this on account of the danger of perforation of the small intestine. A subcuticular layer of continuous sutures of an absorbable material should be laid before the skin is closed with interrupted horizontal mattress sutures of monofilament nylon. It is important that the animal receives aggressive antibiotic treatment until 10 days when the

DOI: 10.1079/9781800623576.0011

sutures if clean and dry can be removed. If there is any doubt, they should be left in place and further antibiotic treatment should be given.

Medical Conditions of the Urinary Tract

Nephritis and nephrosis occur in SACs. The presenting sign will be general malaise and low-grade abdominal pain. It is rarely painful enough to be termed colic. The most common bacterium isolated is *Escherichia coli*. Yeasts, namely *Candida albicans*, have been isolated on rare occasions. Nephrosis is a distinct clinical entity in young crias, between 2 and 4 weeks of age. They will stop sucking and yet appear to be thirsty as they will stand over the water supply. The cause is unknown. Clinicians may be asked to examine these cases post-mortem. They may be mistaken for clostridial disease. Indeed the condition may be as a result of an unknown toxin. There is no treatment.

Prostatitis is seen in young male SACs, particularly when stressed at weaning. Signs will look like cystitis/bladder stones. Indeed, struvite crystals will be seen in the urine, which is usually alkaline with a pH of 9. However, the presence of struvite crystals is difficult to interpret as they are seen in normal urine that is allowed to stand. Long-term antibiotic treatment with penicillin and non-steroidal anti-inflammatory drugs (NSAIDs) should be given. Glycosaminoglycans might be used in treatment following the model of idiopathic cystitis in other animals.

Surgical Conditions of the Male Urinary Tract

Introduction

In SACs the urethra is long and narrow, with a sigmoid flexure and a small cartilage projection at the tip of the glans. Gelded males appear to be more susceptible to obstruction than entire males. Obstruction is virtually unheard of when the animals are at grass but can be seen rarely in animals fed dried food. The animals will be seen to strain. The urethra can be felt pulsating just below the anus. No urine will be passed and the hair near the tip of the prepuce will be dry.

Surgical treatments have a low success rate and have welfare implications and so preventative measures are very important. They should be based on reducing calculus formation. The most common types of calculus seen in animals on a cereal-based ration are phosphates, usually calcium or magnesium salts. They form in the kidney medulla. They are often found at post-mortem as incidental findings. However, as soon as they start to obstruct the flow of urine they start the development of clinical signs. If they block a single ureter this will cause nephrosis, which will remain subclinical as the second kidney will compensate. There is a danger of pyelonephritis in this diseased kidney. The animal then will become ill with a raised rectal temperature. However, if both become blocked the animal will quickly become clinically ill, anorexic, have a hunched gait and painful kidneys.

Urethral obstruction has the signs described above. These will quickly turn to bladder or urethral rupture, renal failure and death. Early diagnosis is very important and can be aided by ultrasonography. Images of the abdomen and bladder can be readily obtained using a 5 MHz sector transducer connected to a real-time, B-mode ultrasound machine. Scans can be recorded using a thermal printer or digital recording equipment. These scanners can be used to examine the abdomen, although the depth of field is limited to 10 cm. The bladder of a normal male is contained within the pelvis, and therefore cannot be visualized during ultrasonographic examination; a bladder that extends for up to 10 cm or more over the brim is considered an abnormal finding. Every effort must be made to prevent the formation of calculi. One of the main problems is the excretion of phosphorus in the urine. Naturally there are differences between individuals. Obviously the mineral content of the diet is important. Cereal diets are high in phosphorus and low in calcium. Additional phosphorus must not be fed. Normally in prepared SAC diets a good regular supply of magnesium is very important. However, in this instance the diet should not contain more than 0.2% of magnesium. Magnesium is absorbed more than twice as efficiently from a concentrate diet when compared to a roughage diet. High magnesium predisposes to urethral blockage. Calcium has a direct link with phosphorus so extra calcium needs to be fed to make sure the calcium:phosphorus ratio is greater than 2 to 1. This will lower phosphorus excretion in the urine.

Another part of the problem is the nature of the diet. High roughage diets require chewing. This stimulates saliva flow. Phosphorus is excreted in the saliva, which then is swallowed allowing phosphorus to be lost in the faeces rather than excreted by the kidney and hence to the urine. If roughage is fed *ad libitum* the amount of phosphorus in the urine is halved. Even feeding pellets rather than a coarse mix of concentrates has an adverse effect as loose concentrates increase saliva and hence increase faecal loss of phosphorus. Apart from the effect on phosphorus excretion, a high concentrate/low roughage diet has an effect on the excretion of urinary mucoproteins. These act as a nidus for phosphorus calculi formation in the kidney medulla.

Urinary volume has a direct effect on calculi formation. The higher the flow of urine the less likely are calculi to form. Urinary volume is obviously linked directly to water intake. SACs must have a constant supply of clean water. This may well be compromised in sub-zero temperatures. The moisture content of the food has an effect. However, what is more important is the frequency of feeding. Intermittent feeding triggers a renal response, so that urine production is decreased and hence urine concentration is increased. *Ad libitum* feeding of roughage stimulates urine production, which in turn stimulates thirst.

Abrupt weaning will reduce both fluid intake and urine excretion. Both will be halved at weaning. High water intake and hence high urine output has a high heritability. It is linked to the potassium composition of the red blood cells. So certain individuals will have a higher urine output and therefore will be less at risk. The normal SAC urine from animals fed on an *ad libitum* roughage diet is alkaline. On the other hand a high-cereal diet lowers the pH, making the urine acid. This effect is beneficial to the animal as an acid diet lessens the formation of calculi. The SAC keeper therefore has a balancing act to perform as high-cereal diets are not necessarily going to have an adverse effect, i.e. they will cause the urine to be acid but will increase the level of phosphate in the urine.

Key factors to prevent urolithiasis

- Ensure an *ad libitum* supply of fresh clean water from accessible drinkers.
- Wean crias that are suckling from their mothers when they are still on grass or outside on roots etc., rather than straight on to a cereal diet.
- Do not supply free access to minerals containing phosphorus to castrated animals except at grass.
- Add calcium carbonate, calcium chloride or calcium sulfate to the cereal diet to maintain a calcium:phosphorus ratio that is greater than 2:1.
- Feed palatable forage *ad libitum*.
- Do not feed pellets.
- Acidify the urine by adding ammonium chloride to the feed at the rate of 1 g per head.
- Add salt to the diet at the rate of 2 g per head to encourage water uptake.
- Give access to urea blocks to encourage water uptake, provided they do not contain phosphorus or high magnesium.
- If there has been a problem of water supply do not handle animals or move them violently as this may make a formed calculus move into an obstructive position.

Treatment of obstructive urolithiasis

The welfare of the animal must be at the forefront of the clinician's mind. Equally very careful consideration must be given before undertaking surgery, which may cause painful urine scalding and the risk of fly strike. Sadly the use of muscle relaxants is extremely rarely successful. Also catheterization without severe damage to the urethra is impossible. Therefore, retrograde flushing is also impossible. Obstruction can occur at three points, which influence the surgical procedure. This must be performed as soon as possible on welfare grounds. Bladder rupture will occur within 48 h. Urethral rupture with urine escaping into the tissues may occur sooner than that.

At the sigmoid flexure there are three options for surgery

URETHROSTOMY This can be performed under a general anaesthetic (see Chapter 8) or sedation and local anaesthesia. The penis is located just below the anus. A linear incision is made over the penis and it is drawn through the incision by blunt dissection. The penis is then incised and the urethra is located within. The urethra is then sutured to the skin with multiple small sutures leaving an orifice of at least the size of a pencil. Urine will flow out and the bladder should be flushed with warm sterile water to remove any further stones. The animal should receive antibiotics and NSAIDs daily and the wound should be cleaned.

MARSUPIALIZATION   In theory this surgery could be performed under sedation and local anaesthesia. However, in reality this would be very difficult and both welfare and sterility would be compromised and therefore a general anaesthetic must be advised. The animal is placed in dorsal recumbency. A linear incision is made through the skin and abdominal muscles just anterior to the preputial orifice towards the umbilicus. The full bladder is drained by puncture through a sterile needle attached to a sterile piece of tube to the outside of the abdomen. The rostral end of the bladder is then drawn to just in front of the prepuce and anchored to the peritoneum, musculature and skin. A very small hole is pierced in the bladder and this is stitched with many small sutures to the peritoneum, musculature and skin. It is very important that there is a seal between the bladder and the peritoneum so that urine cannot leak into the peritoneum. The rest of the abdomen and skin is then closed in the normal manner. On recovery the animal should be draining urine through the small hole in the skin, which should be at the animal's lowest point on the ventral body wall.

SURGICAL TUBE CYSTOTOMY   This has been described by workers in India (Malik *et al.*, 2010). It is a minimally invasive technique through the left paralumbar fossa, which can be performed in lambs or kids. A catheter is placed in the bladder lumen through a metallic cannula and fixed to the skin with a stay suture. The surgery can be performed either standing or in right lateral recumbency. With acidification of the urine the urinary crystals are dissolved leading to the restoration of full urethral patency in successfully treated animals within a few

days. No hospitalization is required. The catheter is removed after normal urination occurs. No recurrence of the condition was noted by the workers in a 6-month follow-up. There would appear to be no reason why such a technique should not be used in SACs.

At the glans penis

Penile amputation has been described by other authors (Hay, 1990). The perineal area from the anus to the scrotum is clipped and prepared for surgery. The tail is held upwards and out of the way by an assistant or by anchoring in position to the pelvic fleece. A 4–5 cm vertical incision is made in the midline from the level of the tuber ischii downwards. Using blunt dissection the incision is deepened until the penis is identified as a firm, smooth, yellowish organ 1–2 cm in diameter. By blunt dissection and manual traction, isolate the penis and pull it outwards through the skin incision. Sever the penis at the lower end of the incision, but above any area of urethral obstruction, making sure that the proximal stump will be long enough to be fixed outside the wound, particularly in fatter animals. Non-absorbable simple interrupted stitches are used to suture the periurethral tissues to the dorsal end of the skin wound. Care must be taken not to puncture the urethra with sutures, or to occlude it by excessive dorsal flexion of the stump.

Tumours of the Urinary System

Adenocarcinomas are seen in the kidneys of SACs. They are highly malignant and will metastasize not only locally but to other organs throughout the body.

Congenital and Hereditary Conditions in SACs

Introduction

These conditions are common not only in the Andes but also in countries that have imported SACs. The gene pool is small in both situations as travelling in the Andes is not easy (Cubero *et al.*, 2002). In fact SACs have the highest incidence of newborns with congenital/genetic defects of any domesticated animals. Failing absolute proof, if the incidence of the condition seems unusually high as compared to other species, the chances are it is genetic. Clinicians should advise clients that just because a breeding pair produces a congenital abnormality they do not have to stop breeding them, as any breeding pair might produce a congenital abnormality. However, if either or both are again involved in producing the same abnormality chances are it is genetic and culling should be considered. The main reason why genetic abnormalities are likely to be high in SACs is because the gene pool was nearly annihilated by the invading Spaniards. Also the numbers exported to the USA, Europe and Australia have not been large. There are 71 known defects (see Table 11.1) (Johnson, 2009). A further factor is phenotypic inbreeding prompted by the show ring or fibre quality resulting in further increasing the chances of undesirable gene pairing to produce abnormalities. There is no evidence to demonstrate that defects are more or less common in alpacas compared with llamas.

Atresia ani

This may be linked with a recto-vaginal fistula. Practitioners should make a careful evaluation. Surgery is simple (see Chapter 9) and can be carried out immediately if the atresia is just of the anus. If a fistula into the vagina is involved surgery may be delayed until the cria is older as it will be more complicated. Atresia recti cannot be left. Animals will need to be humanely destroyed or complicated surgery will need to be undertaken.

Cardiac abnormalities

These are not common but appear to be more common in SACs compared with the numbers in other domestic farm animals. The most common are septal and valve defects. Heart murmurs in neonatal SACs should be noted and investigated with ultrasonography at a later date. It is not advisable to breed from a male with a heart murmur. Arrhythmias will be heard in stressed animals, which may well not be evident when the animal is less stressed. Three-chambered hearts have been recorded. Patent ductus arteriosus and a persistent truncus arteriosus will often explain weak crias.

Choanal atresia

Non-patency of the choanae can be bilateral or unilateral. The former will result in the cria mouth breathing and has a hopeless prognosis and so euthanasia is advised. Unilateral cases can survive, but as the condition is very likely to be inherited animals should not be bred from. It can be differentiated from a cleft palate by visually looking in the mouth and also because milk comes down the nose when a cria, with a cleft palate, sucks. This does not happen in choanal atresia.

External abnormalities

These are rarely life threatening but should be recorded. Ears may be fused or short. Blue eye animals may be deaf but this is difficult to ascertain. Congenital cataracts are recorded. Blocked tear ducts are relatively common. The normal site for the blockage is near the nasal puncta. Under general anaesthetic a piece of nylon suture material can be pushed down the tear duct from the eye and then can be felt at the nasal puncta. The suture material should then be grasped and a very small incision made to allow it to be exteriorized. It should be left *in situ* for 10 days to prevent refusion. Practitioners when carrying out pre-purchase examinations are warned about persistent papillary membranes. This is an extremely rare defect. Fused toes or even extra toes are seen (see Fig. 11.1). Absence of toes and leg deformities are seen (Fig. 11.2). Luxating patellas are seen and carry a poor prognosis as surgery is unlikely to be successful. Undershot jaws are relatively common as opposed to overshot jaws, which are rare. Wry nose is also extremely rare. Short or crooked tails are not that rare. Scoliosis, kyphosis and lordosis all occur. Extra teats are rare. Testicular hypoplasia is reported as are rigs, but both conditions are rare.

Table 11.1. All the congenital and hereditary conditions seen in SACs.

System	Defect	Occurrence	Comments
Muscular	Umbilical hernia	Common	Genetic and possibly acquired
Muscular	Inguinal hernia	Rare	Genetic and possibly acquired
Muscular	Diaphragmatic hernia	Rare	Likely acquired at parturition but …?
Muscular	Schistosomas reflexus	Rare	Unknown, usually combined with arthrogryphosis
Reproductive female	Segmental aplasia	Common	Genetic and occurring at all levels
Reproductive female	Uterus unicornis	Occasional	Genetic; most commonly missing is the right horn
Reproductive female	Double cervix	Occasional	Genetic
Reproductive female	Cervical agenesis	Rare	Likely genetic
Reproductive female	Imperforate hymen	Occasional	Genetic/should be thin tissue
Reproductive female	Fusion of the vulval lips	Rare	Genetic
Reproductive female	Ovarian hypoplasia	Occasional	Genetic
Reproductive female	Ovarian aplasia	Rare	Genetic
Reproductive female	Freemartin	Occasional	Associated with mixed sex twins usually resulting in agenesis of the female tract
Reproductive female	Intersex	Occasional	Likely genetic but…?
Reproductive male	Hypogonadism	Common	Genetic
Reproductive male	Ectopic testicle	Occasional	Genetic/located along prepuce
Reproductive male	Cryptorchidism	Occasional	Genetic
Reproductive male	Crooked penis	Rare	Genetic?/may be acquired
Reproductive male	Penile hypoplasia	Rare	Genetic
Reproductive male	Persistent frenulum	Occasional	Genetic…?
Reproductive male	Hydrocele	Occasional	Genetic…?
Skeletal limbs	Angular deformities	Common	Genetic/nutritional/uterine positioning…?
Skeletal limbs	Patella luxation	Occasional	Genetic if *in utero*/dystocia induced…?
Skeletal limbs	Carpal ankylosis	Rare	Genetic/uterine positioning…?
Skeletal limbs	Arthrogryphosis	Rare	Genetic/teratogenic
Skeletal limbs	Scoliosis	Rare	Unknown
Skeletal limbs	Talus rotation	Occasional	Genetic
Skeletal limbs	Polydactyla	Occasional	Genetic
Skeletal limbs	Syndactyla	Occasional	Genetic
Skeletal limbs	Tail agenesis	Occasional	Genetic
Skeletal limbs	Crooked tail	Occasional	Genetic
Skeletal limbs	Hemivertebra	Rare	Genetic
Skeletal limbs	Contracted tendons	Occasional	Unknown/nutrition/uterine positioning…?
Skeletal limbs	Tendon laxity	Occasional	Unknown/nutrition/prematurity…?
Skeletal head and face	Choanal atresia (CA)	Common	Genetic, based on high incidence
Skeletal head and face	Campylognathia	Common	Genetic and related to CA? (Wry face)
Skeletal head and face	Cyclopia	Rare	Teratogenic/genetic
Skeletal head and face	Cleft palate	Occasional	Genetic
Skeletal head and face	Brachynathism Prognathism	Common	Genetic
Skeletal head and face	Retained deciduous teeth	Common	Developmental
Nervous	Arhinencephaly	Common	Genetic/associated with CA
Nervous	Cerebellar hypoplasia	Rare	Genetic/BVD…?
Nervous	Hydrocephalus	Rare	Genetic…?

Continued

Table 11.1. Continued.

System	Defect	Occurrence	Comments
Nervous	Intention tremor	Rare	Central nervous system anoxia/ BVD...?
Nervous	Hypermetria	Rare	Central nervous system anoxia/ BVD...?
Digestive	Atresia ani	Occasional	Genetic/teratogenic...?
Digestive	Atresia coli	Rare	Genetic/teratogenic...?
Digestive	Mega-oesophagus	Occasional	Likely acquired but...?
Integumentary	Ichthyosis	Rare	Genetic/conjunctivitis
Integumentary	Epitheliogenesis imperfecta	Rare	Genetic
Integumentary	Crooked toenails	Occasional	Genetic
Integumentary	Supernumerary teats	Occasional	Genetic
Integumentary	Teat agenesis	Occasional	Genetic
Cardiovascular	Ventricular septal	Common	Genetic
Cardiovascular	Atrial septal	Occasional	Unknown
Cardiovascular	Ductus arteriosus	Occasional	Unknown
Cardiovascular	Tetralogy of Fallot	Rare	Unknown
Cardiovascular	Persistent right aortic arch	Rare	Unknown
Cardiovascular	Transplantation of great vessels	Rare	Unknown
Urinary	Cystic kidney	Occasional	Genetic...?
Urinary	Renal agenesis	Occasional	Genetic/associated with gonadal agenesis
Urinary	Persistent urachus	Occasional	Likely acquired but...?
Eyes	Cataracts	Occasional	Genetic if at birth
Eyes	Entropion	Rare	Genetic
Eyes	Ectropion	Rare	Unknown
Eyes	Blue eyes	Common	Genetic/associated with deafness
Eyes	Blindness	Occasional	Dysmaturity or unknown
Eyes	Blocked nasolachrymal duct	Common	Genetic if at birth but...?
Ears	Gopher ears	Occasional	Genetic/frozen?
Ears	Crossbred ears	Occasional	Huarizo
Body as a whole	Dwarfs	Rare but increasing	Genetic

Fusion of the vulval lips

This is quite a common finding (Fig. 11.3). If it is total it will be observed after 48 h as a fluid-filled swelling below the anus. A small bleb of local anaesthetic should be inserted over the position where the vulva should be (see Fig. 11.4). Then an incision should be made with a scalpel. Urine will pour out. The incision may have to be enlarged slightly with a pair of straight scissors. Suturing is not required. Often the labial fusion is not complete so that urine will be seen to come out of a small hole in a thin stream. Occasionally the condition will not be observed until the first mating. The correction is similar to that carried out in neonates.

Genetic female abnormalities

Because of inbreeding in the past both in South America and in other countries where SACs are kept there seem to be a large number of genetic female abnormalities. These include:

- True hermaphroditism.
- Segmental aplasia.
- Hypoplastic gonads. This condition is often diagnostically challenging. Arroyo *et al.*

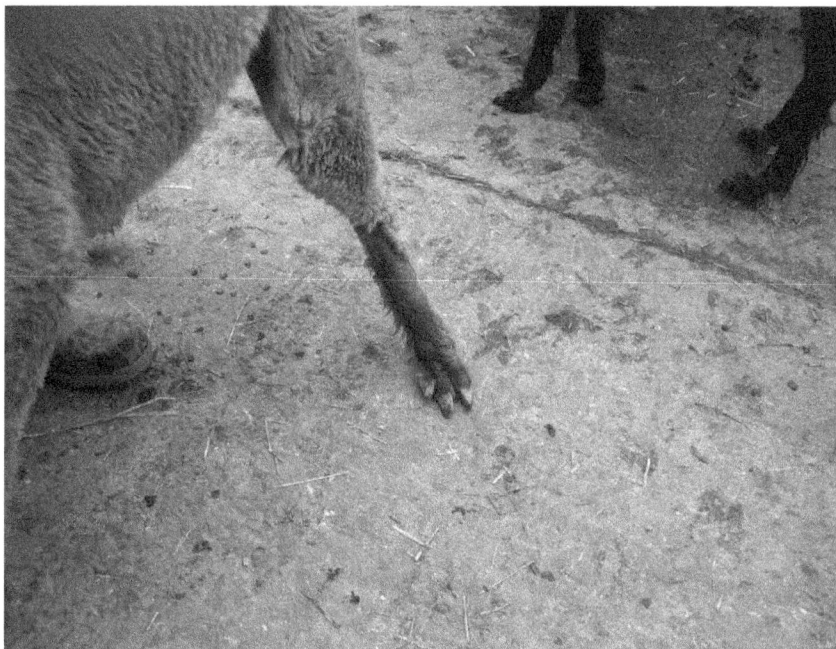

Fig. 11.1. Extra toes are seen.

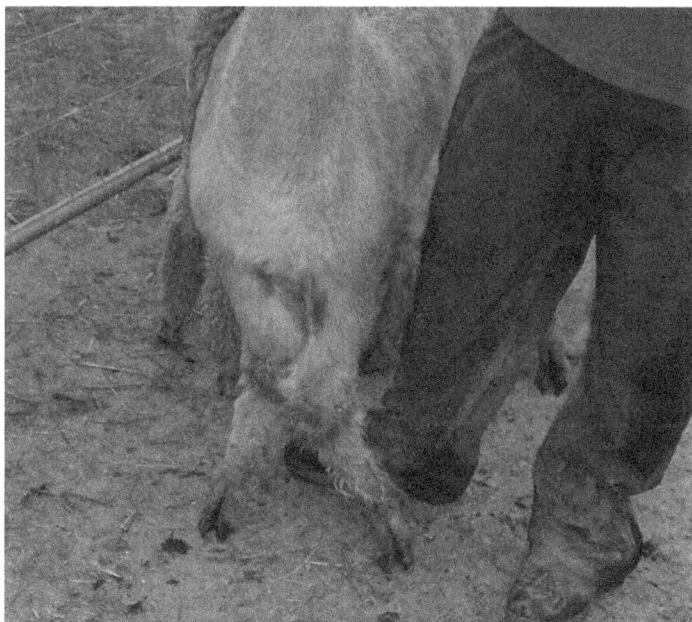

Fig. 11.2. Leg deformities.

(2022) presented a study to describe the clinical, ultrasonographic and histological feature of the syndrome in five female alpacas. Additionally, serum anti-Mullerian hormone (AMH) levels were compared between five female alpacas diagnosed with ovarian hypoplasia/dysgenesis and a group of 11 reproductively sound females. The syndrome was suspected based on the presence of an infantile uterus and lack of ovaries by ultrasonography and laparoscopy. All females had a normal female karyotype (n = 74 XX), but one presented a minute chromosome. The ovaries from these cases

showed three main histological classifications: hypoplasia (n = 2), dysgenesis (n = 2) and dysplasia (n = 1). Serum AMH levels in affected females were significantly lower (P < 0.05) than those of reproductively sound control females. In conclusion, serum AMH level may be helpful in the rapid diagnosis of ovarian hypoplasia/dysgenesis syndrome in alpacas. Furthermore, this syndrome in alpacas presents a variety of histological features. Different mechanisms may be involved in the derangement of ovarian differentiation. Further studies are needed to elucidate the cause of the syndrome.

- Uterus unicornis.
- Persistent hymen.
- Double cervix.
- Vaginal stricture.

Medical Conditions of the Reproductive System

Acquired infertility in females

There is often a very short length of time between parturition and subsequent mating, so any problems are significant. Vaginal infections

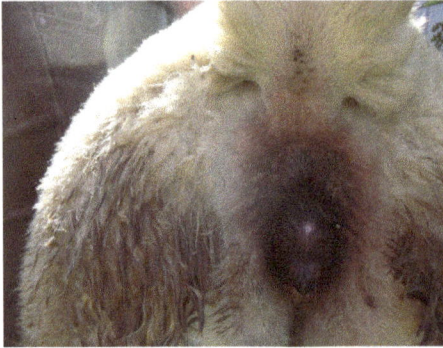

Fig. 11.3. Labial fusion of the vulva.

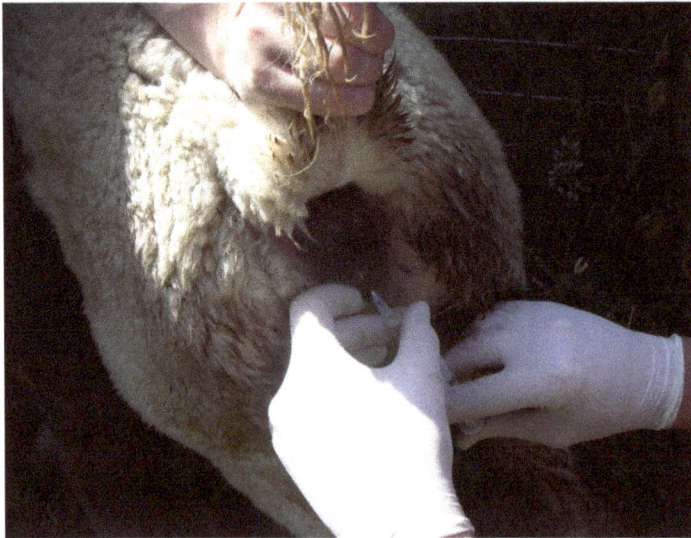

Fig. 11.4. A small bleb of local anaesthetic should be inserted over the position where the vulva should be.

as a result of trauma at parturition will require aggressive antibiotic treatment. Penicillin is the antibiotic of choice. Metritis cases may require antibiotics both parenterally and dissolved in warm sterile isotonic saline as a uterine wash. After such wash outs, 20 IU oxytocin should be injected intramuscularly. Sexual rest should be advised with small doses of prostaglandin given by intramuscular injection.

Cystic ovaries are very rarely seen on ultrasonography. They should be treated with gonadotropin-releasing hormone (GnRH) injections not only before mating but after service. Manual popping of cysts should be avoided on account of the danger of trauma to the rectum and of possible haemorrhage from the ovary. The latter can be life threatening or can lead to adhesions rendering that ovary unable to deliver eggs.

Causes of abortion

As in all species the cause of abortions is rarely diagnosed and so most spontaneous abortions are thought to be non-infectious. Twins definitely play a part as they only extremely rarely come to term. Other causes may be:

- Thermal stress.
- Physiological stress.
- Anaphylaxis.
- Allergies.
- High dietary levels of toxic chemicals, e.g. nitrates, selenium and arsenic.
- Deficiencies of vitamins A or E, copper, iodine or selenium.
- Various poisonous plants (see Chapter 16). The most notable is the ponderosa pine *Pinus ponderosa*. The needles whether fresh or dry have definitely been indicated as a cause of abortion.
- Clostridial disease vaccination (this has also been implicated in abortion in sheep. However, it is thought in sheep to be due to the stress of handling rather than the vaccine itself. This may well be the case in SACs).

A list of infectious causes of abortion might well include:

- *Campylobacter foetus foetus.* This organism will cause abortions, stillbirths and weak crias. The placentitis is easily seen.
- Chlamydiphilosis. This organism is rare in SACs; it will cause abortions in late pregnancy. In-contact female SACs could be given a long-acting dose of oxytetracycline to try to limit the number of abortions and reduce the excretion of organisms.
- *Escherichia coli.* This organism has been isolated in pure culture from SAC aborted fetuses.
- Leptospirosis. *L. harjo* of cattle origin has been isolated from SAC aborted fetuses.
- Q fever. This has been diagnosed in SACs in the UK and elsewhere in the world but not in New Zealand. The organism is shed intermittently in the milk, faeces, vagina and placenta. The latter has a gritty feel. There are abortions normally within 6 weeks of the expected parturition date. There are stillbirths and weak crias. The organism can stay in the environment for a considerable length of time. The problems are seen mainly in the first pregnancy. Prophylactic antibiotics do not seem to be helpful. The best diagnostic tools are a PCR and an ELISA. The complement fixation test is unreliable.
- Toxoplasmosis. This condition is extremely rare in SACs. However, there is a fairly long window during pregnancy when the SAC dam can become infected. Infection occurs from cat faeces on the food. Up to 2 months of pregnancy the SAC will appear to have absorbed the fetus and be barren, but from then on until the tenth month of pregnancy the dam will either abort or have a stillborn full-term cria (Buxton, 1989).

The following organisms are likely to cause abortions in SACs but as yet there have been no published isolates in the UK:

- Blue tongue virus.
- Brucellosis spp.
- *Salmonella* spp.
- Listeria monocytogenes.
- Infectious bovine rhinotracheitis (IBR).
- Bovine virus diarrhoea (BVD). This has been widely reported in the USA. The virus can be readily found in the saliva and in the salivary glands. Antibody positive animals are readily found in infected herds with occasional persistently infective (PI) crias being seen. These are defined as virus positive but antibody negative despite repeated

tests. These crias may be slightly underweight and woolly looking but are impossible to definitely detect clinically. Some PCR-positive animals have become positive only at 15 weeks of age. This implies that it is possible that not all animals identified as PIs are persistently infected, but instead are slowly developing an antibody response and combating the disease. True PIs may show reduced growth rate and be prone to infections or sudden death. In the USA the virus in SACs is related to diarrhoea but in the UK respiratory signs are more common.

- Equine herpes virus 1 (EHV1). This has only been isolated when there is very close proximity to equines.

Clinicians should be aware that infectious abortion is very rare and therefore animals should not be vaccinated unless the cause is proven and the owners have signed a disclaimer. Blue tongue virus vaccination caused some concern in the UK but no vaccination reactions have been implicated. Obviously owners should be counselled in any SAC abortion of the danger to other SACs, other species and to humans. However, a large number of abortions are unlikely. Whole fetuses and some membranes should be submitted to a laboratory. Paired serum samples should be taken from the dam.

Embryonic death

Causes are largely unknown, but these are some of the considered likely reasons for embryonic deaths:

- Polyspermia.
- Gamete ageing.
- Infection. There is no recognized bacteria but streptococci, staphylococci, coliforms, Clostridia, *Actinobacillus pyogenes*, *Peptostreptoccus* spp. and *Bacteroides* spp. have been isolated.
- Endocrine imbalance. This may be an oestrogen/progesterone imbalance.
- Stress of lactation. This may be because of too early postpartum breeding.
- Poor nutrition. This is unlikely; however, mouldy feedstuffs or feedstuffs with a high oestrogenic activity may be responsible.

- Age or more likely parity.
- Uterine crowding. Twins are extremely rare in SACs.
- Thermal stress.
- Physiological stress.
- Genetic incompatibility.
- Immunological incompatibility.

In sheep and goats approximately only 25% of embryos are lost. A larger percentage is expected to be lost in SACs. However, there is approximately a 50% loss in embryos in alpacas in Peru. This loss needs to be investigated, as such a large loss is not acceptable.

Male infertility

The majority of infertility cases in male SACs are actually immaturity rather than infertility. No SAC should be said to be infertile or even subfertile until it is over 3 years of age. Sperm needs to mature in the male so although there is adequate libido and intromission takes place pregnancy does not necessarily follow. However, given a few more months such males will become fertile.

There are certain physical congenital problems that will cause infertility in unproven males:

- Persistent frenulum;
- Corkscrew penis;
- Preputial stricture;
- Hypospadia;
- Hypoplastic testicles;
- Cystic testicles.

There are other physical problems that will cause infertility in previously fertile males:

- Preputial tears;
- Scarring strictures;
- Haematomas;
- Adhesions.

Heat stress and diseases causing pyrexia will cause transitory infertility for some weeks but fertility normally returns after 3 months.

When clinicians are asked to evaluate a stud male for infertility they should carry out a full clinical examination and record a history not only of the breeding records but also any history of illness, stress, movement, etc. Then the mating behaviour should be observed, including libido, mounting, intromission and ejaculation. Post-breeding observations are important regarding discharges from the prepuce or from the vulva. Breeding records of frequency of services, duration of service and records of abnormal behaviour should be studied as well as the pregnancy rates.

Practitioners may have to resort to a short intramuscular anaesthetic (see Chapter 8) for a detailed physical examination of the penis. The most common cause of infertility is the inability to extend the penis because of trauma and lacerations to the prepuce and the glans penis.

Obviously during this anaesthesia electro-ejaculation can be carried out to assess the semen quantity and quality. If this is unsuccessful another means can be used at a later date, e.g. an artificial vagina or intravaginal condom or just vaginal retrieval. None of these methods is consistent and therefore observations on the semen can only give a picture, not a definitive result. Evaluation of viscosity and motility is extremely difficult. At least 50% of individual spermatozoa may be motile and yet there will be no overall motility. Probably the best assessment will be from individual spermatozoa. At least 50% should be normal after staining. Clinicians should be aware that occasional elliptical-shaped red blood cells will be present as contaminants and these may give the impression of spermatozoa with no tails.

Hormone values (e.g. testosterone) can be monitored on a daily basis. One single sample will be of no relevance. Figures are available for the effect of GnRH on levels of luteinizing hormone and follicle-stimulating hormone in male SACs, which can be tried when all other avenues have been exhausted. Testicular biopsy and epididymal aspirates are very invasive and controversial techniques and should be avoided.

It should always be remembered that mating in SACs is a drawn out affair. Semen volume is low and so are sperm counts. There is no storage of semen and so males should not be used more than twice daily.

Ovarian tumours

These will occur and are normally related to lymphosarcomas throughout the abdomen. However, dysgerminomas occur extremely rarely.

They will be seen on ultrasonography. They can be confirmed on laparotomy with removal possible but difficult. Teratomas are found on the ovaries of young adult animals, which on ultrasound will look like ovarian abscesses. Removal by either a flank or midline approach is possible but difficult.

Semen collection

There were problems that limited the wide use of artificial insemination (AI) in SACs. These included inadequate methods of semen collection, poor post-ejaculation spermatozoa motility and lack of standard technique for freezing semen. These have largely been overcome. Good pregnancy rates are now being obtained in several centres in several countries. Embryo transfer has also been perfected thanks to successful collection and transfer of SAC embryos, excellent herd health and reproductive management of the donor, recipient and the male.

Males need to be over 2.5 years of age as before this the sheath may adhere to the glans. Males have a prostate and a pair of bulbo-urethral glands but no vesibular gland. Testicles should be approximately 6 × 3 cm. The penis is a fibroelastic type with a sigmoid flexure, which when extended measures approximately 40 cm. Half of this length (i.e. 20 cm) is beyond the prepuce. When relaxed the penis points caudally. It has a very short cartilaginous process.

There are the following methods of semen collection:

- Electroejaculation;
- Intravaginal device (condom, sac or sponge);
- Vaginal aspiration;
- Artificial vagina;
- Surgically from the male reproductive tract (normally from the epididymis).

Electroejaculation is only carried out under general anaesthesia using intramuscular ketamine, xylazine and butorphanol (see Chapter 8). However, there is actually no need for this as electro-ejaculation has been carried out in the bull and the ram by the author without any ill effect. Welfare considerations have been studied carefully and although the animals appear to be distressed, they readily accept further ejaculations.

Electrical stimulation can be carried out with a well lubricated 12 V ram electroejaculator. The success rate is variable and could not be used for routine semen collection. Obviously this method gives no indication of the mating ability or the libido.

The use of an artificial vagina is a much simpler method, particularly with trained males. Males, particularly animals with a high libido, only require two or three training sessions with a receptive female on hand to be trained. However, certain males will not accept the artificial vagina. This method does give some indication of libido and mating ability. It can be carried out regularly by one person and the quality of the semen is not influenced.

Semen can be used for AI and conservation as well as assessment of sperm morphology and concentration. It should be remembered that camelid semen is of low volume (1–2 ml is the norm) and low density (1×10^5 to 500×10^6). Compared to this the semen of a ram is 2000–5000 $\times 10^6$. It contains highly viscous mucopolysaccharide secretions from the prostate and bulbourethral glands. It liquefies in a day so evaluation of motility is difficult as there is no wave motion. The spermatozoa oscillate and will be seen to move as the semen liquifies. To be considered as normal, 60% of the spermatozoa must be seen to be normal on a stained preparation.

Tumours of the genital tract

These are rare but more common than in other farm animals. Primary uterine adenocarcinoma, leiomyosarcoma and trophoblastoma have been diagnosed. As with ovarian tumours, lymphosarcomas will invade the genital tract.

Surgical Conditions of the Reproductive System of the Male South American Camelid

Normal castration

The testicles are present in the scrotum at birth, and therefore the option of castration before sexual maturity is possible, and indeed castration is vital in hand-raised crias in order to prevent

those becoming aggressive, imprinted adults. However, SAC owners are reluctant to castrate animals below the age of 18 months because they perceive that animal will not mature to its full potential. Practitioners are therefore normally asked to castrate animals between 18 months and 3 years of age.

The simplest method of castration is an open method performed under local anaesthesia. The animal is restrained ideally in a standard sheep trailer with its rear end pushed up to the 'jockey door'. It will then be in the 'kush' position with its body 75 cm above the ground. The scrotum is cleaned with chlorohexidine. A volume of 5 ml of local anaesthetic is injected in a line along the scrotum and into the cord over each testicle. The animal is injected with antibiotics, NSAIDs and tetanus antitoxin (TAT). This can be given on a weight basis but it is sensible to give half the equine dose of TAT. After further cleaning, the scrotum is incised over the testicle. An open castration technique is performed in a similar manner to that carried out on calves. The testicle is pulled and twisted so that the cord is severed by tension high up in the abdomen (see Fig. 11.5). Any scrotal fat which is

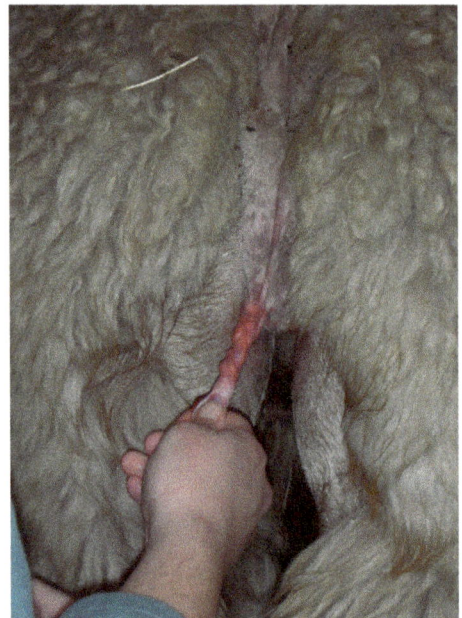

Fig. 11.5. Pulling and twisting the testicle.

present is also removed. The area is sprayed with an antibiotic spray after the second testicle has been removed. The animal is allowed to rise and kept out at pasture. If the surgery is performed during the 'fly' season, fly repellents are applied.

In certain situations it may be preferable to perform a closed method under a general anaesthetic. This can be performed under a xylazine/ketamine combination injected intramuscularly (see Chapter 8). The animal should be placed in dorsal recumbency with the hindlegs drawn forwards, which allows good access to the site. After standard presurgical preparation a closed castration is performed through a single incision in the midline raphe, just cranial to the scrotum, large enough to allow the testicles to be squeezed through. The penis should be palpated to avoid exteriorization or accidental incision, and the testicle is pulled through the incision and sufficient tension applied to expose as much of the spermatic cord and fat as possible. A large pair of artery forceps is applied as high up the spermatic cord as possible near to the inguinal ring. A transfixing ligature of '0' 'Polyglactin' is applied above the forceps. The cord is then severed distal to the forceps. This is repeated for the second testicle. The wound is then closed with a subcuticular layer of continuous suture of '0' 'Polyglactin'.

Castration of animals with a retained testicle

Before any attempt at surgery is contemplated a very thorough examination of the whole inguinal area should be carried out. Clinicians will often be surprised at the strange positions of testicles that are outside the scrotum but are also outside the abdomen and under the skin. Surgery on these animals is relatively easy. However, surgery of rigs is not so easy. The left testicle is more commonly retained than the right. Luckily the condition is very rare. The testicle is normally intra-abdominal. It is rarely visualized on ultrasound. If there are adhesions over the scrotum the practitioner cannot be certain whether the testicle has been removed or if there has been an abortive attempt at removal. The scar should be examined carefully under general anaesthetic. If the scar is only skin deep the inguinal ring needs to be investigated. If a testicle is located it should be removed as well as the

testicle in the scrotum. If it cannot be found the practitioner has a dilemma. The scrotal testicle can be removed and the animal can be left for a minimum of 1 month. It is vital that the practitioner records the testicle that has been removed. Then a rig test can be performed. If that is negative all is well. If it is positive then a further general anaesthetic must be given and the abdominal testicle must be located and removed.

There are three possible approaches for this search. The standard midline approach in dorsal recumbency is not recommended as it is difficult to make the incision caudal enough to follow the gubernaculums to the kidney. A flank incision also has this disadvantage as well as causing damage to the fleece, which may not be acceptable in show animals. The paramedian approach is recommended by the author as this allows a good enough approach caudally. The closure of the abdomen is also more secure than a midline approach. An approach through the inguinal ring should not be attempted on account of the difficulty in closure and the danger of herniation.

The future may well be a laparoscopic approach. However, this is outside the author's experience.

Rig test

This should only be performed if there is no testicle palpable on either side. A blood sample is taken to give a baseline level of testosterone. The animal is stimulated to produce testosterone by either an injection of 750 IU of human chorionic gonadotropin or 10 µg of GnRH. Two further blood samples are then taken at 30 and 120 min. A cryptorchid is likely to show some basal level of testosterone but will normally respond with a minimum of a twofold increase from the baseline level in 30 min (the 120-min sample can then be discarded). A fully castrated male is likely to have a negative baseline level of testosterone, which will show no increase after 30 or 120 min.

Hormonal castration

This has been attempted using canine gonadotropin-releasing factor. Although there was a temporary reduction in testosterone concentrations and testicular width the overall conclusion was that the response was inconsistent and short-lived. There was no evidence of meaningful reduction in sperm production.

Surgical Conditions of the Reproductive System of the Female SAC

Ovariectomy

The indications of ovariectomy in SACs include prevention of pregnancy, to treat ovarian tumours, which are extremely rare, and to provide 'jump females' for semen collection. Teratomas have been reported. The method of choice for ovariectomy would appear to be laparoscopically through a ventral abdominal (Rodgerson *et al.*, 1998). This was easily accomplished and led to no complications on an 18-month follow up.

Reproductive ultrasonography

Normal females

In camelids, ovarian and uterine status can be readily assessed by transrectal ultrasonography, using a real-time linear array scanner with a small 5 MHz transrectal transducer. Follicles appear as distinct black (non-echogenic) circular structures 3–12 cm in diameter and corpora lutea have a dense echotexture, frequently with a central dense white (echogenic) area, 4–14 mm in diameter.

As follicles develop on the ovaries, the female becomes sexually receptive. Generally, only one follicle, on one of the ovaries, reaches maturity (9–13 mm in diameter) and can remain at this stage for about 8 days. If mating occurs at this stage, ovulation will be induced. If mating does not occur the follicle will regress over a period of 3 days at the same time as another follicle is enlarging, usually on the opposite ovary. Because of this overlapping, sexual receptivity will be shown for 1–2 months. There will then be a period of non-receptivity, which may be mistaken for pregnancy. There is a marked variation in individuals, so that there is no normal cycle length assigned to camelids. Lactation is associated with depressed follicular development.

Ovulation is induced by copulation and occurs 1–3 days after mating. Some individuals require a second mating to induce ovulation, so it is wise to allow a second mating a day later. Ovulation can be induced by injecting human gonadotropin (HCG) or GnRH (D. A. Bourke, personal communication). After ovulation the cells around the collapsed follicle proliferate to form a corpus luteum (CL), which secretes progesterone, which in turn suppresses sexual activity. Unless pregnancy occurs, the CL regresses in 10–13 days and another follicle develops.

In 90% of cases, follicles are single, and in 10% there are twin ovulations; however, twin births are extremely rare. Camelids are non-seasonal breeders and will breed all year.

Early pregnancy events

The CL is first visible transrectally at 6 days post-breeding, i.e. 4 days post-ovulation. The initial diameter is 8–10 mm, which will increase to 13–14 mm 20 days post-ovulation. The conceptus may be visible as early as 10 days post-ovulation. Uterine contractibility and embryo motility can be observed up to 35 days.

Pregnancy diagnosis

There are dangers in carrying out rectal pregnancy diagnosis using a rigid guide for the rectal probe. However, it can be carried out at 30 days post-service. In the UK the Veterinary Defence Society (VDS) do not advise the practice, having lost a test case in the courts. It is safer to delay pregnancy diagnosis until 60 days when it can be performed transabdominally using a 3 MHz probe. After 90 days a 5 MHz probe is more useful. Lubricant can be used but most operatives prefer isopropyl alcohol as this is much less messy. Surgical spirit should not be used as this will damage the probe.

The probe should be pressed firmly high up in the inguinal region (see Fig. 11.6). The left or right side may be used at this stage. After locating the bladder, the uterine bifurcation should be visualized. The skull can be seen in a pregnant animal but the vertebrae will not be seen until 67 days. By 83 days the skull can be measured, and the ribcage can be seen. Twins are extremely rare. However, they can reach maturity and be viable.

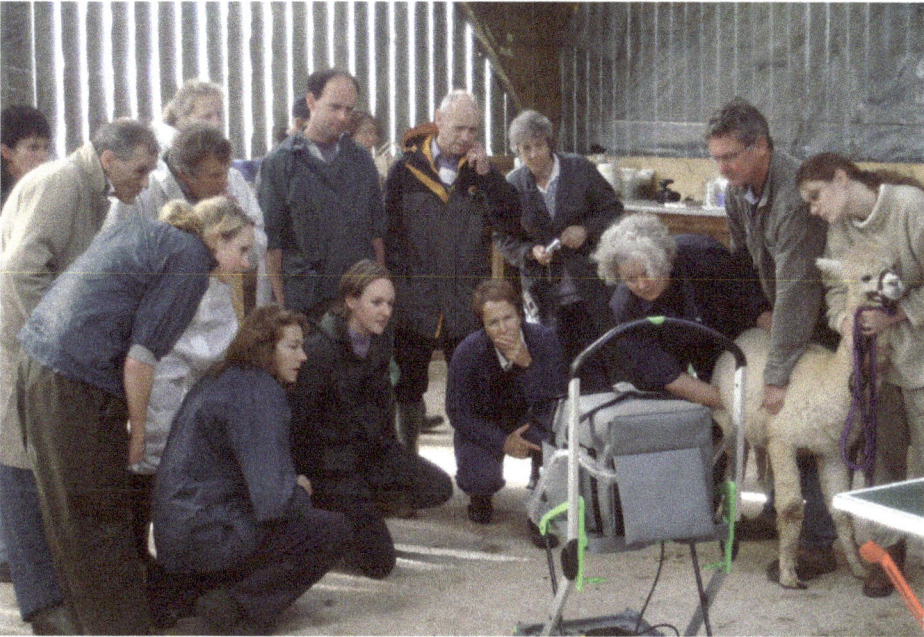

Fig. 11.6. The probe in the inguinal region.

If transrectal ultrasonography is used the normal non-pregnant uterus will appear as mid-echogenic dense tissue with no fluid and an indistinct lumen. The uterus in a case of 'muco-metra', usually caused by a persistent hymen, will be fluid filled without membrane folds or a fetus. It will have a 'snowy' appearance. A 'pyo-metra' will have a thick uterine wall without membrane folds or a fetus. It will have a 'cloudy' appearance.

A heartbeat should be visible from day 25. The cross-sectional horn diameter will be 8–10 cm at 60 days. Fetal loss is high. Fertilization rates are high with 85% of ovulating females having an egg fertilized. Only 50% of embryos survive after 30 days. About 10% of confirmed pregnancies are lost up to day 45. The 'normal' abortion rate is around 5%.

Pregnancy can also be confirmed with a progesterone assay. Ideally blood should be collected 20 days after breeding and again 30 days after breeding. Any value over 1 ng/ml on both occasions is likely to be positive. Some pregnant animals will have progesterone concentrations as low as 0.5 ng/ml (Whitehead, 2017). Oesterone sulphate can be used to indicate early pregnancy if there are accurate breeding records. In a non-pregnant animal the basal blood level is 1 ng/ml. This rises to a peak of 45–50 ng/ml between 21 and 27 days after a successful mating. It then falls to a basal level until it rises again in the last two months of pregnancy. Oesterone sulphate levels in urine are not reliable.

Infertility investigation

This has to be carried out *per rectum*. However, it is prudent for practitioners to require owners to sign a disclaimer. The probe should be inserted into the rectum using plenty of lubricant. Unless the animal has just urinated, the bladder should be easily located as a fluid-filled ball. Moving slightly more cranially the body of the uterus should be visualized. Rotation of the probe will reveal the horns. In maidens the uterus is just above the bladder. However, in older animals it will be more cranial. The normal diameter of the uterine horn of a maiden SAC is between 25 mm and 30 mm. A diameter of 20 mm would indicate immaturity and would not necessarily indicate hypoplasia unless the animal was over 3 years old. The normal ovaries should be round.

Ovarian hypoplasia is very difficult to evaluate on a scan. It is easier to take a blood sample 5 days post-mating to measure progesterone levels. This can be repeated in another 5 days for further confirmation. In maidens the most common abnormality is either a persistent hymen or vaginal aplasia. Both of these conditions will be seen on ultrasound as a mucometra. Surgical correction of a persistent hymen is relatively straightforward (see below). However, vaginal aplasia cannot be corrected.

Uterine cysts are much more common than uterine tumours. Differentiation is difficult. Animals will get pregnant with a uterine cyst in the wall of the uterus. Ovarian cysts are much more common than ovarian abscesses. Differentiation on scan is difficult. Size is the only differential between a follicle and a cyst. A female with a follicle in excess of 4 mm in diameter is worth mating. A follicle up to 13 mm might be normal. Mating should be carried out with an injection of GnRH given 30 h after service. If the follicle/cyst is still present after 10 days it is likely to be a cyst. Mating again should be carried out with 1500 IU of chorionic gonadotropin given intravenously on the day of service.

Practitioners should be aware that in rare cases pregnancy will be achieved with a cyst on one ovary. Also, rarely females will accept the male when pregnant.

Persistent hymen

This should be suspected in any maiden that exhibits pain on service. This may even be violent on repeat service. Diagnosis can be confirmed by gentle digital examination of the vagina to a depth of 7.5 cm. The hymen lies cranial to the urethral opening and can be digitally enlarged. It can be visualized by using a small canine speculum.

Prolapse of the vagina

This is an extremely rare condition but it will occur not only in the pregnant SAC but also in the non-pregnant animal. Initially the pink mucosa of the vagina may be noticed protruding slightly between the lips of the vulva in an animal lying down, only to disappear from view when she stands up. Later the vagina fails to return to its normal position when the animal stands and the prolapse progresses until the vagina is completely everted and the cervix is visible. Initially the vaginal mucosa is pink, moist and smooth but, if not treated, the vagina becomes swollen, oedematous and congested. It is very susceptible to injury. After prolonged exposure, the dried vaginal mucosa becomes rough and haemorrhagic. The animal is now constantly straining as the urethra is kinked and the bladder is full and may even lie inside the prolapse. Trauma at this stage may lead to vaginal rupture, prolapsed bowel and death.

All vaginal prolapses should be treated. With the animal in the 'kush' position a sacrococcygeal epidural anaesthetic should be administered (see Chapter 8). In the pregnant animal, after replacing the vagina and cervix the lips of the vulva should be sutured with a single 'Buhner suture' of uterine tape. A long Seton needle is inserted into the skin at the ventral end of the vulva. It is pushed carefully in a dorsal direction subcutaneously and slightly laterally to emerge ventral to the anus. The tape is threaded and withdrawn. This is repeated for the other side of the vulva. The two ends are tied with a bow so only two fingers can be inserted into the vulva. The owner is advised to untie the bow but not remove the suture if the animal is thought to be parturient. If this is the case the cria can be drawn and the suture removed as the condition should not reoccur in the non-pregnant animal. However, if the cervix is closed and the animal is not parturient then the suture should be retied as the condition will reoccur until parturition has occurred. The animal should not be bred from as the condition will reoccur at a subsequent pregnancy.

If the condition occurs in the non-pregnant animal the prognosis is guarded. Under epidural anaesthesia the vagina should be cleaned and replaced and then a 'Caslick's' operation as in the mare should be performed. A strip of mucosa should be removed from both sides of the vulva including the dorsal end. The lips should then be sutured with single interrupted sutures of monofilament nylon. A small orifice should be left at the ventral end of the vulva to allow for urination. The animal should be given antibiotic cover and pain relief with NSAIDs for 10 days, when the sutures can be removed.

Prolapse of the uterus

This condition is rare. It will occur immediately after parturition and should be treated as a real emergency. Normally the animal will be in the 'kush' position. She should be allowed to remain in that position. It is important than no attempt is made to stretch out her hindlegs as is advocated in cows. This is very painful for SACs. The uterus should be protected with a clean sheet underneath it. The afterbirth should be removed and the organ should be cleaned with warm very dilute chlorohexidine solution. An epidural anaesthetic should be given together with antibiotics and NSAIDs. The organ should be replaced into position. This is normally relatively easy to accomplish. It is vital that the uterus is totally returned to its normal state. Then 30 IU oxytocin should be given intramuscularly. The author favours using a Buhner suture as described for vaginal prolapse (see above). However, in theory if the uterus has been correctly placed this should not be necessary. Antibiotics and NSAIDs should be continued for 5 days. Irrigation with 2 l warm isotonic saline twice during this period is beneficial. Further oxytocin should be given after each irrigation. There is no evidence available to give advice on the likelihood of a reoccurrence at a subsequent pregnancy. However, prudence suggests further pregnancies would be unwise.

Normal Parturition

Dystocia in SACs is relatively uncommon with less than 5% requiring any assistance. Dystocia may be defined as failure of transition from stage 1 to stage 2 of labour or when little or no progress is made for 30 min or more after the start of stage 2 of labour. Stage 1 of labour for a veteran female will not last more than 4–6 h but may last for up to 24 h in a maiden.

Normal delivery occurs from the standing position between dawn and noon (Fig. 11.7). Before parturition the dam makes no effort to

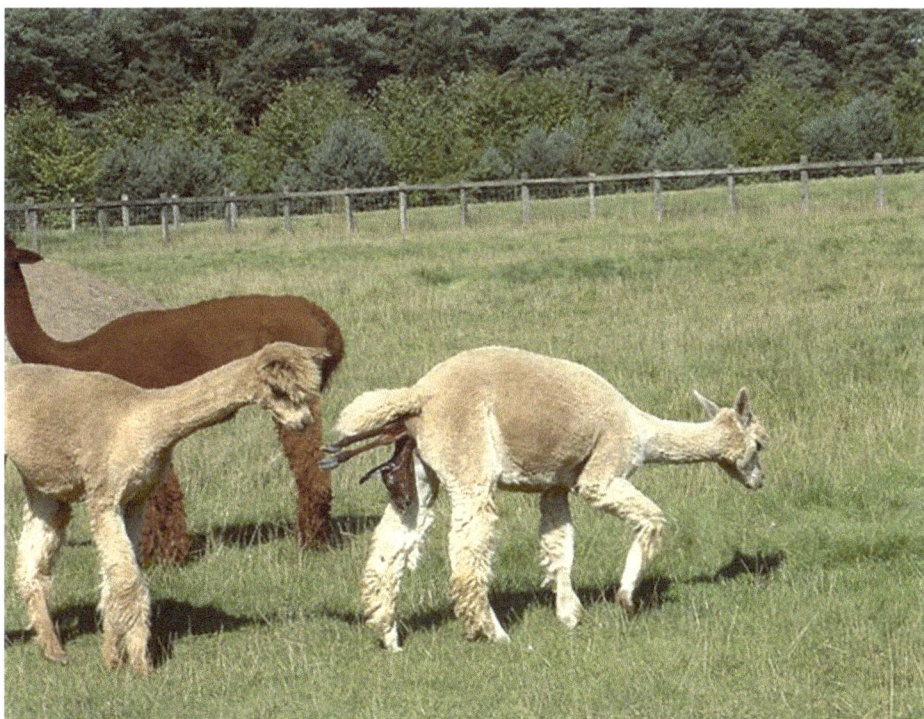

Fig. 11.7. Normal parturition.

leave the herd. The dam tends to show little in the way of mothering behaviour while being watched but can be surprisingly aggressive if she thinks the cria is being threatened (Fig. 11.8). Spring-born crias in the northern hemisphere are stronger, grow faster and have fewer hypovitaminosis D problems. The reverse is the norm in the southern hemisphere. Supervision should not be too intense or the mother will become distracted. However, it is important that the cria suckles as soon as possible as the cria needs to consume 10% of its body weight of colostrum within the first 24 h. Most crias will get up and be steady on their legs within 2 h. Equally the placenta is normally shed in 2 h. Some mothers are reluctant to allow the cria to suckle until the third stage of labour, i.e. voiding of the placenta, has been completed. Owners should not interfere with crias in this time if possible (Fig. 11.9). An injection of 10 IU oxytocin may be given at this time subcutaneously. Normally a placenta is said to be retained if it has not been shed in 6 h (see below). Owners should interfere before 2 h

if the weather is bad or if a maiden is being crowded out by curious older females. The placenta is not consumed in SACs.

The navel of the cria should be dressed only after 2 h if the parturition has been unassisted. Iodine or tetracycline spray should be used. If the cria has not been seen to suck after 2 h the mammary gland should be checked for mastitis. The wax plugs are *normal* and should be left *in situ*. They will act as an indicator that each individual teat has been sucked. The meconium should be passed in 36 h. If not, the cria should be given an enema. There are several human preparations freely available.

SACs have a very small milk cistern for each teat so that frequent sucking is required. This is normal and does not necessarily mean a female does not have enough milk. It is normal for the cria to keep moving between teats. Sucking is good for the dam as it will stimulate the production of endogenous oxytocin, which will aid uterine involution. Exogenous oxytocin can be given in small doses (i.e. 10 IU) to aid milk

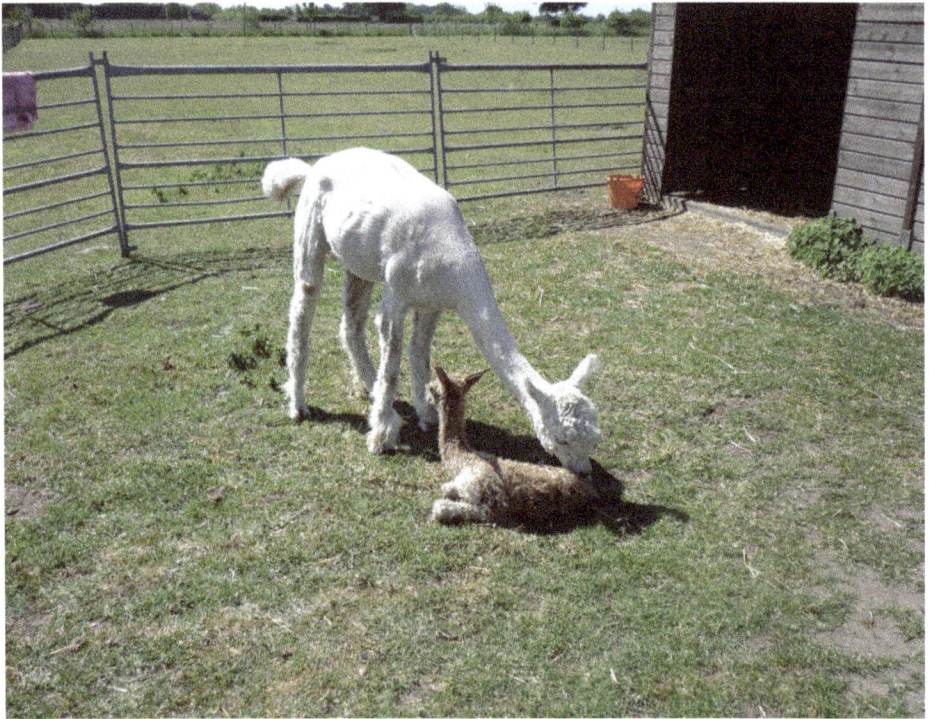

Fig. 11.8. Mothering behaviour.

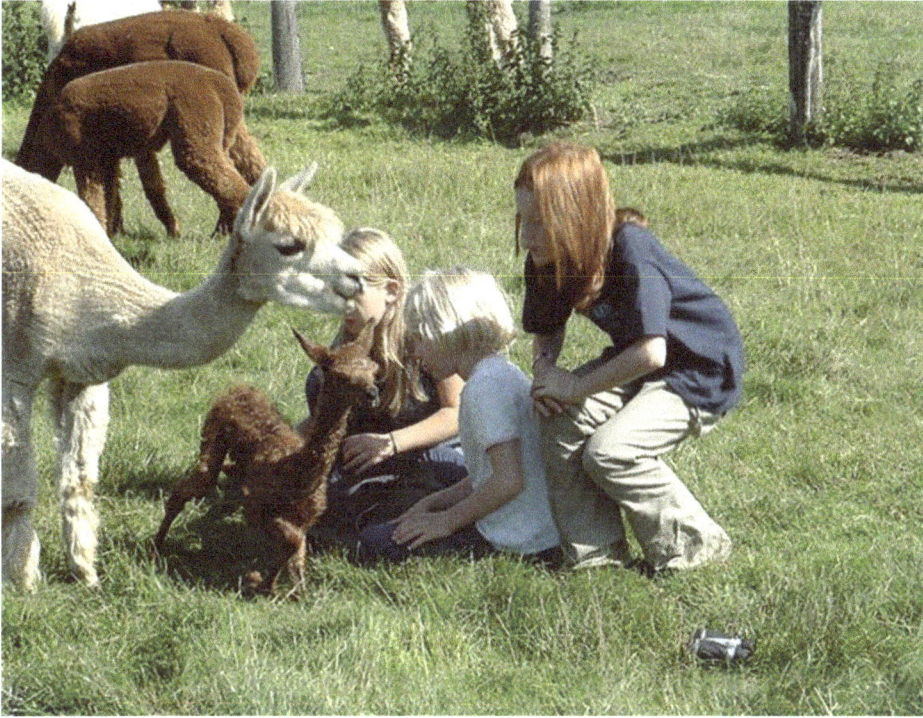

Fig. 11.9. Owners should not interfere too early.

let-down. There is a drug donperidone that is available in paste form in the USA and tablet form in the UK. The dose is 1 mg/kg orally.

Dystocia

General

As with all species the decision to treat the dystocia *per vagina* or by Caesarean section can be difficult even for experienced clinicians. These are guidelines for when a Caesarean section should be carried out:

- If the cervix is inadequately dilated or the pelvis is of an inadequate size to extract the fetus.
- If the pelvis is too small to allow a hand to be introduced to manipulate the fetus.
- If the uterus has insufficient room to grasp and manipulate the fetus.

- If there is insufficient room for a fetotomy to be performed on a dead fetus.

The most common cause of dystocia is fetal malpositioning. Relative fetal oversize is an extremely rare occurrence. Poor cervical dilation similar to ring womb in sheep is also extremely rare. Pelvic problems (e.g. fractures, tumours and abscesses) can cause problems.

Uterine torsion

Uterine torsion, which is actually torsion of the anterior vagina, will occur. It is much more common in SACs than in sheep. This should be corrected by rolling. At least three people will be required (Fig.11.10). The animal should be rolled in the direction of the twist and allowed to get up immediately. If the twist has been corrected but the cervix is only partially dilated the practitioner should not delay but apply traction after making sure the fetus is in the correct position.

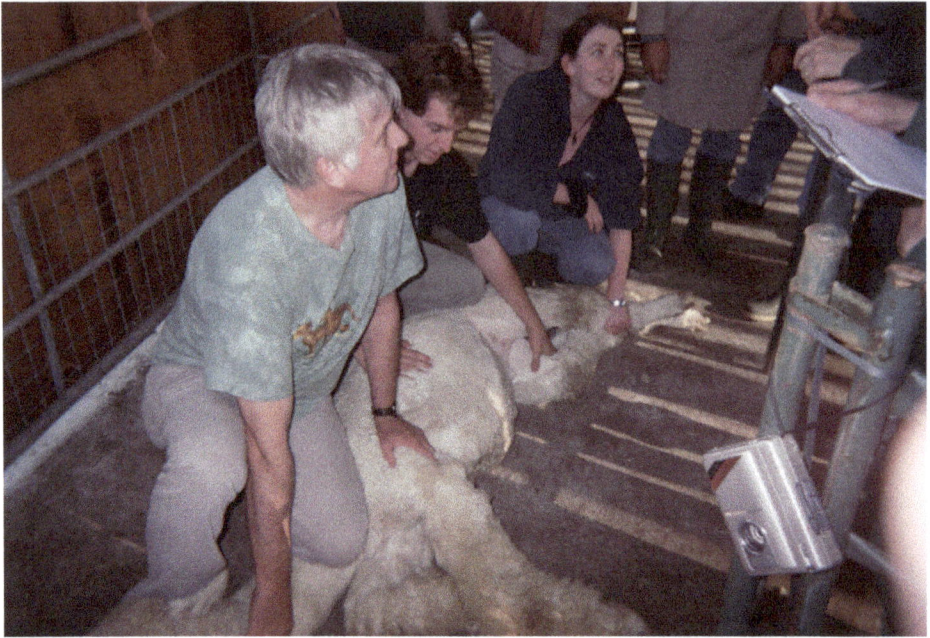

Fig. 11.10. At least three people are required to roll a SAC.

This traction will naturally dilate the cervix. If the practitioner delays, the cervix will become indurated and fail to dilate and Caesarean section will have to be performed.

Uterine torsion can also occur in the last third of pregnancy and not at parturition, as in the mare. This is a true torsion of the body of the uterus and not the anterior vagina. Diagnosis is difficult as it is inadvisable to perform a rectal examination. The presenting sign will be colic. As most SACs are very stoical this will not be very violent. However, in any cases of colic in pregnant animals well on in their pregnancy uterine torsion should be suspected.

Rolling could be tried in an ad hoc manner. The most likely direction is clockwise, so this should be tried first. The animal should be allowed to stand for 10 min to access any improvement in pulse rate and pain. If there is no improvement rolling in the opposite direction should be tried. Failing improvement, a left flank laparotomy should be carried out to ascertain a diagnosis. If there is torsion of the spiral colon this will not be affected by rolling but it will be discovered promptly. Obviously if there is a uterine torsion it should be corrected, leaving the fetus *in situ* to come to term.

Retained placenta

As the SAC has a diffuse placenta this rare condition is more acute than in the ewe or doe. Removal with 30 IU oxytocin given intramuscularly should be attempted within 6 h of parturition. Antibiotics and NSAIDs should also be given. If the placenta is still *in situ* in a further 6 h, uterine irrigation and more oxytocin should be given. This should be repeated in a further 6 h. Gentle traction will then normally accomplish removal.

Endometritis

This is a relatively common condition in camelids. It will commonly occur after any assistance at parturition. Regular washouts of sterile saline preferably with an indwelling catheter is a reasonable treatment. There is little evidence to advise the use of antibiotics unless such a treatment is unsuccessful, and a sensitive bacterium has been cultured. The author has no experience of flushing blocked oviducts.

Embryotomy

In cases where the cria is putrid and rotten, the vagina will be dry and swollen. The cria will be emphysematous and cannot be delivered *per vagina*. Caesarean section carries a very poor prognosis and therefore a decision is likely to be made to destroy the animal on welfare grounds unless a simple embryotomy can be performed.

The animal should be given antibiotics and NSAIDs. Her tetanus status must be checked. If the cria is in anterior presentation, using a large amount of obstetrical lubricant or 'J lube' a rope should be put around one carpus and the leg should be drawn out as far as possible. An incision should be made with a scalpel on the medial side of the leg to allow insertion of a disposable embryotomy knife. The knife should be put up as far as possible to cut the skin up into the axilla and if possible over the shoulder joint up to the top of the scapular. All the attachments of the shoulder blade to the chest wall should be broken down with an outstretched hand pulling the leg constantly. The whole front leg can then be removed after cutting the remaining skin. This process should be repeated on the opposite side. A rope is then placed on the head and the whole of the rest of the cria can be removed.

In cases of a 'hung cria', i.e. when the head is out and the legs cannot be felt, it is vital to make 100% certain that the cria is dead. In these cases the head can be cut off as near to the body as possible to allow the forelegs to be located and extended. The cria can then be drawn. If the cria is alive it is usually possible to repel the head, after putting a rope over the poll and into the mouth, and locate the legs. It is best if both legs are extended before drawing the cria. However, if one leg is in extension and the other is totally back against the body it is normally possible to draw the cria. If the cria is in a posterior presentation it normally can be drawn. If it is dead and emphysematous an embryotomy may be required. The hocks should be brought caudally and sectioned with embryotomy wire just distal to the hocks. The ropes can then be attached to the hock joint and the cria can be drawn using a large amount of lubricant.

Caesarean Section

In dystocia, if the uterus or cria is not accessible or the cervix is closed immediate Caesarean section is indicated. Damage to the cervix or uterus is more likely when trying to force manipulation of the cria when there is inadequate space or cervical dilation. Uterine laceration is more likely to occur in SACs compared with sheep. If the size of the dam precludes transvaginal examination a Caesarean section should be performed. Delay in the decision to perform surgery may result in death of the cria or even the mother. However, in the author's experience there appears to be an adequate amount of room even in small alpacas.

Caesarean section is most easily performed via the left paralumbar fossa or ventral midline laparotomy. Clinicians should use whichever technique they are comfortable with. The thin, tense abdominal musculature and friable linea alba present problems. General anaesthesia allows a midline approach and leads to good relaxation and repair but decreases the chances of the survival of the cria. Not only is the cria depressed by the drugs used, but it then receives no immediate attention from the dam as she needs time to recover. A recovery area heated to 90°F (32°C) should be prepared for the cria.

The author favours a paralumbar fossa approach. If there are good handlers, sedation is rarely required. If needed, 0.1 mg/kg xylazine and 0.1 mg/kg butorphanol can be given in the same syringe intramuscularly in the quadriceps.

Lignocaine without adrenaline is then filtrated at the proposed incision site. This should be kept to the minimum as an overdose can be toxic. No more than 4 mg/kg should be given. This is 15 ml of a 2% solution of lignocaine for a 75 kg alpaca. Systemic antibiotics and NSAIDs should be given and the tetanus status checked.

An oblique (30° from vertical) skin and then muscle incision should be made, following a line between the tuber coxae and the angulation of the ribs. This follows the aponeurosis of the internal abdominal oblique muscle and also mimics the line of the uterus, making it easier to exteriorize. The incision does not need to be long, only the width of a hand. If possible the uterus should be exteriorized to lessen contamination. It is usually possible as 95% of pregnancies are in the left horn.

After removal of the cria and feeling to make sure there is no twin (under 0.1% chance), if the placenta is beginning to separate it can be removed before closing the uterus, otherwise it can be left *in situ*. However, it needs to be peeled away from the incision in the uterus to allow easier suturing. Toxic metritis as seen in horses is not a feature in SACs, nor is prolonged retention as in cattle.

The uterus should be closed with a single inverting layer of Lembert sutures using synthetic absorbable suture material. If the uterus is oedematous and friable a second layer should be put in. Obviously clinicians should be mindful of subsequent pregnancies. The uterus is more vascular than in the ruminant but there is no need to place an inner blanket layer as in the horse. An intramuscular injection of 20 IU oxytocin should be given after replacement of the uterus. Intra-abdominal antibiotics should be instilled before abdominal closure with two layers of continuous sutures of synthetic absorbable suture material. The deepest layer must include the peritoneum. The skin should be closed with single interrupted mattress sutures of monofilament nylon.

Antibiotics should be continued for 5 days and NSAIDs for 3 days.

Induction of Parturition

This intervention should not be encouraged as often service dates are unreliable. If owners insist, it is best achieved with a prostaglandin injection of 187.5 µg of cloprostenol (equivalent to 0.75 ml of the standard solutions) intramuscularly. This should be followed by 125 µg of cloprostenol (equivalent to 0.5 ml of the standard solution) injected 24 h later. Fluprostenol 40 mg intramuscularly can also be used to induce parturition in SACs within 10 days of their due date. Parturition will occur on average in 21 h (Bravo *et al.*, 1996). Neonatal survival is not affected. Neither dexamethasone nor oxytocin is suitable to induce parturition in SACs.

Diseases of the Mammary Gland

Removal of supernumerary teats

SACs have four teats and rarely have extra teats. They should not be removed unless clinicians feel they will interfere with crias sucking. A small amount of local anaesthetic should be injected into the base of the teat to be removed. Practitioners would be well advised to check with the owners to make 100% certain that they are removing the required teat. A pair of small 'Burdizzos' is placed at the bottom of the spare teat and clamped shut. After 30 sec they are removed and the spare teat is removed by cutting with a pair of curved scissors along the clamp line. The tetanus status of the animal should be checked and fly control should be implemented.

Mastitis

Mastitis is a very rare condition in SACs. It is often brought on by trauma, e.g. dog bites or jumping out of pens soon after parturition. A variety of organisms can be involved. Treatment with antibiotics and NSAIDs is required. SACs will develop peracute mastitis immediately after parturition if there is failure of sucking. The organism is either *E. coli* or *Klebsiella pneumonia*. The condition is more likely with human interferences, e.g. hand stripping. Owners should be urged to be hygienic. The condition has a poor prognosis and if the animal is severely shocked and toxic with a low rectal temperature, euthanasia should be carried out. If clinicians feel that there is a chance of recovery, treatment should be aggressive, i.e. hospitalization, warmth, intravenous fluids, NSAIDs and appropriate antibiotic treatment for gram-negative organisms.

Mycobacterium bovis has been found to cause mastitis in an alpaca (Richey *et al.*, 2011). The 8-year-old animal had a period of ill-thrift with respiratory signs before developing a discharging sinus involving the left quarter of the mammary gland. Gross post-mortem examination identified multiple caseous lesions in the lungs, liver, lymph nodes, kidney, omentum and pericardium. The udder contained multiple variable-sized abscesses. The supramammary lymph nodes and accessory superficial lymph nodes were enlarged with multifocal caseous material. *M. bovis* was isolated. This demonstrates the potential for direct exposure to *M. bovis* via milk and possible spread to other herds via movement of crias before the development of clinical signs. Obviously this has zoonotic implications (see Chapter 17).

Mammary neoplasa

This condition is extremely rare but any swelling in old females that is not painful or associated with mastitis and continues to enlarge should be investigated and monitored. If it is a squamous cell carcinoma, euthanasia may be the only option particularly if the local lymph nodes are involved. Welfare must be paramount in any decision making.

Udder oedema

This is common in first lactation camelids. It is only a problem if the dam resents nursing by the cria. If udder oedema is present before parturition, the gland should not be milked out as this increases the risk not only of mastitis, but also hypocacaemia. NSAIDs are helpful, given by injection.

Poor milkability

This is seen in first lactation females particularly after giving birth to a premature cria. Should a normal cria at parturition not gain weight, lack of milk should be suspected. However supplementing milk from a bottle may exacerbate the problem. It is important to make sure there is no mastitis. The milk should be checked. Camelid milk contains more protein, sugar and calcium and less fat, sodium, potassium and chloride than cows.

Failure of passive transfer

The aim is for crias to receive 12% of their body weight of colostrum in the first 12 h of life.

However, if it receives 10% within 24 h it will probably have received sufficient.

Failure of passive transfer (FPT) occurs with weak crias or ineffective nursing from blocked teats, mastitis, poor milk production and poor maternal instincts. It can be monitored by measuring the birth weight and reweighing at 8 h. Milk secretion should be checked and effective nursing (a white moustache) should be observed. The passage of meconium and urine by the cria is encouraging. Post-partum blood samples compared with 18–24 h later is ideal as a practical assessment of FPT. The PCV of the cria should have dropped and the total protein in the blood should have risen. The treatment of FPT is to give plasma collected from a healthy animal in the same environment. The argument against intraperitoneal transfusion compared to intravenous is that it is not so effective and might cause peritonitis. However, intraperitoneal transfusion is much less stressful for the cria and is much quicker as administration can be done in 10 min after careful aseptic preparation. Plasma can be given orally but as it only contains one-fifth of the immunoglobulin G (IgG) level of colostrum it is not very efficient. It is always worthwhile giving more colostrum as although no IgG is absorbed after 24 h, local immunity in the intestine will be enhanced. Antibiotics orally should be avoided as they tend to upset the gut flora. Antibiotics can be injected to prevent septicaemia. However, they will in no way replace good colostrum within 24 h of birth nor will they be as effective as giving plasma either intravenously or intraperitoneally.

FPT may be the fundamental cause of neonatal mortality, which is under 3% in the USA but is approximately 12% in Peru.

Treatment of premature or dummy crias is difficult. Rather than tube these crias several times a day it is better to place an indwelling nasogastric tube in crias that are either unable or unwilling to suck their dams or a bottle. In this way colic and bloat can be avoided. A volume of 10% of the body weight of the cria should be given daily, ideally on an hourly basis.

Collection of plasma

Ideally this needs to be done in advance and then the plasma is stored in a deep freeze on the client's holding. The plasma can be stored safely for a year provided it is kept deep in the freezer, i.e. not near the door where it might defrost. Obviously power cuts are a problem but they would be the owner's responsibility. If really cold temperatures (i.e. lower than −20°C) can be found, then the plasma can be stored for 5 years. The veterinarian should charge for the collection and giving of the plasma. Disease control problems are avoided by using the owner's own animals for plasma collection. The temptation to use plasma from another holding should be resisted as any problems would be a legal nightmare.

Ideally a large healthy well-handled gelding should be used for collection. A 70 kg alpaca can donate 500 ml of blood. A large llama can donate twice that figure. The double bags available in the UK normally take 500 ml. It is important not to exceed the amount of blood or there is a danger of clotting, through lack of anticoagulant. The blood, unlike equine blood, needs to be centrifuged. With the double-bag system 500 ml of blood should yield 300 ml of plasma. This would be sufficient for one cria.

After the plasma is separated and the bag is tied off, it is advisable to place an elastic band around the bag to form a waist. After freezing, the elastic band can be removed. This will give the practitioner a warning if the bag has become defrosted in the freezer as the waist will be lost. It is very important that the plasma bags are handled with care as the plastic becomes brittle when frozen. Double wrapping them with the label on the outside is a prudent precaution.

Giving of plasma

Cross matching of plasma is not required as SACs have only one blood group with one factor.

The plasma needs to be defrosted very slowly in a water bath at 37°C. This will take 20 min. A microwave should not be used as there is a danger that some of the proteins will be damaged. Plasma can be given intravenously or intraperitoneally. Clinicians must use their judgement. Intravenous administration will be more stressful for the cria. However, this procedure is likely to be carried out in weak crias and so this fact may not be so significant. More IgG is absorbed intravenously so more plasma has to be given if the intraperitoneal route is chosen. Either way strict surgical antisepsis precautions should be taken. If the intravenous method is used, a blood administration set should be used with a filter to remove any cryoprecipitates. The jugular or the cephalic vein can be used. It is prudent to give the plasma slowly at one drop a second for the first 10 min to check for any adverse reactions. After that the rate can be sped up to almost a steady stream. Even so the transfusion will take over 1 h for an alpaca cria and obviously more for a bigger llama cria. If there is a mild reaction dexamethasone can be given intravenously at 0.1 mg/kg. This is approximately 0.25 ml of a 2 mg/ml soluble solution. This dose can be massively increased if there is a bad reaction or 1:1000 adrenaline can be given at 0.01 mg/kg. Hypertonic saline would be useful and obviously oxygen if it is available. Such reactions are rare and therefore if this procedure is being carried out on the farm there is not a need to transport bulky oxygen cylinders.

Commercial plasma service

In the UK there is a transfusion service run by Pet Blood Bank UK. Details can be obtained from their website www.petbloodbankuk.org. They also have prepared a useful 90-minute webinar.

12

Medicine and Surgery of the Neurological System

Neurological Diseases

Congenital conditions

These may be inherited or acquired. Prolonged parturition may lead to hypoxia and brain damage. Damage to crias by poor parturition technique is very rare.

Atlanto-occipital malalignment

This condition may be iatrogenic from rough correction of a neck deflection at parturition. It is important that practitioners place the head-rope behind the ears and through the mouth like a bit rather than around the neck. Animals can have Atlanto-occipital malalignment without any interference at parturition. The prognosis is extremely guarded. Clinicians should be aware of welfare issues.

Hydrocephalus

This condition is rare and is thought to have a hereditary element. Unlike in cattle the skull is rarely large enough to cause parturition difficulties. The condition will be seen by the owner after birth. Euthanasia is the only option.

Kyphosis

This is mainly seen in premature fetuses. It could be an inherited condition but that is unlikely. Humane euthanasia should be carried out promptly.

Degenerative conditions

Spondylosis

This is a condition of geriatric animals. The pathology is the formation of excess sponge-like bone in the lumbar area of the spine. This has a slow onset. The excess bone pinches on the nerves as they emerge from the spine. The most common chronic manifestation is the animal will drag the toes of its hindlegs. The condition does not seem painful but is progressive. Non-steroidal anti-inflammatory drugs (NSAIDs) are often given but they rarely appear to be beneficial. In certain cases the extra bone, the spondyle, may fracture. This will cause acute lameness with pain and even crepitus over the area. However, the animals can recover as this small fracture can repair. Clinicians must use their judgement on whether euthanasia should be performed.

Infectious diseases

Abscesses

Any abscess either in the brain or the spinal column will give serious neurological signs.

© Graham R. Duncanson 2023. *Veterinary Treatment of Llamas and Alpacas*, 2nd Edition (G.R. Duncanson)
DOI: 10.1079/9781800623576.0012

Borna disease

This virus has been found in the brains of llamas and alpacas that have died showing neurological signs of ataxia and recumbency. NSAIDs caused some short-lived improvement. Liver enzymes showed raised levels but there were no other diagnostic signs. The main differential must be rabies. The diagnosis can be confirmed by polymerase chain reaction (PCR) and immunohistology. It is a very rare condition.

Clostridial myositis

This is caused by *Clostridium chauvoei* and is called 'blackleg' in cattle. It can occur from a wound over a muscle that does not drain, or by trauma that becomes infected. It can be caused by poor intramuscular injection technique. The animal will be acutely lame and very ill. There is often marked swelling. Treatment with high doses of penicillin is rarely effective. Animals should be covered by adequate clostridial vaccination.

Equine herpes virus

Equine herpes virus (EHV) is exceptionally rare in SACs. It has been reported in SACs running with zebra. EHV 1 was the virus type isolated (Rebhun *et al.*, 1988). The zebra did not show any marked signs but the SACs were very ill with acute neurological signs. These included blindness characterized by dilated unresponsive pupils and funduscopic evidence of varying degrees of vitritis, retinal vasculitis, retinitis, chorioretinitis and optic neuritis.

Listeriosis

This is a rare condition in SACs compared to sheep mainly because SACs are rarely fed silage. The disease normally has an acute onset with a marked fever and severe neurological signs including seizures. Diagnosis can be confirmed with a cerebrospinal fluid (CSF) tap. This will show a raised protein, a raised creatine kinase and a large number of monocytes. Tetracycline or florfenicol is the antibiotic of choice for treatment. These should be coupled with NSAIDs and careful nursing.

Louping-ill

This virus certainly occurs in SACs. It manifests as ataxia, seizures, opisthotonous and sudden death. Diagnosis can be confirmed by virus isolation. There is a PCR test available.

Otitis media

Ear conditions are very rare in SACs. Foreign bodies (e.g. barley awns) may cause problems as can functional narrowing of the ear canal. The tympanic membrane is very difficult to visualize in SACs. Ear ticks can cause infections as can misplaced ear tags and microchips. Equally, infection can come up the Eustachian tubes from upper respiratory conditions caused by a variety of organisms including *Actinomyces* spp., Group D *Streptococcus* spp., *Listeria monocytogenes*, *Proteus* spp. and *Pasteurella* spp. There may be a head tilt and facial nerve deficits, e.g. flaccidity of ear and lip with a deviation of the muzzle. The condition is normally painful. Treatment should include parenteral antibiotics and NSAIDs, which will need to be given long term. If surgery is considered the animal should be at least radiographed. Computerized tomography scanning is appropriate if finances allow.

Protozoal meningitis

A cryptococcus has been found in a CSF tap in an 8-year-old alpaca in Australia that died showing neurological signs (Goodchild *et al.*, 1996). It is likely that this is not a primary pathogen.

Rabies

This disease will be seen in SACs in endemic areas. It will be caused by a bite from a carnivore. The SAC is the end host and so there is very little likelihood of the SAC having virus in its saliva. However, practitioners should take care. The history will probably give the diagnosis. SACs may become aggressive but that is rare. Once neurological signs are apparent the prognosis is hopeless and euthanasia should be carried out.

Septic bacterial meningitis

This is seen mainly in crias below 1 year of age. The invading organism is usually *Escherichia coli*. The antibiotic of choice is a combination of penicillin and gentamicin. Other authorities suggest florfenicol.

West Nile virus

West Nile virus (WNV) is an arthropod-borne flavivirus. The vector is the mosquito. There is some debate as to whether there is a suitable vector in the UK. Dead birds found in the UK have been shown to have seroconverted to the virus but no live virus has been found in the UK. However, an outbreak may occur in the UK in the future as it is on mainland Europe and of course extremely widespread in the USA. The disease is primarily spread by birds and then from them to humans, horses and SACs. The horse and the SAC are the end hosts. They cannot spread the disease. Humans can actually spread the disease to horses and SACs. In horses and perhaps in SACs the virus is common but very rarely causes disease. However, when there is disease it is very serious with up to 35% mortality. The clinical signs are ataxia, general weakness and general torpor. Treatment can only be supportive. Control is through vaccination, which is very effective in horses and may well be very effective in SACs, and by controlling mosquitoes. More radical measures include draining swamps and killing birds.

Metabolic diseases

Hepatic encephalopathy

Advanced liver disease will lead to hepatic encephalopathy, which carries a very poor prognosis. The animal will show acute neurological signs indicating pain, e.g. head pressing. Liver enzymes will be raised. A liver biopsy will show how advanced the condition has become. Practitioners cannot be faulted for encouraging euthanasia. However, in a few instances remarkable cures have been recorded after hospitalization and fluid therapy including large doses of vitamin B.

Hypocalcaemia

This is a metabolic condition of the lactating female (see Chapter 2).

Hypoglycaemia

This is a condition of the newborn cria. It is mainly seen in premature crias (see Chapter 11).

Hypomagnesaemia

This metabolic condition is extremely rare in SACs (see Chapter 2).

Uraemic encephalopathy

This neurological condition is the terminal condition of several other syndromes, e.g. intestinal volvulus or ruptured gastric ulcers. There will be ulcers in the mouth and there will be a strong smell of urea on the breath. There is renal shut down and the prognosis is normally hopeless. Obviously the animal needs to be put on to intravenous fluids and the primary cause of the condition needs to be addressed. However, euthanasia is likely to be the most humane option.

Miscellaneous

Deafness

Deafness is well recognized in camelids. The incidence is unknown. It is normally congenital. There is a link with blue eyes and white hair. The mode of inheritance is unknown. Deafness can occur secondarily to nerve conductive problems in the middle ear or due to sensorineural injury in the cochlear nerve.

Facial paralysis

This sign of damage to the facial nerve is normally seen immediately after trauma. However, it can be seen with a slower onset as a result of the development of a haematoma. There is a danger that this will become infected and so make the condition worse. Antibiotics and NSAIDs should be given.

Heat stroke

This is not common in the UK but is seen in Australia and the USA. SACs must be given adequate shade and water. Shearing at the correct time of the year is helpful. Rectal temperatures will be very high. The animals will show tachypnoea and tachycardia. Recumbency carries a poor prognosis. The animals need to be immersed in ice cold water until the rectal temperature returns to normal. This should be carried out immediately. No time should be lost while a drip is set up. Intravenous corticosteroids are helpful. While an ice bath is being prepared ice packs should be placed in the groin and axilla. Some authorities suggest an enema of ice cold water. However, this is hazardous on account of the danger of rectal tears. Hosing down is a better immediate treatment.

Hypothermia

This is a condition of young crias born in the winter or very early spring left in exposed conditions. Obviously it should be prevented. However, if it does occur in crias over 24 h of age it is vital that they receive a glucose enema before they are warmed up otherwise the central nervous system will die through lack of glucose. If the cria is under 24 h, of age it should be tubed with colostrum. Obviously the crias need to be warmed up. However, the use of hot air blowers should be avoided as initially they cause a drop in core temperature as a result of the latent heat of vaporization.

Mega-oesophagus

This condition is rare (see Chapter 9).

Polioencephalomalacia

The actual cause of this disease as in cerebro-cortico-necrosis (CCN) in sheep and goats is unknown. It certainly responds to treatment with thiamine (vitamin B1) injections ideally 15 mg/kg intravenously at 6 h intervals, but these can also be given subcutaneously. The prognosis is good provided the SAC is not recumbent. It is mainly seen in 1-year-old or young adult animals following a change of diet or overfeeding of concentrates. Animals are blind and wander away from others. They are depressed but will eat if the food is in front of them. Their rectal temperature, heart rate and respiratory rate are normal. They may have diarrhoea as a result of the dietary changes.

Tumours of the brain and spinal cord

These tumours are extremely rare. However, they will occur more frequently in SACs than in some other animals because SACs are allowed to become geriatric. The most common are metastases from other sites, e.g. malignant melanomas or adenomas of the adrenal glands. Gliomas and meningiomas will be found in the brain of crias.

Musculoskeletal

Bilateral luxating patellae

This condition is probably present at birth but is only noticed by the owner as the cria grows and becomes more mobile. Diagnosis is not difficult. However, surgical repair is extremely difficult and likely to be unsuccessful. As the condition is inherited euthanasia is a more humane option.

Gait abnormalities

There is no end to the different gait abnormalities shown by young crias. Rarely is the cause known. There have been some remarkable improvements shown so even quite serious abnormalities should be monitored before euthanasia. However, clinicians should always be mindful of welfare. Normally if the condition deteriorates to recumbency the prognosis is hopeless.

Hip problems

The hip joint in SACs is well formed. Dislocations are extremely unlikely. Correction may be accomplished but the joint will never be stable, and therefore early euthanasia is advocated.

Peripheral nerve damage

Peripheral nerve damage can occur to any nerve. Clinicians should always check for loss of sensation and for motor reflexes. The most important condition is radial paralysis, which will give the impression of forelimb fracture. However, if the leg is placed for the animal it can bear weight without pain. It is miraculous how in 6–10 weeks they will learn to flick the foreleg forward and appear normal. Sensation may or may not be recovered. The nerve will only regrow at 1 cm/month.

Parasitic diseases

Meningeal worms

These worms are contracted in North America from the 'white tailed deer', *Odocoileus virginianus*. As the name suggests this deer was first found in the state of Virginia. The deer is mainly found in the eastern USA. It is the migrating larvae of *Parelaphostrongylus tenuis* that causes the problems. These are ingested by the SACs by eating infected snails, which in their turn have eaten the worm eggs. It takes over 1 month for the SAC to develop the signs. These cause an interference with the gait starting with the hindlegs. These signs may lead to ataxia and recumbency. Occasionally the brain will be affected and the animal deteriorates rapidly. Obviously, the sooner treatment starts the better. Recumbent animals have a poor prognosis. The specific therapy is fenbendazole at 50 mg/kg for 5 days. However, symptomatic treatment is also required. This needs to be aggressive if the animal is recumbent. The definitive diagnosis is made by a CSF tap. The CSF will show an eosinophilia and a raised protein. In many areas in the USA where the disease is common veterinarians will advise monthly prophylactic treatment for meningeal worm. There are no reports of resistance to anthelmintics; however, with such regular usage there is likely to be resistance built up in bowel nematodes.

A nematode worm has been reported in the CSF of an alpaca in Europe (Michaely *et al.* 2022). The suggested species was *Baylisascaris procyonis* found in raccoons on the same farm. The diagnosis was only made after death at post-mortem. Only supportive treatment had been attempted.

Toxicities

Botulism

This condition, as in sheep and goats, is very rare. Animals will drool and may become recumbent. The pathognomic sign is the flaccid anus when the temperature is taken. These animals may recover with good nursing. Penicillin and NSAIDs should be given.

Ionophone toxicosis

These drugs are very toxic to SACs. Toxicity normally occurs if animals gain access to food destined for chicken feed. Animals will be recumbent and then show convulsions. These may be controlled with intravenous barbiturate but they will soon return. In theory compartment one of the stomach (C1) should be emptied and flushed. However, such treatment has not been recorded.

Rye grass staggers

This toxicity is caused by an endophyte that grows on rye grass, particularly in dry weather. The main sign in SACs is ataxia and a head tilt. This will occur in several animals. Normally animals recover if moved to a new unaffected pasture (see Chapter 16).

Tetanus

This is a potential threat in SACs. Vaccination is advised. Tetanus antitoxin should be given at half the horse dose in high-risk situations (see Chapter 6).

Tick paralysis

This condition is an acute, progressive, ascending motor paralysis caused by a salivary neurotoxin produced by certain species of ticks. *Ixodes* spp. and *Dermacentor* spp. have both been involved in causing the condition in the UK. These and other species have been involved in other parts of the world. The first signs seen are normally hindleg paralysis. Normally there is a serious tick infestation. The ticks should be killed and removed as soon as possible. Antibiotics should be given as there is often sepsis at the site of the tick bite. Animals will normally recover with supportive treatment. If they are quadriplegic, recovery is less likely, particularly if there is drooling of saliva.

Traumatic conditions

Cerebral hypoxia

This occurs with a delayed parturition. Crias will not lift up their heads and certainly will not make any effort to get up. Euthanasia is indicated. Mild forms will just appear dazed. If they can get up and suck they may manage to survive. Great care needs to be taken at weaning.

General trauma

Any SAC found dead or moribund with neurological signs should be examined carefully for signs of trauma. This seems more common in SACs than in sheep and goats. Fractured vertebrae in the neck are commonly reported. It can occur at parturition but is extremely rare as relative fetal oversize is not a problem in SACs. Crias may be attacked by dogs, predators or very rarely male SACs. Mis-mothering and aggression by females does not seem to occur.

Vertebral body fracture

If these are diagnosed rapidly with radiographs these cases may survive with good neck support. However, normally they are fatal or require immediate euthanasia.

Vertebral body subluxation

Prompt treatment with realignment under general anaesthetic may be successful if the subluxation is in the neck region and a supportive collar can be kept in place for 6 weeks. Radiographs should be taken to rule out a fracture.

Eye Disorders and Visual Defects in General

As in all conditions a good history is vital. Eye disorders and visual defects may appear to have an obvious cause but the clinician must endeavour to make not only an actual diagnosis but also to find out the underlying cause of the condition. A corneal ulcer may appear obvious but treating the ulcer without curing the entropion that is causing the ulcer will be at best a waste of time and at worst a welfare issue resulting in the loss of an eye. Practitioners must be mindful that if an eye condition cannot be treated satisfactorily and is causing long-term pain, the eye should be removed.

The history should obviously include the age and the number of animals affected. A record should be kept as to which eye is affected. Indeed if both eyes are affected that needs to be noted. If the eyes appear normal both from a normal visual examination and from an examination with an ophthalmoscope, then there is likely to be an underlying central lesion. Obviously the examination should include the eyelids and the other structures around the eye. The lens and the retina may well help with diagnosis, but oedema of the optic disc does not appear to be a useful sign in SACs. There is therefore no indication given of intracranial pressure by studying the optic disc. The visual pathways can be tested for integrity by the menace response or lack of it. This blink test needs to be carried out with care. It must be remembered that if there is air movement the animal may well blink even if it cannot see in that eye. The swinging light test can be used to test brain to eye pathways. A light shining in one eye will make the pupil in that eye contract. It will also make the pupil in the other eye contract but to a lesser degree. This will be reversed if the light is moved to the other eye in a normal animal. If there is a defect the pupil will not contract. It should be remembered that there is a crossover of the optic nerves. Where the lesion is situated will determine whether there are effects seen in the opposite eye or in the same eye.

Eye Disorders and Visual Defects in Neonatal Crias

Cataracts

Congenital cataracts may be seen in premature crias or in full-term crias. They may be inherited. There is no treatment. If the cria has some vision, it is reasonable to wait to see how it will adapt. However, if it is totally blind, euthanasia should be performed.

Entropion

This condition is extremely rare in SACs. It should be corrected surgically by carrying out a 'cake slice op'. After putting in the local anaesthesia, the area around the eye needs to be clipped and prepared for surgery. A small slice of skin is then removed. The wound is then sutured with fine interrupted simple sutures. The eyelid is then permanently in the correct position. The sutures need to be removed in 10 days. Owners should be urged not to breed from these crias.

Eyelid hypogenesis

There are various manifestations of this extremely rare condition. Clinicians need to use their own judgement on surgery, leaving alone and euthanasia.

Non-pigmented iris

This condition is not rare. The affected animals do not seem to be bothered by this condition throughout their lives.

Eye Disorders and Visual Defects in Older Crias and Adults

Causes of blindness without visible visual defects and no other illness

Sudden onset of blindness will occur in older crias and even adults without visible visual defects and with no other illness. Vital signs will all appear normal. The animals will eat food presented to them or in the case of crias will suckle when shown the teat of their mother. In the author's experience the cause is never found even on post-mortem. The condition appears to be irreversible. The author has considered vitamin A deficiency but this seems very unlikely as all the cases seen occurred at grass.

Causes of blindness without visible visual defects but also showing some signs of illness

Cerebro-cortico-necrosis

With cerebro-cortico-necrosis (CCN), the animals will be severely depressed and show ataxia.

They will have a papillary light reflex (PLR) but will appear blind. This condition is going to have a sudden onset. Any cria that is recumbent, blind, and showing strabismus and opisthotonous is likely to have CCN. There will be no pyrexia. Response to intravenous thiamine at 10 mg/kg is the best pointer to a correct early diagnosis. A heparinized blood sample can be taken for transketolase estimation. This is a specific test for CCN. Thiaminase can best estimated in a faecal sample or in C1 contents if the animal has died. The pathognomic sign at post-mortem is seen in the brain. The cerebral hemispheres will macroscopically show a yellow discoloration and fluoresce under ultraviolet light (see Chapter 15).

Coccidiosis

A very severe neurological type has been described. There will be a PLR (see Chapter 9).

Gid

As yet this parasite has not been recorded in SACs. There is likely to be a head tilt and a PLR in at least one eye (see Chapter 9).

Keto-acidosis

There is normally a severe energy deficit and hypoglycaemia. There will be a PLR (see Chapter 2).

Meningitis with or without hypopyon

The animals will be very ill with a raised temperature. Normally they would have a PLR. In adults *Listeria monocytogenes* should be suspected. In crias other organisms may be involved.

Trauma to the head

The animals will have fixed dilated pupils. The head should be very carefully and gently examined. Radiographs will be useful.

Various plant poisons

Among other plant poisons, aflatoxins, bracken, brassicas and deadly nightshade will cause blindness. A PLR will not be present (see Chapter 16).

Various poisons

Lead, sulfur, salt (caused by water deprivation), arsenic, mercury and antifreeze will cause blindness. The animals will have a PLR (see Chapter 16).

Vitamin A deficiency

The animals have fixed dilated pupils. In advanced cases they will be ataxic and may show head-pressing. The condition is irreversible.

Tumours of the eyelids

The most common are squamous cell carcinomas of the third eyelid. These have a good prognosis if they can be removed before the tumour has invaded the conjunctiva. Surgery is straightforward as the eyelid can be removed with a pair of scissors under anaesthesia. Haemorrhage is minimal and suturing is not required.

13

Medicine and Surgery of the Locomotory System

Conditions of the Limbs

Introduction

Crias need adequate amounts of calcium, phosphorus, protein and vitamin D for their skeletons to grow properly. While there will always be occasional animals that accidentally break a leg there are certain problems that increase the risk of fractures. If practitioners have the slightest doubt about the presence of a fracture (this is particularly important in crias, which are very stoical) they should splint the affected limb. Welfare is paramount. Radiographs should be taken and treatment should be carried out promptly.

Increased risks of fractures may develop over long periods of time. The bones may become increasingly fragile. Severe copper deficiency has been reported to cause fractures, as copper is needed for development of a normal framework within the bone. Long-standing parasitic infections, particularly intestinal nematodes, also predispose to fractures because damage to the gut wall prevents the young animal absorbing enough phosphorus. Where animals are kept in areas of old lead mining the continual daily intake of small amounts of lead as they graze makes the bones liable to fracture. With all three conditions the young animals will be ill-thriven. Problems with rickets are well documented in SACs, particularly crias. It is thought that SACs

bred up in the Andes rely on high levels of sunlight to make vitamin D. This is denied them in other areas of the world particularly the UK. Therefore supplementation of vitamin D either by mouth or by injection is required regularly in crias, particularly those crias born later in the year in the northern hemisphere.

Abnormal 'kushing' in neonates

Neonates are often shaky when born and have difficulty getting into the 'kush' position. They are in danger of being trodden on by their mothers and other animals. It is important that they are separated until they have become stronger. Owners should assist them to 'kush' normally.

Angular limb deformity

Angular limb deformity (ALD) is common among llamas and alpacas. It is normally seen in neonates but may be seen later in life. It may be congenital or acquired. Hypovitaminosis D is the most common cause, but the condition definitely has a high heritability. Injuries may play a part when the other three legs are forced to take more weight. Careful clinical evaluation should

© Graham R. Duncanson 2023. *Veterinary Treatment of Llamas and Alpacas*, 2nd Edition (G.R. Duncanson)
DOI: 10.1079/9781800623576.0013

be carried out. Extensive hair growth may hide ALD so that it is only revealed at the first shearing. ALD is described by the joint most affected by the angulation and by the direction to which the limb distal to the angulation is deviated (valgus = lateral deviation, varus = medial deviation). When surveyed, the occurrence of the condition showed no difference in male or females.

Radiography is vital to assess the clinical findings. Paul-Murphy *et al.*, (1991) published a useful paper on radiographic findings in young llamas with forelimb valgus deformities.

Carpal valgus originating at the level of the distal radius is the most common ALD requiring surgery in affected camelids. It is vital that it is carried out before nine months of age before the growth plates stop growing. The ideal age is three to four months. There are three surgical options: periosteal stripping, transphyseal bridging and corrective osteotomy. The author only has experience with periosteal stripping, which is relatively simple to perform and has a good success rate.

Contracted tendons in adults

This is rare and is often of unknown aetiology (Fig. 13.1). Application of a splint can be tried with considerable care taken to avoid pressure necrosis. Sectioning of the superficial flexor tendon under general anaesthetic may be the ultimate treatment.

Dropped pasterns

Hyperextension of the metacarpal-phalangeal joint is a condition of llamas. It is rarely seen in alpacas. It is mainly a condition of old animals but can affect young llamas. The condition has been linked with raised serum zinc levels and decreased copper levels. However, a direct causality has not been established. Most affected llamas can live normal lives but there are concerns over the wisdom of pregnancy. There is no treatment.

Flying scapular

This is a very rare condition that may occur in SACs, normally after weaning but before maturity. The muscles securing the scapular to the ribcage become weak and rupture to some extent so that the ribcage drops. The spine is then lower in the thoracic area compared to the lumbar-sacral area. The animal is still mobile. The condition is irreversible.

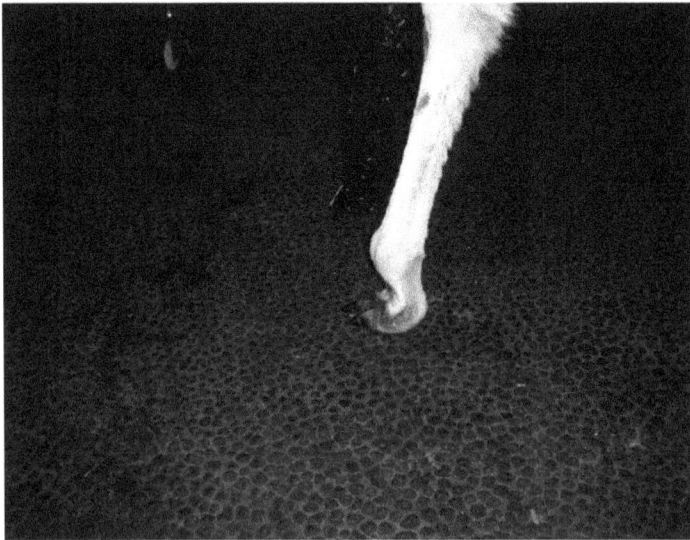

Fig. 13.1. Contracted tendon.

Fractures

Fractures occur in SACs and are particularly a concern on account of the length of their long bones. Crias are most at risk. Practitioners need to be particularly vigilant on account of the stoical nature of SACs. Fractures are particularly easy to dismiss. Many types of repair have been described in the literature: intramedullary pins, screws and plates, external fixation pins as well as external splints and casts. Very great care has to be taken with external casts on account of the dangers of pressure necrosis (Fig. 13.2). Even amputations have been carried out without compromising the welfare of the individual.

Certain old SACs may suffer from osteoporosis. The cause is unknown but they will often develop multiple fractures. Euthanasia is indicated.

Luxating patellas

This not uncommon fault is often not noticed until after weaning. It is an inherited defect and has nothing to do with early castration or rickets. Obviously there are various grades of the condition. Surgery is unwise and euthanasia is indicated if the condition becomes worse.

Scapulo-humeral joint luxation

This luxation in alpacas has been reported by a group of authors in the USA (Rousseau *et al.*, 2010). Only ten cases have been reported throughout the USA so this is by no means a common condition. It is much more common in males. Various surgical options were pursued with varying results. It should always be considered in cases of forelimb lameness in SACs.

Sequestrations

These can form in the bones of young growing animals from a week onwards. The common presentation is peracute lameness. Radiography will not reveal a fracture and at this stage there are no other radiological signs but these will develop later. Clinicians should radiograph these limbs in a further 2 weeks. Dead bone fragments will then be seen. There is no known definite aetiology of this condition. The most likely explanation is septic necrosis in the diaphyseal region of the bone. Sadly, high doses of antibiotics on day 1 do not seem to help the condition. Once a diagnosis has been made surgery appears to be the only worthwhile treatment. Antibiotics and

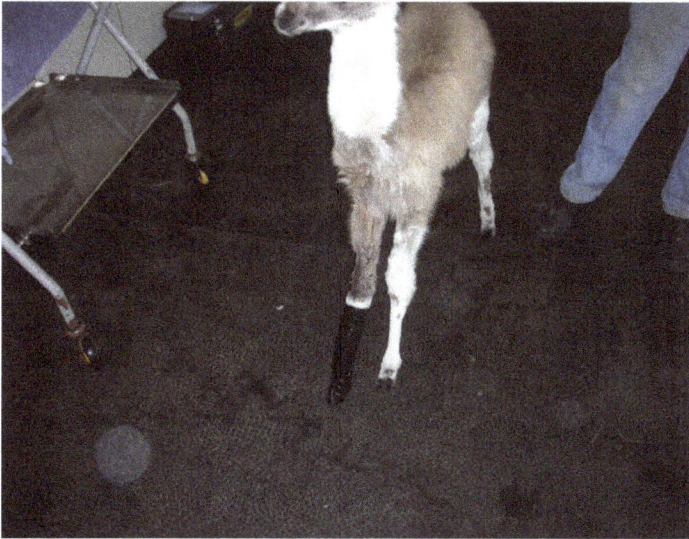

Fig. 13.2. External cast.

tetanus antitoxin should be given prior to sur-gery. Surgeons should cut down on to the se-questrum and remove it. There is no need to splint or bandage the leg but the cria and its mother should be kept separate from the rest of the group.

Total spasticity of the limbs

This condition seen in neonates looks very similar to the 'spider lamb' syndrome in sheep. The outcome is hopeless if the animal is quadriplegic. However, if the animal can use its front legs normally but it is only paralysed behind, time and good nursing may bring about a recovery.

Foot Problems

SACs have a soft pad and a terminal toenail. The pad may look eroded and pitted, especially in wet weather (Fig. 13.3). Footrot is extremely rare. Treatments with formalin or zinc sulfate do not seem to be effective. Animal husbandry methods must be used to keep the feet dry. Copper sulfate is not only ineffective but dangerous on account of the toxicity.

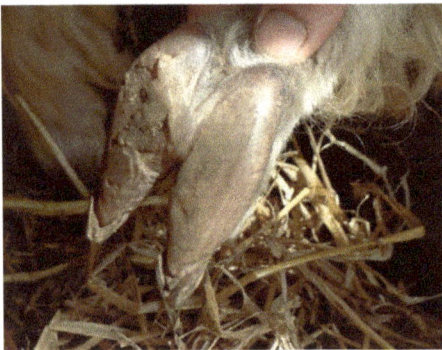

Fig. 13.3. Eroded pad.

Overgrown toes are common in SACs out-side of South America when they are kept on soft ground. They should be trimmed regularly.

Surgical Removal of the Digit

Septic pedal arthritis does occur in SACs. How-ever, it is rare. Antibiotic treatment even if pro-longed is rarely successful. Welfare must always be considered. Euthanasia is certainly an option to relieve further suffering. Full drainage of the distal phalangeal joint with subsequent arthrod-esis may be considered. However, this will result in a long period of severe pain. Surgical removal of the digit is a more humane option. However, it is vital that this surgery is not attempted if there is sepsis in the proximal joints as pain will per-sist. If clinicians are in any doubt, radiography should be carried out.

Regional anaesthesia can be used (see Chapter 8). The distal limb can be cleaned but full asepsis is not required. A length of embryot-omy wire is placed between the digits. The saw-ing direction should be at an angle of 45° above the horizontal. The skin, soft tissue and half the second phalanx should be removed. The foot then should be bandaged before removal of the tourniquet. The animal should be given antibiot-ics and non-steroidal anti-inflammatory drug (NSAID) cover for a minimum of 1 week. The bandage should be removed every third day until clean granulation tissue is seen.

Tumours of the Skeletal System

In SACs bone tumours are exceptionally rare. They are only really seen as a metastasis of a mel-anoma in the mandible. However, tumours of the cartilage of the ribs are not that unusual. Diag-nosis may be difficult as it is often difficult to find out how long the tumour has been present. It may resemble an old fracture occurring as early as at parturition or trauma to the ribs later in life.

14

Skin Conditions

Introduction

When dealing with skin conditions it is important to not only obtain a full history (e.g. what species, age groups and genders are affected, have new animals been brought on to the holding, etc.) but also to carry out a full clinical examination of the animal. Careful observation is required to check for pruritis. It should be remembered that healthy animals may show signs of skin irritation (Fig. 14.1). If pruritis is observed the clinician needs to eliminate ectoparasites before investigating other conditions. Direct visual examination should be carried out with the naked eye and a magnifying glass. Many larger parasites can be visualized. Skin scrapings can be taken from the moister marginal areas of lesions after clipping away the hair or wool. One or two drops of 10% potassium hydroxide solution can be added to soften and clarify the scraping before direct microscopic examination for ectoparasites or fungal hyphae/spores. Culture can be carried out from skin scrapings, plucked hair or moist material from lesions. Direct impression smears can be stained with Gram, Giemsa or a modified Wright's stain such as 'Dif Quik'. Scabs covering active rather than healing lesions can be taken, kept dry and referred for further investigation. It should be remembered that it is dangerous to include scalpel blades with referred samples.

The ultimate diagnostic tool is the skin biopsy. When skin is processed for histopathology some potentially important surface features may be partially lost through the chemical processing. Consequently there should be no surface preparation of the skin prior to collecting a skin biopsy. It is quite acceptable to clip the surrounding hair. If an entire nodule is going to be removed then it should be sent in sufficient formal saline to preserve it. If it is large it should be cut in half to allow the formal saline to penetrate it. If just a biopsy is going to be taken it is best to use a specially prepared 6 mm biopsy punch. Multiple biopsies may be taken and sent. The sites of each biopsy should be recorded. A biopsy may be taken and labelled from normal skin. However, it is best not to include too much normal skin with the biopsy as when the section is prepared it may not be apparent which is normal and which is diseased skin. It is very important to give a full report to the pathologist so that the pathologist is aware of the extent of the diseased tissue and the timescale as to when the changes arose. It is also important to select the pathologist carefully. The pathologist not only needs to be familiar with skin disease but also with SACs.

It should be remembered that some skin disease conditions in camelids may be zoonotic. It is therefore prudent to communicate such diseases to owners and handlers.

DOI: 10.1079/9781800623576.0014

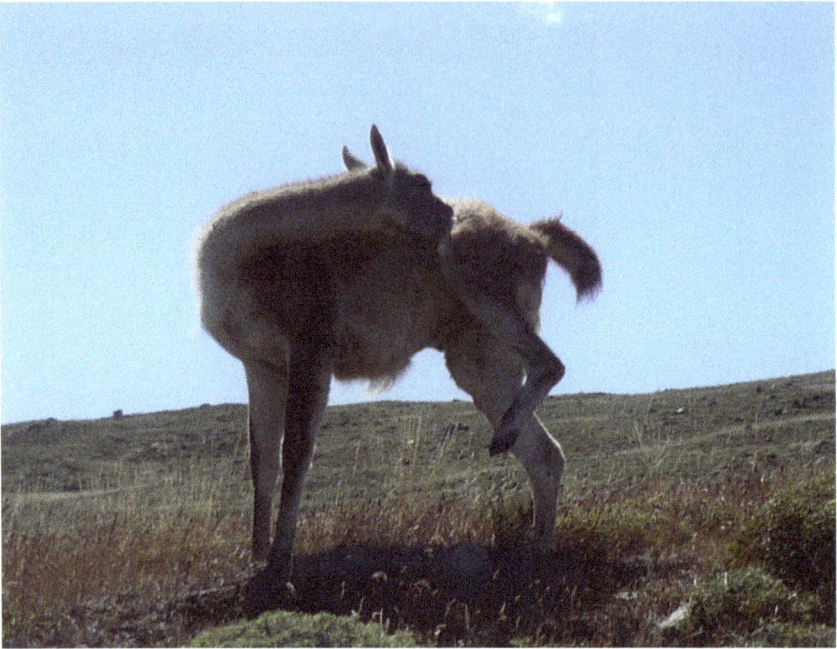

Fig. 14.1. A wild guanaco in Argentina.

Viral Skin Diseases

Blue tongue virus

Blue tongue virus (BTV) causes hyperaemia of the oral mucosa with excoriations of the tongue, lips and gums that become ulcerative and necrotic. There is also a coronitis with hyperaemia and swelling around the coronet leading to obvious lameness (see Chapter 9). It is only included as a skin disease for completeness.

Contagious pustular dermatitis

This is primarily a disease of sheep, however it will affect SACs. It is perhaps the most important viral skin disease of sheep and is called 'orf'. It is highly contagious and is found worldwide. It is caused by a *Parapox* virus. The lesions most commonly occur on the commissures of the lips, muzzle and occasionally on the feet and genitalia. It can manifest as a flock outbreak or can be seen in the lambs in spring and summer. If the crias are still sucking the teats of the

females they will get infected udders with disastrous results, i.e. mastitis.

The initial lesion consists of a number of red papules within which vesicles develop, rupture and a thick scab is formed. Proliferative changes may then occur resulting in papillomatous lesions. Secondary bacterial infection is common with all lesions and in females with mastitis deaths may occur. Difficulty in sucking may cause weight restriction in crias and lesions on the coronary band may result in lameness.

Diagnosis should be straightforward clinically. It can be confirmed by virus isolation. The disease will spread rapidly. Although it is a virus, antibiotics are useful. A blanket dose of a penicillin/streptomycin injection is very helpful. Really bad lesions should be treated with oily creams. Antibiotic aerosols should be avoided as they tend to cause the scabs to harden. When these scabs are knocked off there are large eroded areas underneath.

There is a live vaccine available for sheep. This vaccine should not be used in SACs. It is a live vaccine and very bad reactions have been reported.

Foot-and-mouth disease

Vesicle lesions of foot-and-mouth disease (FMD) are found on the oral mucosa and the coronary band. The condition is included under skin disease for completeness (see Chapter 9).

Malignant catarrhal fever

In the UK, malignant catarrhal fever (MCF) is caused by ovine herpes type 2 virus (Ov-VH2). The sheep is thought to be the natural host. In Africa the natural host is the wildebeest. It is thought to cause cutaneous manifestations in SACs. The lesions are a severe generalized alopecia with granulomatous mural folliculitis. A definitive diagnosis may be made by polymerase chain reaction (PCR). The condition is normally fatal. There is no treatment and so euthanasia is recommended if a definitive diagnosis has been made.

Peste des petits ruminants

Peste des petits ruminants (PPR) is caused by a morbillivirus and is related to rinderpest. PPR will infect camels and has been seen by the author in northern Kenya. It has not been reported in SACs. Clinicians should not be concerned that they will miss this disease as the signs are very obvious. There is high fever with erosions on the mucous membranes of the mouth and eyes. There is acute bloody diarrhoea and also signs of pneumonia. The author would expect whole herds to become infected and the majority to die. There is no specific treatment. However, oxytetracycline injections might reduce the number of deaths. Non-steroidal anti-inflammatory drugs (NSAIDs) may be helpful. No vaccine appears to be available but the literature claims that one has been developed. It is more likely that regulations will require all the animals to be slaughtered as a disease control precaution.

Pseudorabies

This disease is often called Aujeszky's disease. It is primarily a virus affecting swine. It is mainly a neurological disease (see Chapter 12).

Rabies

This virus disease affects SACs. It is primarily a neurological disease (see Chapter 12).

Rinderpest

Hopefully this has been eradicated from the world thanks to the excellent vaccine prepared by Sir Walter Plowright. It is caused by a morbillivirus. The primary host is cattle but camels have been affected. It has never been reported in SACs.

Vesicular stomatitis

This rhabdovirus is very rare. It is really only of relevance as it may cause confusion with FMD. It mainly occurs in other species and has not been reported in SACs.

Bacterial Skin Diseases

Actinobacillosis

This condition commonly occurs in SACs. It is normally associated with the head and neck but it has been reported on the body in Norfolk in the UK. It is characterized by thickening of the skin with multiple granulomatous swellings often associated with the lymphatics. These swellings are unrewarding to lance as the pus is only in small pockets. The actual organism is *Actinobacillosis lignieresi*. This is thought to gain entry either through wounds in the skin or the mucosa of the mouth. Treatment with penicillin is unrewarding. However, prolonged daily dosing with streptomycin is normally effective. A minimum of 10 mg/kg for 10 days is suggested.

Actinomycosis

This condition is really a disease of cattle called 'lumpy jaw' or if it occurs in the soft tissues of the mouth it is called 'wooden tongue'. The syndrome is seen in SACs quite frequently. *Actinomyces* spp. form firm nodules on the face.

Lancing is unrewarding as they are granuloma-tous and only release small amounts of yellow-ish white granules. Treatment with penicillin is unrewarding. However, prolonged daily dosing with streptomycin is normally effective. A min-imum of 10 mg/kg for 10 days is suggested.

Anthrax

This is normally a systemic disease in SACs. It can be manifest as a cutaneous form like that seen in humans (see Chapter 17). It takes the form in camels of a malignant pustule, normally on the face, but the author has seen it in the groin. Smears made from the lesion will reveal the bacteria on staining with old methylene blue. The disease in the UK is notifiable and is ex-tremely unlikely to be seen. However, the author has treated cases in Africa that have responded well to 5 days of procaine penicillin.

Caseous lymphadenitis

Caseous lymphadenitis (CLA) is caused by *Coryne-bacterium pseudotuberculosis*. It occurs in sheep and goats throughout the world. It was first isolated in the UK in 1990 (Baird, 2003) from an importation from Germany. Studies have revealed that all cases in the UK have come dir-ectly from that case. There has been no official action as control was thought not to be feasible. The disease could affect SACs.

Abscesses would be likely to develop in the lymph nodes under the skin but could also occur in internal organs, e.g. in the lungs. It will then manifest as a respiratory condition (see Chapter 10). Swollen abscessed lymph nodes are easy to see. If incised they would take on an onion-like appearance with concentric rings of fibrous tissue and inspissated pus, or they could be just filled with soft pasty pus. The main spread is from the rupture of abscesses into the environment where the organism can survive for a seriously long time. If there are abscesses in the lungs the disease can spread by the re-spiratory route. The herd can contract the disease by importation of infected animals but can also obtain the disease from contaminated fomites, e.g. clipper blades.

Diagnosis could be made on clinical grounds and confirmed by culture of the organ-ism from an abscess. Culling is the only course of action as there is no effective treatment. Total eradication could be achieved. In theory the or-ganism is sensitive to several antibiotics but penetration into the abscesses is impossible. There is a vaccine available. It is not licensed in the UK and its use has not been reported in SACs.

Clostridial cellulitis

This is often called malignant oedema and can occur in SACs. It is most common in males as a result of fighting wounds. The causal organism is *Clostridium septicum*; *Clostridium sordellii* has also been isolated. Both these organisms are now covered by a licensed vaccine for sheep. This same vaccine is licensed for cattle at double the dose. It can be used in SACs but it should be used at the sheep dose. The higher cattle dose causes adverse reactions in the form of cold abscesses.

It is a very serious condition. The area of swelling is initially hot and painful with crepitus. This then turns cold and gangrenous. Initially the animal has a fever but this rapidly abates before death. Diagnosis should be made on clinical grounds. Confirmation is difficult as there is rapid autolysis after death. However, if smears are ob-tained promptly they will confirm the diagnosis using fluorescent antibody techniques (FAT).

Treatment may be attempted if the disease is caught in the febrile stage. High doses of crys-talline penicillin should be given intravenously together with NSAIDs.

Dermatophilosis

This is often called mycotic dermatitis in text-books, which is a misnomer as it is caused by a bacterium *Dermatophilus congolensis*. It is also called 'fibre rot'. The disease manifests as an ex-udative dermatitis affecting the back and flanks. The disease is progressive. It starts with exud-ation, which then crusts and scabs. The initial penetration is facilitated by prolonged wetting of the fleece during periods of prolonged wet wea-ther. Diagnosis may be made on clinical grounds and confirmed by Giemsa stain of the scabs.

Treatment in severe cases is parenteral antibiotics and antibiotic cream on the raw areas. Most mild cases will heal spontaneously.

Morel's disease

This disease is clinically very similar to CLA. It is seen in goats in Europe in Poland, Germany and France. It has also been seen in Africa and Asia. However, the causal organism is *Staphylococcus aureus* ssp. *aerobius* not *Corynebacterium pseudotuberculosis*. It has a shorter incubation period of 3 weeks, rather than months with CLA. The abscesses are not as closely related to the lymphatics as in CLA. Initially it has a morbidity of 70–90%. This falls to 10–20% as it becomes endemic. It could occur in SACs. It would only be differentiated from CLA by culture. In goats, antibiotic treatment appears to be ineffective. Autogenous vaccines do not offer protection. It must be assumed that SACs would follow the goat model.

Necrotic dermatitis

This condition is caused by *Pseudomonas aeruginosa*. It is a very serious condition as not only is it very difficult to treat but also it predisposes the animal to myiasis. Preventive measures need to be stepped up. It appears to follow prolonged rainy conditions, particularly within 6 weeks of shearing. However, the exact trigger mechanism is not known. Animals can become very ill if the area of the affected skin is large. The local lymph nodes will become swollen. The diagnosis can be confirmed on culture. Treatment is parenteral broad-spectrum antibiotics together with local creams containing miconazole nitrate, prednisolone acetate and polymyxin B sulfate.

Nocardiosis

This disease was first reported in goats by Peter Jackson at Cambridge (Jackson, 1986). It is very rare in the UK although it seems to be widespread in central Asia. Abscesses are common in central Asia but the actual bacteria involved appear to be similar to those seen in the UK. There is a very rare bacteria *Actinomadura madurae*,

which causes granular pus in similar abscesses all over the body. This condition is also called actinomycetic mycetoma. In theory it could occur in SACs. Treatment in goats is unrewarding. High daily doses of streptomycin are recommended over a period of at least 1 month.

Peri-orbital eczema

This condition is thought to be bacterial and is likely to be caused by a *Staphylococcus*. The condition characteristically affects trough-fed SACs. The early lesion is seen as a small inflamed and scabbed area on one or other of the bony prominences of the face or less commonly on the nose. This extends, usually around the eye, hence the name, to give an alarming scabbed, discharging sore. The condition is not serious except in the rare occasions when the infection spreads actually to the eye. Most cases are self-limiting and do not require treatment. However, severe cases may require aggressive antibiotic treatment. The author recommends daily injections for 3 days with amoxicillin with clavulanic acid and local treatment with the same antibiotic, which is available as an intramammary preparation for cows.

Scald

This is also called benign footrot in lambs. It mainly occurs in warm moist conditions with animals on lush pastures. It only occurs in crias that are kept on the same pasture as affected lambs. The interdigital skin becomes inflamed and painful. Normally there is no separation of the horn or suppuration. There is no smell as in typical footrot. The bacteriology is not straightforward. Certain strains of *Bacteriodes nodosus* are involved. Normally *Fusibacterium necrophorum* is not present.

Individual cases respond well to antibiotic aerosols. If large numbers are affected then foot bathing in 0.5% zinc sulfate is helpful.

Staphylococcal dermatitis

This may actually be the same condition as peri-orbital eczema, as it occurs on the face and nasal bones in SACs. However, it also occurs on the limbs, vulva and prepuce. It is a suppurative condition that takes 4–6 weeks to resolve. The causal organism is a beta-haemolytic *Staphylococcus aureus*. Treatment would be the same as for peri-orbital eczema.

Staphylococcal folliculitis

This is a benign condition that affects young crias. It is normally a condition associated with housed animals. The clinical signs are normally mild with small pustules on the lips, muzzle and nostrils. Diagnosis should be made on clinical grounds. However, it can be confirmed on the isolation of *Staphylococcus hyicus* or histologically as a pyogenic folliculitis with ulceration of the epidermis. The condition will normally resolve without treatment in a few days.

Fungal Skin Diseases

Aspergillosis

This is a rare disease caused by *Aspergillus fumigatus*. It has been found in vicuna kept in captivity. The condition shows the form of ulcerating nodules in the groin. It is refractive to treatment. As the disease may be contagious, slaughter should be advised. The disease may be diagnosed by culture but false negatives will occur. Histopathology is a safer method of diagnosis.

Cryptococcosis

This is an extremely rare skin disease. The nodules are seen on the head and may become ulcerated. *Cryptococcus neoformans* can be isolated on culture. Treatment is rarely successful. Long-term broad-spectrum parenteral antibiotics and natamycin washes might be helpful.

Malassezia dermatitis

Malassezia spp. may be isolated from the skins of normal SACs. They can be seen on impression smears stained with a modified Wright's stain such as 'Dif Quik'. If very large numbers of 'peanut shaped' yeast organisms are found on diseased skin they may well be significant. Swab samples may be cultured on ordinary Sabouraud's media. The clinical signs will include erythema, scale, hyperpigmentation and malodour. Various baths seem effective, e.g. chlorhexidine, enilconazole, miconazole or selenium sulfide can be used twice weekly for a minimum of 3 weeks and then regularly at weekly intervals until the condition resolves. However, if there is a trigger factor involved this will need to be treated at the same time.

Phaeohyphomycosis

This disease is caused by an opportunist free-living fungus, *Peyronellaea glomerata*. It forms papules and aural plaques on the ears. It may be related to ear tags. It appears to be self-limiting.

Pythiosis

This rare fungal disease is seen in South America in alpacas. It seems that the causal organism, *Pythium insidiosum*, can only affect the skin of wool animals that are exposed to total immersion in water for some hours. The ulcerated plaques will heal if the animals can be kept dry for 3–4 weeks.

Ringworm

This is a rare condition in llamas. It is much rarer in alpacas, where it is normally seen on the non-fibre-covered areas. In llamas it may be found all over the body. The most common organism is *Trichophyton verrucosum*, which is normally caught from cattle. It must be remembered that it is a zoonotic condition (see Chapter 17), therefore the practitioner should warn the owner to take normal hygienic precautions. Washing carefully with soap and water or dilute chlorhexidine is worthwhile. Owners should avoid rigorous scrubbing or strong disinfectants as the skin barrier will be breached, allowing the fungi to penetrate. The other organism isolated from llamas is caught from dogs. It is *Microsporum canis*. *Trichophyton mentagrophytes* has been found in SACs kept with goats. The clinical picture of round crusting lesions is the same for all three species of fungi. Pruritis is more marked with *T. verrucosum* infection. Obviously several animals are likely to be infected.

The areas most commonly affected in llamas include the face, ears and back. In very rare instances the legs and tail head are affected. The lesions are first seen as firm raised plaques attached to the underlying skin, which then become detached to reveal circular raised crusts with local thickening of the skin. Thickening of the stratum spinosum with hyperkeratosis and proliferative dermatitis will be seen on histological sections. However, histology is not normally required to confirm a diagnosis. The organism is readily grown on proprietary plates and will be identified by a red colour change within 10 days. Often there will be secondary bacterial infection. Only debilitated animals will get a bad infection. In normal animals the infection is self-limiting in a few months. If treatment is required for special animals (e.g. showing animals), there are topical fungicides like natamycin and oral antibiotics like griseofulvin. The latter is very effective against *T. verrucosum* and *T. mentagrophytes* but not so effective against *M. canis*. Griseofulvin must not be used in food-producing animals in the UK but could be used in SACs.

Protozoal Skin Diseases

Besnoitosis

This is a disease of llamas in South America. It does not seem to affect alpacas. It is caused by the protozoan *Besnoitia caprae*. Diagnosis is difficult as it causes large areas of thickened skin, which is very similar to scabies. Diagnosis can only be made from skin biopsies. The condition is refractory to treatment. Euthanasia is advised.

Leishmaniosis

This disease has not been recorded in SACs. It is seen in sheep in South Africa. If SACs were imported into South Africa it is possible that they might become infected.

Sarcocystis capricanis

This organism, which causes skin disease in goats, has been reported in central Asia although in fact it occurs throughout the world. The author found the organism in goats with severe alopecia in Mombasa in Kenya. However, demodectic mange was present at the same time and so the cause of the alopecia was in doubt. The organism has not been recorded in SACs. However, SACs may act as secondary hosts to intestinal *Sarcocystis* spp. found in carnivores in South America.

Parasitic Skin Diseases

Blowfly strike

Myiasis is rare in SACs high in the Andes. However, it can occur in all other temperate, subtropical and tropical areas. Most blowflies are secondary strikers, i.e. there has to be a wound first for the maggots to invade the skin (Fig. 14.2). There are three genera of flies involved: the blue bottle, *Calliphora* spp.; the green bottle, *Phaenicia* spp.; and the black bottle, *Phormia* spp. In the Americas there is a primary striker, *Cochliomyia hominovorax*. This is a screw worm and will invade healthy skin. It has largely been eliminated in North America. Once a SAC has been struck, the area of skin under the fleece that is involved will be permanently damaged, ruining the animal for show and lessening the fibre production. The condition if advanced can be life-threatening and so treatment needs to be aggressive. The animal should receive antibiotics and NSAIDs immediately. If it is in severe shock the author gives dexamethasone at up to 4 mg/25 kg intravenously in place of the NSAIDs. If the animal is cold it is warmed up with hot water containers under blankets. The area around the strike is trimmed of fibre and cleaned. *All* the maggots are removed with warm salty water. If this is difficult the author uses a hairdryer. Cypermethrin in a 1.25% w/v non-aqueous liquid is applied to all the affected parts at the rate of 2.5 ml per

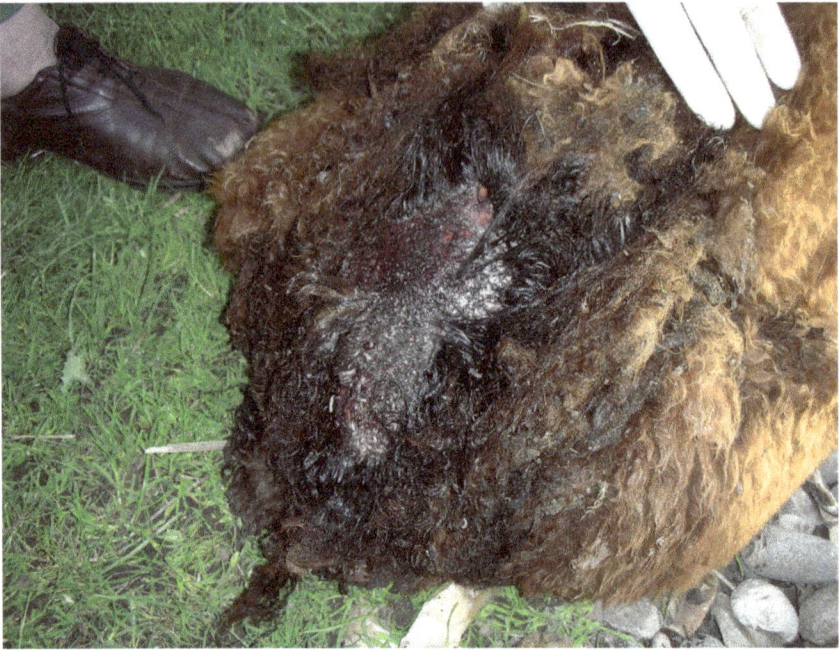

Fig. 14.2. Blowfly strike.

100–150 cm² (roughly the size of a hand). The whole wet area is dressed with oily cream, normally a mixture of acriflavin and benzene hexachloride. The tetanus status of the animal is checked. The animal's progress is monitored. The antibiotics and anti-inflammatories are repeated at the correct intervals.

At the present time the author considers the risk of blowfly strike too low to warrant the routine application of synthetic pyrethrums to alpacas in the UK.

Lice

These are easily diagnosed by their shape and the fact that they cause pruritis. This in turn leads to matted fibre and eventually alopecia. Because they can readily be seen by owners and handlers it should be noted that lice are generally host-specific. They do not cross species lines very easily. Therefore, you are not likely to pick up lice from your alpaca and llama, and if you do they will not stay on you more than a few hours. Lice infestation (pediculosis) is most common during winter months presumably because temperature, crowding and feeding management are optimal for spread and proliferation of these pests. Further, louse infestations are more severe in debilitated animals such as those suffering malnutrition and intestinal parasitism (D. E Anderson, personal communication). All stages of louse live on the host, but they can be rubbed off into the environment and transmitted over short periods of time. The life cycle can be as short as 2 weeks or as long as several months. Adults live up to 6 weeks. Adults cement their eggs onto hair shafts and these eggs will hatch in 1 to 3 weeks. The egg casing remains attached on the hair shaft and this empty nest is what is seen at shearing. There are two types found in SACs worldwide. Sucking lice *Microthoracius* spp. are found on the fore end of the SAC mainly on the head, neck and withers. They can be treated with injectable avermectins. Oral avermectins are ineffective. Biting lice *Bovicola breviceps* are found all down the spine from the neck to the tail head.

Neither injectable nor oral avermectins are effective. They require topical applications. However, they need to be used with care as some spot-on and all pour-on products may damage the skin and the fibre. The safest is fipronil put on as a spray or cypermethrin diluted as a spray. All the treatments for lice require a repeat treatment in 10 days to control the unhatched eggs. *Bovicola breviceps* is the only louse confirmed in the UK (Foster, 2008). A light infestation reported in llamas was reported to be of little clinical significance by authors in the UK (Twomey *et al.*, 2010b).

Treatment of the environment is usually impractical.

Mites

Chicken mites

Both the Northern fowl mite (*Ornithonyssus sylvarium*) and the red mite (*Dermanyssus gallinae*) have been accused of causing pruritis in SACs kept in close proximity to chickens. Removal of the chickens and thorough cleansing of the environment is the best course of action. Treatment of chickens is constantly being reviewed and so any treatment being used on chickens should not be used on SACs without careful evaluation.

Chorioptes mites

These are the most common mites found in SACs in the UK. There is some doubt as to the naming of the species. However, at the present time it is *Chorioptes bovis*. It causes mild pruritis, alopecia and scaling. Lesions are commonly found on the head, ears, feet and perineum but can also extend to the limbs and ventral abdomen. A high prevalence has been reported (D'Alterio, 2005) in the south-west of England. Over 20% of alpacas were affected and mites were identified in 40% of these cases. Of animals that actually had no skin lesions, 55% were found to be harbouring mites. The most likely area to find mites was in the interdigital space.

The commonly used treatment is the injection of doramectin at 1 ml/33 kg given every 3 weeks. This does not seem to be very effective and leads to resistance in internal nematodes. Even weekly treatments have been tried on the whole herd without lasting cure. Certain individuals may well show an allergic response. Orthoparakeratosis and parakeratosis with thickening are seen in these individuals (Fig. 14.3). It has been postulated that this is linked with a zinc deficiency. However, although zinc levels have

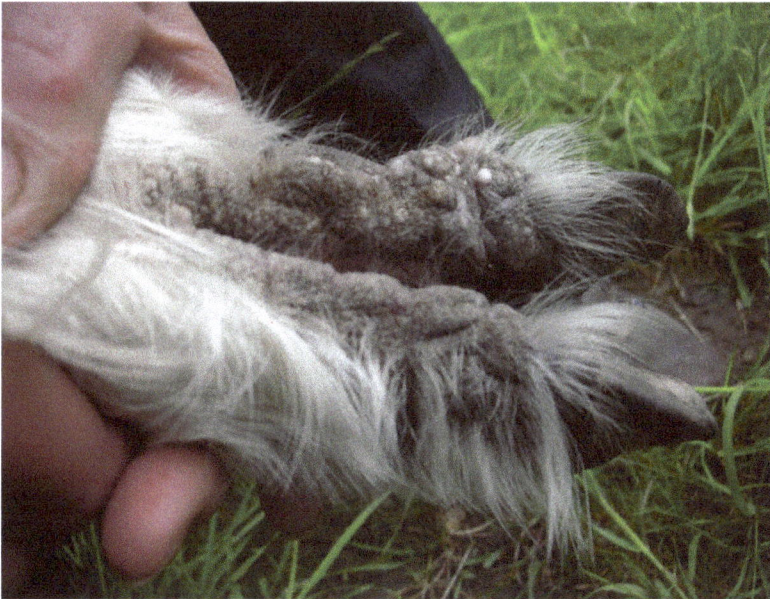

Fig. 14.3. Chorioptic mange.

been shown to be low in certain individuals, levels do not correlate with infection. Equally individuals do not respond to zinc supplementation.

Some owners do manage to clear up the condition with very persistent treatment. This treatment is based on topical application of either eprinexin diluted with dimethyl sulfoxide (DMSO) to affected areas weekly for three months or fipronil spray applied weekly for a similar length of time.

Demodex mites

These rarely cause problems but may be seen without clinical manifestation. They are commonly seen in the ear canal without causing problems. Practitioners should warn owners of the danger of instilling any ear preparations into the ears of SACs. Before any treatment for demodectic mites is undertaken on the body of animals, it is vital to rule out any other causes of dermatitis and to examine healthy animals to try to see demodectic mites. Weekly treatments with 2% povidone iodine scrubbing followed by 0.05% amitraz have been advocated.

Harvest mites

These are *Thombicular* spp. They may cause temporary pruritis. However, they are an environmental mite and do not reproduce on SACs, so any infestation will be self-limiting. Owners should not spray SACs without careful investigation.

Psoroptes mites

The mites found on SACs are indistinguishable from those causing sheep scab and so it is to be expected that SACs become infected from this source. Equally it is likely that SACs can harbour the mites and spread them to healthy sheep. They are also indistinguishable from the mites affecting rabbits. It is very likely that *Psoroptes ovis* and *Psoroptes cuniculi* are the same species. They can infect all areas of the animal. However, they are particularly likely to be found on the ears and in the ear canal. Treatment with injectable avermectins three times at weekly intervals is normally successful.

Sarcoptes mites

These mites may well be more common than was previously thought as differentiation from

C. bovis is not easy. The mite that has been found on SACs is *Sarcoptes scabiei* var. *auchinae*. It should be remembered that this mite is a potential zoonosis. It causes more intense pruritis than *C. bovis*. Mites can be found all over the body. There will be hyperaemia, papules and pustules with crusting. As the mite seems to burrow deeper than *C. bovis*, treatment with regular avermectins by injection seems to be effective.

Vitamin and Mineral Related Skin Diseases

Cobalt deficiency

Deficient animals will have a rough brittle haircoat or wool. Other deficiency signs (e.g. weight loss) may be severe.

Copper deficiency

The other signs of copper deficiency are much more important (see Chapter 2). However, black SACs will show a lack of pigment. Fibre animals will show a lack of crimp.

Iodism

Alopecia and scaling will be seen in SACs if they are fed foods very rich in iodine (e.g. seaweed) over long periods of time.

Sulfur deficiency

This is extremely rare but has been reported in SACs. It is more marked in fleece animals as there is fleece biting and alopecia. Diagnosis can be made from serum or liver samples.

Vitamin A deficiency

It is extremely rare for SACs to be fed a diet deficient in vitamin A. The coat will show a generalized seborrhoea. However, the main sign is an irreversible retinal atrophy causing blindness.

Vitamin C deficiency

This deficiency has been recognized in SACs. It is non-pruritic and shows marked alopecia and some scaling. It may not be a true deficiency but rather a vitamin C responsive alopecia.

Vitamin E deficiency

This condition is seen in SACs. It is not a real deficiency but rather a vitamin E/selenium responsive dermatosis. The animals appear healthy and are non-pruritic but lose their hair.

Zinc deficiency

This is rarely a zinc deficiency but usually a zinc responsive condition. There is marked scaling and crusting. Clinicians should remember that any blood samples for zinc levels must be taken into bottles without rubber stoppers or erroneous results will be obtained. It is a very over-diagnosed condition. The majority of camelid feeds have adequate zinc levels.

Physical Causes of Skin Disease

General

Clinicians should never forget commonplace trauma. Air gun pellets will cause abscesses, normally on the flank. They may be found when lanced or confirmed quite simply with a rectal linear ultrasound scanner. Tethered animals will develop tether galls or bell strap galls. Working llamas may get saddle sores. These are welfare issues and owners should be counselled carefully. Chronic foot lameness in the front legs will result in excessive kneeling and the formation of hygromas on the carpi. Burn cases will often result in keloids and crusty nodules.

Frostbite

This condition has been seen in SACs when outside in extreme weather conditions. It is normally the ears that are affected. The skin will slough. The animals should be given antibiotics to prevent secondary bacterial infection and NSAIDs to lessen the pain. Obviously the animals should be brought inside until the weather improves.

Photosensitization

Sunburn will cause crusting in photosensitized animals. This condition occurs because of the presence of photodynamic substances in the skin capable of causing severe dermatitis in the presence of sunlight. Such agents release energy obtained from the light in hyperoxidative processes harmful to the skin. This may be primary as a result of a photodynamic agent (for example a plant, e.g. St John's wort *Hypericum perforatum*; see Chapter 16) or a photosensitizing drug (e.g. phenothiazine), or secondary due to impairment of liver function resulting in failure to denature chlorophyll and build-up of the photodynamic agent phylloerythrin in tissues. The plant bog asphodel *Narthrecium ossifragum* has been implicated in this secondary type (see Chapter 16).

The clinical signs typically occur in non-pigmented areas of the animals free from fibre in alpacas and anywhere on llamas. Diagnosis may be made on clinical grounds with confirmation by showing raised serum levels of phylloerythrin and, in the case of hepatogenous disease, raised levels of serum liver enzymes. Animals should be housed and any severely affected areas treated with oily creams. The condition is often first seen when animals are turned out on to lush green pastures (e.g. silage aftermaths), having been on poor pasture. The liver is unable to cope with the increased amounts of dietary chlorophyll.

Sunburn

The harmful effects of ultraviolet radiation from direct sunlight in shorn alpacas should not be forgotten as a potential cause of skin damage particularly in areas where there is no shade. Encrustment of the non-pigmented skin with ultimate necrosis of the epidermis, upper dermis and superficial sebaceous glands may occur. Animals should be housed and oily creams applied to the affected areas. Antibiotics and NSAIDs may be required in severe cases.

Trauma

SACs can obviously be burnt by either a naked flame or a hot piece of metal. There are some more unusual forms of trauma, e.g. attacks by magpies. Shearing wounds are sadly rather common.

Toxic Causes of Skin Diseases

Milk toxicity

Crias will develop toxicity similar to photosensitization when suckling on dams that are suffering from hepatic toxicity from eating certain poisonous plants, e.g. Sacahuista bear-grass (see Chapter 16).

Tick toxicosis

This occurs sporadically. Several species of tick have been incriminated. The tick, usually a pregnant female, produces a toxin that causes a systemic disease. All the fibre falls off leaving a thickened, reddened skin. The animal will recover if kept out of the sunlight and given antibiotics parenterally to prevent secondary infection. The animal should have all the sore areas covered with oily cream.

Neoplastic Conditions

The malignant tumours that may occur in the skin anywhere on the body are histiocytomas, lymphosarcomas, malignant melanomas and squamous cell carcinomas. The latter occur in the conjunctiva, on the third eyelid, on the penis and on the vulva. Melanomas are not restricted to white SACs. They can occur in animals of other colours.

Skin Diseases of Uncertain Aetiology

Munge

This a condition described in camels. Its correct name is idiopathic, necrolytic, neutrophilic, hyperkeratotic dermatosis. It can only be diagnosed by taking skin biopsies. Invariably chorioptic mites will be found. It is an over-diagnosed condition. Practitioners should be careful before considering taking skin biopsies as the damaged skin may not heal.

Pemphigus foliaceus

This condition causes a diagnostic challenge for the clinician. It is an autoimmune mediated disease (Fig. 14.4). Bacteria, fungi and even parasites may well be found as secondary invaders. If the skin condition persists after treatment for these conditions the practitioner should suspect pemphigus. It can be confirmed by a biopsy. The main presenting signs include a generalized severe pustular eruption involving most of the body. Treatment is difficult as all the secondary bacteria, fungi and parasites have to be removed before regular steroid treatment is carried out. Although in theory dexamethasone should not be effective if given orally, that has not been the author's experience. The dose is 2 mg/kg given every other morning throughout the summer in temperate countries. Normally the condition calms down during the winter months only to flare up again in the spring.

Wool slip

This condition is associated with winter shearing. It seems to affect animals in poor conditions. There may be a link with either low copper levels or secondary low copper as a result of high molybdenum levels. This alopecia is non-pruritic and the underlying skin appears normal. There is no treatment. Prevention can be carried out by raising the nutritional level at times of stress, e.g. changing the time of shearing/housing.

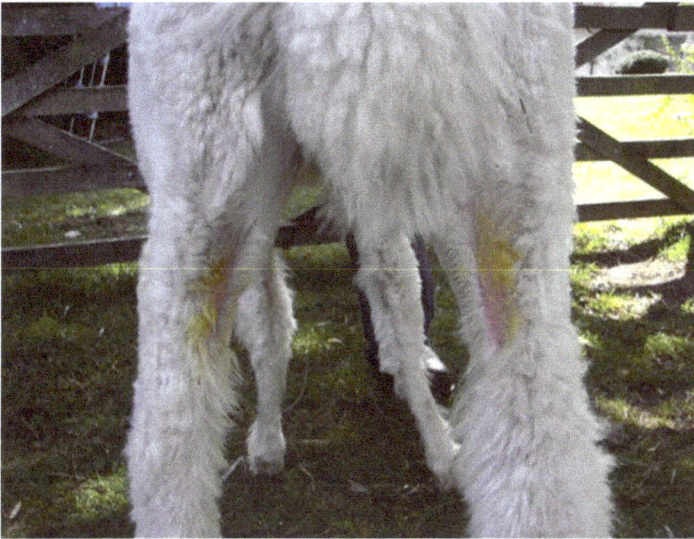

Fig. 14.4. Pemphigus foliaceus.

15

Cause of Sudden Death and Post-Mortem Technique

Survey of Medical Conditions of Concern on Alpaca and Llama Farms

A survey carried out by Stephanie J. Mitro (personal communication) requesting the top five to ten diseases or problems encountered on alpaca and llama farms revealed a broad spectrum of concerns that vary significantly in some respects among farm owners and the veterinarians that care for these animals. The survey, having been sent out over a camelid internet list-server, yielded a total of 78 responses, 50 of which were owners and the other 28 comprising veterinarians. Responses from various geographic regions included Australia, Italy, Argentina, Canada and 24 states in the USA. Sadly there were none from the UK, Eire or New Zealand.

The top medical concerns among owners were parasitism, illness and defects in crias, reproductive problems, skin disorders, nutritional imbalances, and gastrointestinal disorders. Veterinarians, on the other hand, noted oral health as the number one medical concern followed closely by reproductive problems, parasitism, illness and defects in crias, skin disorders, and nutritional imbalances. These top six categories listed for each group comprised approximately 64% of the owners' and 61% of the veterinarians' main concerns in overall camelid health.

Of the owners that responded to the survey, 16.9% noted endoparasites as well as some ectoparasites as a major concern on their farms. Parasites of particular concern included meningeal worms, coccidiosis, liver flukes, tapeworms, and the ectoparasites of mites, lice and ticks. Only 10.1% of veterinarians compared to 16.9% of owners noted parasites as high on their list of priorities. Although parasites were still among the top five in priority, oral health ranked number one with 12.3% of veterinarians noting the importance of dental maintenance of camelids. Only 4.7% of owners, interestingly, noted oral health as a high priority. Problems noted within this category included abscessed teeth, long incisors and mandibular disease. As one can see there are varying ideas between owners and veterinarians as to the areas of major consequence in camelid health and management. A breakdown of the disease problem categories between owners and veterinarians has been provided in Table 15.1 for reference in comparing the two groups' concerns with each area. The percentages highlighted in bold are areas of major concern for both owners and veterinarians for easier comparison of the two.

Among complaints with crias, ranked second among owners and fourth among vets, were the following: failure of passive transfer, weakness, diarrhoea, congenital anomalies and deformities, septicaemia and poor weight gain. Reproductive problems noted included uterine infection, dystocia, abortion, uterine torsion,

© Graham R. Duncanson 2023. *Veterinary Treatment of Llamas and Alpacas,* 2nd Edition
(G.R. Duncanson)
DOI: 10.1079/9781800623576.0015

prolapsed uterus and vulvular discharge. Skin disorders comprised primarily those of idiopathic origin and zinc deficiency. Obesity, various deficiencies as well as toxicities from the soil of certain geographical regions, and the problem of keeping weight on some animals comprised the category of nutritional imbalances. Of most concern with gastrointestinal (GI) problems were ulcers and diarrhoea; however, peritonitis, GI obstructions, colic and choke were also noted. Ocular abnormalities included infections, traumatic injuries, corneal ulcers, cataracts and glaucoma. And finally within the 'other' category, owners noted individual cases of a heart murmur, urinary tract infection, ear trauma and mastitis, while veterinarians also noted a urinary tract infection and ear trauma, along with urinary calculi, neurological disease, unexplained fever, mammary adenocarcinoma, management issues, and the threat of foreign animal disease.

Geographic areas represented by owners and veterinarians and their major concerns were the following:

- Within Western USA (states including Colorado (2), Oregon (2), Washington (3) and California (2)) owners noted reproduction, cria illnesses and deformities, parasites, and dermatitis among top concerns, while vets added dental problems and GI illness to this list and showed less concern for parasites as a major problem.
- In the Southern States (Texas (4), Florida, Georgia, Tennessee, New Mexico and Alabama), owners' primary concerns were with parasites followed by dermatitis, cria illness, nutrition, abscesses, and GI disorders. Vets in this area made no note of concern for dermatitis or GI disorders, but tended to agree with the concern about parasites, primarily meningeal worm, and also were concerned with abscessed teeth.
- Owners in the Eastern States (Pennsylvania (2), New York (3), Virginia (2), North Carolina, New Jersey, Massachusetts and Vermont) recognized major problems with cria illness, parasites, namely meningeal worm, nutrition, and lameness. Vets tended to agree with all of these chief concerns with the exception of lameness and expanded on the list, adding abscessed teeth, dermatitis, and foot/nail and reproductive problems.

- Within the Midwest (Michigan (3), Ohio (3), Indiana (2), Kentucky and Kansas) owners noted parasites, lameness, nutrition and GI disorders primarily, while vets' concerns were focused on dental problems as well as meningeal worms.
- One veterinarian from Alaska ranked premature crias, parasites, dermatitis, vitamin D deficiencies, teeth abscesses, osteomyelitis and colic among top interests in camelid health, and an owner from Montana noted zinc deficiencies, strongyle worms, arthritis, and reproductive problems of importance to him.
- Outside of the USA, Canadian owners from British Columbia and Ontario noted lameness, cria diarrhoea, nutrition, and GI disorders of significant concern. The one vet that contributed to the survey from the area also mentioned dystocia, teeth abscesses and osteomyelitis, foot/nail problems, parasites, ocular disorders, and dermatitis.
- There was one veterinarian from Argentina whose concerns included primarily fatalities caused by clostridiosis, but also noted some problems with sarcocystosis, rotavirus infections, bovine herpes virus, and leptospirosis.
- A vet from Italy also noted clostridiosis as a major problem along with parasites, GI disorders, vitamin D deficiencies, heat stress, tooth abscesses, ocular disease and breeding problems.
- Lastly, two Australian veterinarians noted vitamin D and selenium deficiencies, parasite infections (*Haemonchus*) and liver disease to be of major importance along with dermatitis, GI disorders, and heat stress.

In reviewing the differences briefly between the issues of camelid health and management that owners and veterinarians find most pertinent, it is evident that some discussion needs to be initiated between the two groups so as to address both sides' concerns and provide better care for alpacas and llamas. If nothing else, this survey should at least open both owners' and veterinarians' eyes to the major concerns of the other and hopefully stir up some interest to learn more about the other group's concerns and how they need to be addressed to secure more effective management practices leading to healthy animals and financial gain within the camelid industry.

Table 15.1. A survey by owners and veterinarians of their major concerns

Disease problems	Owners	Veterinarians
Parasites	**16.9%**	**10.1%**
Cria illness/defects	**12.2%**	**9.5%**
Reproduction	**9.3%**	**11.2%**
Dermatitis	**9.3%**	**8.9%**
Nutritional imbalances	**8.1%**	**8.9%**
Gastrointestinal	**8.1%**	8.4%
Lameness	6.4%	2.2%
Oral health	4.7%	**12.3%**
Abscesses	4.7%	0.0%
Wasting disease	0.6%	4.5%
Ocular	2.9%	5.9%
Heat stress	2.9%	3.4%
Respiratory	1.2%	2.2%
Arthritis	2.9%	0.0%
Foot/nail injuries	1.7%	2.8%
Liver disease	0.6%	2.8%
Bacterial/viral	2.9%	2.2%
Other	3.5%	5.0%

The fact that the UK, Eire and New Zealand as well as several South American countries did not contribute to this survey does not mean that the results are not pertinent in those countries.

Iatrogenic Causes of Sudden Death

Sudden death is a misnomer. In reality it is found dead since last seen. The owner will very rarely see an animal die. It is even rarer for the clinician to see death. Sadly when such deaths occur it is usually at the time of veterinary treatment. The likely causes of iatrogenic deaths in SACs are shown in Table 15.2.

Anaphylaxis from administration of medicines

This must be a very rare event. It has been reported following the use of the antibiotic tilmicosin, 'Micotil', which is licensed in sheep. This antibiotic has been associated with sudden deaths in SACs and should not be used in this species.

General anaesthesia

General anaesthesia in adult animals is bound to carry a high risk, particularly if the surgery

Table 15.2. Possible iatrogenic causes of sudden death.

Anaphylaxis from administration of medicines
General anaesthesia
Lumbar/sacral collection of cerebrospinal fluid
Massive haemorrhage (this could occur at
    parturition where there is no human involvement)
Intra-arterial injection
Intravenous injection
Sedation

is likely to be long and gaseous anaesthesia is required. The risk can be minimized by careful monitoring and supervision of recovery.

Lumbar/sacral collection of cerebrospinal fluid

Lumbar/sacral collection of cerebrospinal fluid (CSF) is not a hazardous procedure. However, unless clinicians have been adequately trained it is a procedure that does have risks as the spinal cord is actually present at this site.

Massive haemorrhage

This can occur at parturition without human interference. However, it is extremely rare without trauma caused by rough parturition techniques. Very great care should be taken by clinicians when assisting the parturition, particularly in small alpacas. Haemorrhage occurs from the middle uterine artery. This artery may also be ruptured at the time of uterine prolapse.

Intra-arterial injection

This type of injection is always an error. However, it is relatively common with most clinicians admitting that it has occurred when they have been attempting an intravenous injection in SACs. The carotid artery lies just deep to the jugular vein in the caudal third of the neck.

Intravenous injection

There are no licensed medicines in SACs in the UK. Most medicines that are licensed for sheep and cattle can be used in SACs using the cascade principle. There are certain licensed medicines that anecdotally cause collapse and death in cattle and horses when given intravenously. The most notable are potentiated sulfonamides and vitamin B complexes. It is not suggested that these medicines are never given intravenously. However, clinicians should consider carefully before using them by this route and should always inject them extremely slowly. It is well known that magnesium sulfate, which is supplied in a 25% solution, should never be given intravenously to any animal but only subcutaneously. Even the 5% solution should be injected very slowly if given intravenously.

Table 15.3. Causes of sudden death.

Anthrax
Cast on the back
Chemical poisons
Clostridial disease
Drowning (this may occur at dipping or in deep
    water)
Electrocution
Hypomagnesaemia
Lightning strike
Poisonous plants
Ruptured aneurysm
Ruptured uterine artery
Snake bite
Trauma (this is mainly road traffic accidents or
    fighting in males)

Sedation

Although xylazine is widely used as a sedative it should be used with caution. The safety margin is not large. It is prudent to dilute the 2% solution, which is manufactured for cattle, when injecting crias and young growing alpacas. Weights can be deceptive particularly in fleece-covered animals. Accurate weighing is very useful. Very small doses of xylazine are required.

Reasons for Animals to be Found Dead

True sudden deaths are very rare. Possible causes of sudden deaths in SACs are shown in Table 15.3.

Anthrax

This is not easy to diagnose from gross pathology in SACs. As it is so rare clinicians are unlikely to take a blood smear and find the classical bacteria with their capsules. Obviously if an enlarged spleen is found on post-mortem anthrax should be suspected. In cattle, haemorrhages are seen from external body orifices. This feature is not often seen in SACs. However, there will be enlarged lymph nodes with ecchymoses and petechiae seen on the mucosal surfaces.

Cast on the back

This is only a problem in an over-fat, unshorn pregnant female, heavy in the wool, which has rolled into a depression. Animals can survive for many hours and will recover when righted. However, it is vital that the individual is shorn without delay as they often will be cast again in the next 48 h.

Chemical poisons

There are very few chemicals that will actually cause sudden death, as normally quite large quantities need to be consumed. Metaldehyde in 'slug bait' is a possibility, as is nicotine from a pipe smoker's pouch full of tobacco. Both these poisons will be found in compartment one of the stomach (C1). Normally lead poisoning is a chronic toxicity but acute deaths with neurological signs will be seen when animals have ingested paint from old gates or doors. The paint will readily be seen in C1.

Clostridial disease

This is the most likely cause of sudden death in well-fed SACs. *Clostridium perfringens* types A, C and D will all cause sudden death. It is nearly always seen in animals that have access to lush grass. Type D has been seen in animals on high-concentrate diets. There is rapid autolysis. An excess of abdominal fluid and pericardial fluid will be seen. The small intestine will be hyperaemic and ulcerated. Diagnosis can be confirmed by toxin neutralization tests. Glucosuria is only seen in sheep and not in SACs. *C. chauvoei* will cause black leg in ruminants; there is doubt if it has been seen in SACs. Given the circumstances (e.g. a contaminated needle from an injection), it is likely that it would occur. There will be an area of crepitus. Smears should be taken for testing for fluorescent antibodies. *C. novyi*, which will cause 'Black's disease' in ruminants, has not been recorded in SACs. *C. septicum* will cause sudden death in SACs. Oedematous swellings without any gas formation will be seen. *C. botulinum* has not been recorded in SACs but it is certainly likely to occur as it has been seen by the author in camels in northern Kenya.

Drowning

The diagnosis is likely to be obvious, with the lungs being full of water or dip. Inhalation pneumonia from incorrect drenching technique will not cause sudden death.

Electrocution

This is an extremely rare cause of death. It is only likely to occur if an animal gets tangled up in an electric fence powered from the mains. Young animals might chew through electric leads, resulting in electrocution.

Hypomagnesaemia

This condition can occur, though it is extremely rare in SACs. The classic situation for the disease to occur is when the grass has been very heavily fertilized. Actual sudden death is unusual. The area around the carcass should be examined carefully, as often the signs of the convulsions before death will be seen. Normally the animal will be recumbent showing severe neurological signs, which even with magnesium treatment

are irreversible. A serum blood test from an animal that is still alive will be diagnostic. Testing the aqueous humor from a carcass will be helpful. Haemorrhages may be seen on the endocardium but these are not actually diagnostic but only indicate that the animal has died after having convulsions. However, the history will indicate that hypomagnesaemia is a possible cause.

Lightning strike

Diagnosis is likely to be circumstantial. There has to have been a thunderstorm in the last 24 h! The whole body should be examined for signs of burning. Then careful skinning should be performed so that lines of subcuticular haemorrhages are not missed.

Poisonous plants

There are poisonous plants that will cause sudden death in SACs. However, these are rarely consumed in large enough quantities to bring about almost instant death. Diagnosis of plant poisoning can be made by examination of the contents of C1. The plant that is often quoted in the textbooks is yew. This certainly causes sudden death in cattle, which require very little to cause rapid death. The author has seen a case in an alpaca. However, there is considerable doubt now if yew is as toxic to small ruminants as previously thought (Angus, 2010; Scott, 2010; Stevenson and Swarbick, 2010). These authors indicate that certain breeds of sheep and deer are relatively resistant. However, herd and flock owners should still be vigilant, particularly when other feeds are not available, e.g. in snowy conditions.

Llamas are particularly at risk from plant poisoning when tethered on a trek. In this scenario normal feed will be eaten first and then the animals may consume a large volume of a toxic plant. Obviously alpacas and llamas are at risk if they escape from their normal habitat or if they are presented with cut toxic plants on rubbish dumps or compost heaps.

If plant poisoning is suspected then the mouth should be checked to see if there are any parts of the plant still in the mouth. Some plants containing alkaloids that directly affect the heart are so toxic that death will occur instantly. SACs will die very rapidly if they consume laburnum seed pods. The area around the body should be checked for evidence of browsing.

Ruptured aneurysm

Aneurysms can occur anywhere in the animal. If they occur in the brain the animal will be found dead. Diagnosis without multiple histological sections will be very difficult. If the rupture occurs in the mesenteric vessels then the abdomen will be full of blood. This is seen in horses on account of the damage done to mesenteric blood vessels by the migration of large strongyle larvae. This does not happen in SACs so such a rupture is extremely rare.

Ruptured uterine artery

This is a very rare occurrence in SACs and is seldom seen. It may occur while there is an assisted parturition but more commonly the parturient animal is found dead, with the cria alive and well. Obviously on post-mortem the abdomen will be full of blood.

Snake bite

The author doubts that an adder would have sufficient venom to kill an alpaca or llama in the UK. However, in countries where there are more venomous snakes this is certainly a possibility. Normally animals are bitten on the face and so the small puncture wounds should be looked for if the head is swollen.

Trauma

The signs shown from road traffic accidents will be broken bones, subcutaneous haemorrhage and rupture of internal organs. Trauma from fighting in males will be obvious externally and can be checked with careful skinning of the neck. This will reveal the haemorrhages from the bites.

Careful examination of the neck may also reveal a fracture. Very great care will be required opening the neck vertebrae to examine the spinal cord. Samples should be taken for histology.

Post-Mortem Examinations

Equipment required

- Large plastic bucket with disinfectant, warm water, soap and towel;
- Butcher's knife and flaying knife;
- Scalpel and blades that fit;
- Rat-toothed forceps (15 cm);
- Fine forceps (15 cm);
- Blunt-nosed straight scissors (20 cm);
- Bowel scissors;
- Bone cutters, saw and hedge loppers.

Sampling materials

- Plastic trays (50 × 30 × 5 cm);
- Plastic bags of various sizes;
- Sterile universal bottles;
- Plastic jars (1 l);
- Bottles of formalin (kept separate);
- Pots containing 50% glycerol for virus isolation;
- Swabs (plain, transport media and specialized for respiratory pathogens);
- Vaccutainers:
  - Red top – serum – routine serology and biochemistry
  - Green top – heparin – glutathione peroxidase (selenium)
  - Lilac top – EDTA – haematology
  - Grey top – oxidase/fluoride – glucose
  - Blue top – acid wash – special ions, e.g. Zn
- Pasteur pipettes and rubber sucker;
- Clip-board;
- Post-mortem report form, lab submission form.

Sampling

1. If the animal is presented alive and blood is required for examination, then it is better to take it before the animal is killed.

2. If you require examination of the brain then it is better to use chemicals for euthanasia, rather than a humane killer or free bullet.

3. Before sampling it must be decided if swabs are going to be taken and/or bacteriological plates are going to be prepared immediately.

4. Abnormal lymph nodes should be transacted and put into two universal bottles. These must be labelled. One will be kept fresh and the other at a later stage will be filled with 10% formalin.

5. As a rule of thumb there should be ten parts of formalin to one part of tissue.

6. Impression smears should be taken from the cut surfaces of any malignant oedema subcutaneous tissues or muscles and air dried.

7. Individual samples can be put into plastic bags or universal bottles. If histology is required at a later date, 10% formalin can be added.

8. Urine can be collected into a universal bottle (testing for glucose is not useful for the diagnosis in SACs of possible clostridial disease).

9. Milk can be collected into a universal bottle.

10. Faeces can be collected from the rectum.

11. Blood samples can be taken from the heart blood. These would not be useful for biochemistry or haematology. However, certain serological examinations are useful and a zinc sulfate turbidity test is meaningful in young crias.

12. The entire thyroid gland should be dissected out for later weighing.

13. Samples of diseased lung should be taken from the edge of the lesions after swabs have been taken. As antibiotics do not penetrate consolidated lung tissue, samples for bacteriology can be taken from such a site.

14. Samples from abscesses should include scrapings from the interior of the abscess wall.

15. Abnormal heart lesions are often best examined microscopically after swabs have been taken of the heart blood.

16. Swabs should be taken from joint cavities.

17. Muscles can be stored fresh in plastic bags, or bottles and some should be put aside to have 10% formalin added later.

18. Smears can be made from bone marrow and some can be retained to have an addition of 10% formalin later.

19. Swabs should be taken from liver, spleen and kidney.

20. 100 g of both liver and kidney should be retained for toxicology.

Only after these samples have been taken are the intestines examined and opened:

1. Bezoars should be preserved in universal bottles.

2. 1 kg of rumen contents should be taken into a plastic bag for toxicology.

3. The contents of C1 should be examined carefully for the presence of poisonous plants. If they are found they should be stored in plastic bags for identification.

4. The contents of C1 can be tested for thiaminase to diagnose cerebro-cortico-necrosis (CCN).

5. For helminthological studies, the entire contents of C3 and/or the small intestine should be collected into a large jar for washing and sieving later.

6. The contents of affected parts of the small intestine should be collected into universal bottles (minimum 20 ml) to examine for clostridial toxins.

7. 30 g of caecal contents or faeces should be taken into a plastic bag for worm egg counts and bacterial culture.

8. Histological samples are only worthwhile from the intestines if the carcass is absolutely fresh.

Technique for post-mortem when single handed without a trough to hold the SAC in dorsal recumbency

Examine the external surfaces and feel the superficial lymph nodes. Record the breed and sex.

1. Weigh the SAC and note its condition score.

2. Examine its incisor teeth and its eyes. Take a sample of its aqueous humor into a red vaccutainer.

3. Look at its feet and feel its peripheral leg joints for swellings.

4. Examine the udder/scrotum.

5. Place the SAC in lateral recumbency with its right side uppermost.

6. With a knife cut through the skin in the axilla and the muscles of the shoulder so that the whole of the right foreleg can be reflected back to lie on the floor.

7. With a knife make a bold cut through the skin in the groin. Cut through the muscles into the hip joint, cutting the femoral ligament, and lay the right hindleg on the floor.

8. Flay the skin from the front leg caudally along the midline to the incision near the hindleg so the skin can be laid back over the backbone. The inside surface can be used to lay out visceral organs.

9. Flay the skin from the front leg rostrally up to the head so the teeth and mandible are exposed.

10. At the xiphisternum carefully open the abdomen with a pair of blunt-nosed scissors and make an incision along the midline caudally to the pelvis.

11. Make a second incision through the body wall from the xiphisternum along the line of the last rib to the backbone, so that the abdominal muscles can be reflected.

12. Examine the organs *in situ* in the abdomen. Starting at the xiphisternum C2 will just be visible. Caudal to C2, C3 will just be visible below the liver, which will rise up into the thorax and slightly caudal to the last rib (12th). Caudal to the liver will be seen the glandular saccules of C1. Dorsal to these saccules will be seen the caudal sac of C1. Cranial to this is the duodenum. Caudal to the saccules on the body wall will be seen the proximal loop of the ascending colon. The right kidney will be visible on the dorsal surface of the abdomen halfway between the last rib and the hindleg. The rest of the abdomen will be filled with jejunum. (If the SAC had been placed with its left side uppermost, C3 would be seen lying on the ventral wall of the abdomen with the glandular saccules of C1 just above it. Above them would be seen the caudal sac of C1 reaching up to the spine. Behind the caudal sac of C1 close to the spine the spleen would be seen. The rest of the abdomen is filled with the spiral colon. A small section of the descending colon will be seen caudal to the spleen and a small amount of jejunum will be seen just cranial to the ilium.)

13. Cut the diaphragm with a pair of blunt-nosed scissors under the ribs.

14. With the garden loppers cut the ribs either side of the sternum so it can be removed.

15. Cut the intercostal muscles with a knife between every other rib and then break them back over the backbone.

16. The right lung will now be visible cranially with the liver caudal to it.

17. Starting under the mandible elevate the tongue with a knife so that the whole pluck (i.e. larynx, trachea, lungs and heart) can be removed

for examination later after the oesophagus has been tied. Examine the cheek teeth at this time.

18. Examine the lungs, having cut down the trachea. Sample the heart blood and examine the heart.

19. After tying off the rectum the three compartments of the stomach C1, C2 and C3, the intestines, the spleen and the liver can be removed.

20. Examine the whole of the gastroenteric tract and the lymph nodes from the outside.

21. Take samples after examining the liver and spleen.

22. Away from the carcass open up the gastroenteric tract after taking samples and even milking out the small and large intestines separately for parasite examination. Examine the contents and the mucosal surface.

23. The bladder can be examined and a urine sample can be taken.

24. The female or male genital organs can be examined.

25. The kidneys can be removed and examined.

26. After this the head can be removed from the neck and the brain can be removed.

27. The brain should be examined for CCN.

If there is a proper post-mortem table available the post-mortem can be performed with the SAC in dorsal recumbency.

Removal of the brain

This is not an easy procedure. Clinicians should take special care for health and safety reasons. Goggles and face masks should be worn. Rubber gloves should be worn as for all post-mortem examinations. The skin over the head including the ears should be flayed away from the bones of the skull. Using a meat saw two parallel cuts are made through the skull in a rostral-caudal direction laterally to the eyes. A third saw cut is made across the nasal bone just caudal to the eye sockets joining the two lateral cuts. A final fourth saw cut is made across the caudal aspect of the cranium linking the caudal ends of the two lateral saw cuts. The skull can then be lifted off, revealing the brain underneath. This should be examined for gross pathology and then examined under fluorescent light to diagnose CCN. The brain can then be removed to take histological samples after any bacterial samples have been collected.

Post-mortem examinations of neonatal crias and aborted fetuses

1. It should be remembered that mummified fetuses are useless for diagnostic purposes.
2. The placenta as well as the aborted cria can be sent to a referral laboratory if possible.

3. If a fetus cannot be sent then fresh peritoneal fluid, pleural fluid and C3 contents should be sent on ice if possible, together with fresh liver. A totally separate small piece of liver in formalin should be sent.

They will look for *Brucella*, but as practitioners you will be aware it does not occur in the UK. They will also look for *Toxoplasma*, *Chlamydophila*, *Listeria* and *Salmonella* as well as doing general bacteriology.

16

Poisons

_____

Introduction

The first problem with poisoning cases is establishing a diagnosis. If the poison is definitely known, that is obviously very helpful. However, owners in the UK are often very keen to wrongly blame farmers for suspected poisonous sprays, so any history needs to be taken with caution. If there has definitely been a spilled chemical, then the clinician should make sure this fact is used immediately so that any antidote can be obtained while the patient is being brought in. Equally if a plant has been eaten, the clinician should make sure the owners pass on the name of the plant so the toxicity can be checked and treatment can be readied while the animal is being brought in. If a plant has definitely been eaten but they do not know what it is, the clinician should make sure the owners bring some of the plant in with them. It needs to be stressed that the leaves and the fruit and maybe even the roots are required to help identification. Also clinicians should remember to tell the owner to remove any other animals away from the toxic plant or substance.

If the alpaca or llama is seriously ill a full clinical examination should be carried out. Clinicians must not base a diagnosis exclusively on the history of exposure to the poison. If there are no helpful diagnostic signs and the poison is unknown, a drip of normal isotonic saline with

a 16G catheter should be set up. Clinicians should remember that the saline must be warm. Efforts should be made to make sure that the animal itself is warmed up by being not only in a warm place but also having hot water bottles around it. There are commercial coats available for crias, alpacas and llamas. Obviously if the poison is known and there is a specific treatment available, this should be given as a priority. Otherwise the clinician should carry out symptomatic treatment. The practitioner needs to make a careful clinical judgement if the animal is _in extremis_. Welfare must be considered. Euthanasia must be considered. If there are several animals affected it may be kinder to put the really badly affected animals to sleep and concentrate on treating the animals that could possibly survive.

Notes should be taken as poisoning cases often lead to litigation or to insurance claims. It is likely that any animals that have died or are put to sleep will have to be post-mortemed. Careful notes once again should be taken with a full identification. Obviously carefully labelled samples will need to be collected (see Chapter 15).

With animals that are found dead, it is important to try to establish a time of death. The owner may be convinced that it has been sudden but in reality it may be that they have not looked at the animals for a length of time (see Chapter 15).

© Graham R. Duncanson 2023. _Veterinary Treatment of Llamas and Alpacas_, 2nd Edition (G.R. Duncanson)
DOI: 10.1079/9781800623576.0016

Information Required from a Suspected Poisoning Case

- Owner (manager if different);
- Address;
- Contact phone numbers plus fax plus email address;
- Illness in previous 12 months;
- Exposure to other animals in last 21 days;
- Vaccination history with other medications, including wormers and topical medicines;
- Location, e.g. pasture, wood, waste ground, garden, pond and housing;
- Recent change of location, e.g. transport to shows, access to waste, old construction materials, mining, dredging;
- Recent deaths;
- Age, sex, pregnancy, weight loss;
- Size of total herd and size of group (shared feed or water between groups);
- Morbidity and mortality;
- Date of first animal to be seen sick or dead;
- Onset and progression of signs;
- Malicious threats or new staff;
- Recent changes in feed or pasture;
- Weeds or moulds;
- Insecticides, acaricides, anthelmintics, herbicides and rodenticides;
- Outside services, e.g. tree planting, pasture seeding, fertilizing, burning, building construction;
- Changes of diet, including new hay, hard feed, spoilt feed, etc.;
- Pasture type, e.g. bare, lush, weeds present.

Clinical Sign Checklist

- Neurological: ataxia, salivation, blindness, impaired vision, depression, excitement, seizures, head pressing, cerebellar signs, weakness, dysphonia.
- Gastroenteric: anorexia, polyphagia, polydipsia, colic, vomiting, diarrhoea, melena, icterus, tenesmus.
- Respiratory: dyspnoea, tachypnoea.
- Cardiovascular: arrhythmia, bradycardia, tachycardia, anaemia, oedema, haemorrhage, haematuria, icterus, haemoglobinuria, fever, weakness.
- Urino-genital: anuria, polyuria, haematuria, anoestrus, hyperoestrogenism, agalactia, abortion, stillbirth.

Clinical and Post-Mortem Specimens for Toxicology

- Blood: 10 ml in EDTA (purple top vaccutainer) chill and submit on ice if possible.
- Serum: 10 ml (red top vaccutainer) before death or from heart blood after death. Spin remove clot; submit chilled or frozen.
- Brain: send half frozen and half in formal saline.
- Cerebrospinal fluid: 4 ml if possible, chilled.
- Ocular fluid: 4 ml chilled or frozen.
- Contents of C1, C2, C3 and intestines; 1 kg from each should be taken and frozen.
- Injection site: 100 g frozen for drug residues.
- Liver: 200 g frozen.
- Kidney: 200 g frozen.
- Urine: 100 ml, half chilled, half frozen.

Plant Collection

The ideal method of preserving a suspected toxic plant is to freeze it. If this is not possible, it should be partially dried and then placed in a paper bag. This should then be placed in an oven at 150°F (65°C) for 12 h to totally dry the plant. Plants should not be microwaved or refrigerated.

It is very difficult to find plants in hay as they will not be evenly distributed. It is better to examine the area from which the hay or silage was cut.

Diagnostic Criteria

- History;
- Clinical signs;
- Clinical laboratory evaluation;
- Post-mortem picture;
- Chemical evaluation.

Evaluation of Water Drunk by Possible Poisoned Animals

- Salt content;
- Sulfate content;
- Nitrite/nitrate content;
- Algae;
- Hardness;

- Minerals;
- pH;
- Bacteria;
- Temperature.

Treatment

The first effort must be to try to prevent further absorption of the toxin. The clinician should consider trying to empty the first compartment of the stomach (C1). If the animal is very ill and a specific treatment is not being given, the practitioner has very little to lose. A general anaesthetic is not given as a local block is going to be used in the left paralumbar fossa. Entry into C1 may well make a diagnosis by finding the plant in the organ. It is advisable to stitch C1 to the peritoneum of the abdomen so there will be very little contamination. Any remaining plant toxins can be removed by removing the ingesta and flushing C1. The animal can be rehydrated by half filling C1 with electrolytes. A proprietary antacid preparation containing some bicarbonate can be used. If there is a specific treatment then that must be carried out. Also symptomatic treatment in all cases will be useful.

Plant Poisons

Plant poisoning is liable to occur under a variety of circumstances. Obviously if animals are allowed to escape they are in danger of gaining access to toxic plants. Tethered animals or animals on a trek are at risk if they are short of food and only have access to a plant that they normally would not eat, but which is toxic. Llamas and alpacas are at risk from access to garden rubbish or indeed being fed cut toxic plants. Such plants may be presented by mistake as browse or dried in hay or haylage. SACs will find it particularly difficult to reject plants in silage. It is very important to remember that it is a complete myth that llamas and alpacas will not eat plants that are bad for them. SACs originate on the altiplano in South America, which is remarkably free of toxic plants. SACs are therefore particularly prone to ingesting poisonous plants with which they are unfamiliar.

Abrus precatorius (gidee-gidee)

This vine with pink flowers, which turn into curled pods containing red and black seeds, is found throughout the tropical parts of Australia and in the tropical islands to the north of Australia. It is also called the rosary pea or the precatory bean. The seeds are toxic and cause acute enteric signs. The only treatment is supportive.

Acacia berlanderi (guajillo)

This shrub causes poisoning under drought conditions in Mexico. The animals become recumbent but retain their appetite. They will recover with good nursing and a toxin-free diet. Obviously the rest of the flock or herd should be given supplementary feed immediately.

Acer rubrum (red maple)

This tree is found in eastern parts of the USA. It is rarely eaten by SACs except llamas on the trek. It contains an oxidant that will cause haemoglobinuria. If the animals are very anaemic they will need to be given whole blood as a transfusion.

Aconitum napellus (aconite)

This flowering plant of the ranunculus family occurs throughout the world. It is called 'monkshood' in the UK. It takes its name from the dark blue helmet-shaped flowers. It is one of the most poisonous plants in the UK. All parts of the plant are poisonous and contain an alkaloid that causes neurological signs, e.g. recumbency and dilated pupils. These signs lead on to acute depression and death. Treatment including stimulants is ineffective.

Adenium obesum (desert rose)

This plant is found worldwide in hot dry locations. It is sometimes called mock or desert azalea. It is a succulent shrub or small tree with red flowers. It contains cardiac glycosides, but is rarely a problem as it causes vomiting and is not palatable to SACs. The treatment is symptomatic.

Adonis aestivalis (adonis)

There are approximately 35 species of this plant found in Europe and temperate Asia. *A. aestivalis* is found in North America. It was thought to be cardiotoxic and could be ingested in hay. Authors in the USA carried out careful evaluation of its toxicity in sheep (Woods *et al.*, 2011). They concluded that sheep were resistant to intoxication. It is suggested that SACs may also be immune.

Adonis annua (pheasant's eye)

This plant is found in the UK. It should not be confused with *Adonis microcarpa*, which has the same local name in Australia. There has been no record of *A. annua* causing signs of toxicity.

Adonis microcarpa (pheasant's eye)

This annual herb with glossy scarlet flowers is found in the temperate parts of Australia and is grown in gardens in the UK. All of the plant is toxic as it contains a cardiac glycoside. Animals will be found dead. The remainder should be given oral activated charcoal at 5 g/kg with an electrolyte solution by mouth. In theory the cardiac arrhythmias can be controlled by atropine. However, this requires very careful monitoring.

Aesculus hippocastanum (horse chestnut)

This is a very common large tree found in the UK and originated in the Balkans. It contains a saponic glycoside termed aesculin. Harwood *et al.* (2010) reported poisoning in a Cashmere goat. There have been no reports in SACs. The goat showed severe tachycardia and tachypnoea. There was profuse salivation and cyanosis. The main post-mortem signs were respiratory and circulatory. There is no known antidote.

Aesculus spp. (buckeye)

This is a large shrub, which can even grow into a tree, and is found throughout North America.

The young shoots and seeds are particularly poisonous. It causes neurological depression and inflammation of the mucous membranes. Treatment is symptomatic and normally successful.

Aethusa cynapium (fool's parsley)

This herbaceous weed with white flowers occurs in Europe and North America. In the UK it is also known as lesser hemlock. It has a repulsive smell, making it a rare cause of toxicity. It causes recumbency and inappetence. The latter sign aids recovery as normally insufficient amounts of the plant are consumed to cause death. There is no specific antidote and treatment is symptomatic.

Agapanthus orientalis (African blue lily)

This is a tall perennial herb found in gardens worldwide. It is the rhizome that is liable to cause problems in SACs. It causes intense irritation of the tongue and pharynx. The toxin is self-limiting and not dangerous as the symptoms regress in 30 min. Treatment is symptomatic.

Agave americana (American aloe)

This garden plant is found worldwide and may also be called the century plant. Poisoning is self-limiting in SACs as the plant contains irritant oxalates that cause pain and inflammation of the lips, tongue and pharynx. Treatment is symptomatic.

Agave lechuguilla (lechuguilla)

This perennial desert plant is found in the southwest of North America. Large quantities need to be consumed over a few weeks to cause toxicity. This is likely to occur in drought conditions. The plant contains an unidentified liver toxin, which causes photosensitization. The animals need to be brought in out of the sunlight and put on a low-protein diet. Vitamin B injections may be helpful. The plant also contains toxic saponins that can cause abortions. There is no preventative treatment.

Agrostemma githago (corn cockle)

This annual plant is seen in cornfields throughout the world. However, it is rapidly disappearing thanks to improved agricultural methods. The growing plant is avoided by SACs. The only possibility of poisoning is when the seeds are mixed in with grain, which is then fed to llamas or alpacas. The saponins in the seeds cause haemoglobinuria, acute diarrhoea, tachypnoea and death. Blood transfusions are indicated. There is no specific antidote.

Agrostis avenacea (blow-away grass)

This grass occurs in subtropical and temperate areas of Australia. It is also found in New Zealand, New Guinea and on many Pacific islands. There is a complex toxicological process, which results in convulsions and death, called 'floodplain staggers'. The toxic principle is a corynetoxin, which is produced by Rathayibacter toxicus, a bacterium in the seed head nematode galls on the grass. There is a hope to develop cyclodextrin, a toxin binding agent, to be an antidote, but as yet trials have not been successful.

Aleurites fordii (tung oil tree)

This tree used to be grown for its oil on farms in south-eastern USA. It is now found wild in woods and is also grown in gardens. All parts of the tree are toxic. It causes acute bloody diarrhoea, dehydration and death. There is no specific treatment but supportive fluids should be tried.

Allamanda cathartica (golden trumpet)

This is a climbing perennial found in tropical areas of the Americas. It contains lethal alkyl-iridoid terpenoids. Luckily it is very irritant and SACs will not eat sufficient to cause major toxic signs. A llama would require 2 kg to cause major signs and possible death.

Allium spp. (onions)

In theory onions should be toxic to SACs as they are to cattle in large quantities. SACs do not seem to be able to ingest a sufficient quantity to cause toxicity. Wild onions are found in woodlands but do not seem to be eaten by SACs. The species are Allium ursinim, A. vineale and A. oleraceum. They are actually garlics and do not appear to be toxic.

Aloe barbadensis (Curacao aloe)

This succulent herb is also called the Barbados aloe. It is found in the tropical and semitropical parts of the Americas. The young succulent leaves are the most dangerous to SACs as they are attractive and contain high levels of an anthraquinone glycoside, which causes severe diarrhoea. Treatment is symptomatic.

Alstonia constricta (quinine tree)

This tree is found in Queensland and northern parts of New South Wales. The leaves and the fruit are toxic to SACs. They contain indole alkaloids. These cause titanic spasms of the skeletal muscles. Treatment consists of heavy sedation with alpha-2 agonists.

Amaranthus retroflexus (redroot pigweed)

This plant occurs in North America. SACs will eat it if there is no other food available. It causes hindleg paralysis and eventual death. There is no antidote.

Amianthium muscaetoxicum (stagger grass)

This is a perennial herb found in acid soils on the eastern seaboard of North America. It is not normally touched by SACs unless there is absolutely no other food available. Such an occasion might be a on a trek. It causes death by respiratory depression. There is no antidote. The animal should be destroyed if in extremis.

Ammi majus (bishop's weed)

This herb is found in the temperate areas of Australia, where it causes problems. It originated in the Nile valley. It contains furano-coumarins, which cause photosensitization and the more serious corneal oedema. The animals should be brought in to the dark. Non-steroidal anti-inflammatory drugs (NSAIDs) should be injected and put as drops into the eyes.

Anabena spp., *Aphanizomenon* spp. and *Microcystis* spp. (algae)

Algae cause poisoning by high concentrations of specific species of blue-green algae in the drinking water. It is often a problem in still inland lakes, e.g. the Norfolk Broads in the UK. The acute form of toxicity will kill the animals within 1 h. The presenting sign is cyanosis. In more chronic cases there is photosensitization shown on the faces of white-faced llamas as crusty lesions. All animals will show raised liver enzymes. The diagnosis is made by collecting the algae for the laboratory. The treatment is supportive, obviously removing the animal from the contaminated water and providing clean water is vital.

Apocynum spp. (dogbane)

This is a large perennial herb found in open woods throughout North America. The toxic glycoside, which it contains, causes dilated pupils and congested mucous membranes. Symptomatic treatment with intravenous warm isotonic saline may be successful.

Arachis hypogaea (peanut hay)

This should not be fed to SACs as it will cause an acute respiratory syndrome, similar to fog fever in cattle. There is a specific antidote, which is methylene blue at 10 mg/kg given slowly intravenously. The best approach is to set up an intravenous drip of warm isotonic saline and then slowly add the methylene blue. The prognosis is poor.

Arctotheca calendula (cape weed)

This annual herb originated in Cape Province in South Africa, hence its name. It is now found in California and southern parts of Australia, not only in gardens but in the wild. It causes nitrate poisoning if large amounts are consumed rapidly. There is vasodilatation and shock. The antidote is intravenous 1% methylene blue at the rate of 5 mg/kg.

Argemone spp. (Mexican poppies)

These are found in all areas of North America, throughout Australia and in gardens in Europe. They are an ornamental thistle-like plant with yellow flowers. The seeds, which contain iso-quinoline alkaloids, are toxic. The toxic signs are cardiovascular with ventral and submandibular oedema, collapse and death. There is no known antidote. The seeds if crushed are detoxified by sunlight.

Arum maculatum (cuckoo-pint)

This plant is found in hedgerows in the UK and in northern Europe. It is also called 'lords and ladies'. It is very bitter and therefore extremely rarely eaten by SACs. Crias are attracted to the bright red berries, which are extremely poisonous. They cause acute gastritis and violent diarrhoea. Poisoning is likely to be fatal unless intravenous fluids can be given immediately.

Asclepias spp. (milkweed)

This is a well-documented poisonous plant for rabbits. It is found in North America. SACs will only eat it when it is dried and hidden in hay. It is rare for animals to ingest enough to cause problems. Initially there is gut stasis followed by diarrhoea. There is no specific antidote but NSAIDs are helpful.

Astragalus spp. (locoweed)

This plant is found in the western states of the USA. It is called 'milk vetch' in the UK. It is a perennial leguminous herb. It contains the toxic alkaloid swainsonine, which causes tetanic convulsions, dilated pupils, dyspnoea, coma and death. It is a cumulative poison so that unless large quantities are available, SACs are rarely poisoned. The first appearance of toxicity is that the animal will appear to have very dull eyes. It will cause abortions. There is no specific antidote. The convulsions should be controlled with diazepam. Intravenous fluids are helpful.

Atropa belladonna (deadly nightshade)

This plant, which is found in hedgerows in the UK, is also found throughout Europe. It now is also found in North America. It is often confused with the more common woody nightshade. Woody nightshade is not nearly as toxic as deadly nightshade. Normally animals will not touch deadly nightshade when it is growing. The only cases reported have been when it has been included in hay (Hubbs, 1947). As the name suggests the plant contains some atropine that gives the signs of poisoning, i.e. enlarged pupils and ileus. However, the more toxic principle is an alkaloid hyoscamine. The specific antidote is neostigmine at 0.01 mg/kg given subcutaneously. The ileus should be treated with isotonic saline and flunixin intravenously. More old-fashioned treatments include strong black coffee and alcohol per os.

Baptisia spp. (wild indigo)

There are several species of these herbaceous perennials, e.g. false indigo and yellow indigo. They grow in the north-eastern areas of the USA and are dangerous in the spring when they are green. They contain various alkaloids that cause neurological signs and acute diarrhoea. SACs rarely eat enough to cause severe symptoms. Treatment is symptomatic and deaths are unlikely.

Beta vulgaris (sugarbeet)

The tops of this crop are often fed in the UK quite safely. However, toxic signs of acute diarrhoea and recumbency may be seen in alpacas that are suddenly given large quantities. The treatment that is often successful is vitamin B preparations and 20% calcium borogluconate, both given slowly intravenously. The dose of the 20% calcium borogluconate is 80 ml.

Brachiaria spp. (signal grass)

This grass is found in tropical areas in Asia and Australia. It contains steroidal saponins and causes abortion and photosensitization. Animals will recover if brought in, but abortion is rarely prevented.

Brachyachne spp. (native couch grass)

This grass found in the interior in Australia causes cyanide poisoning when large amounts of the grass are consumed rapidly. Animals are likely to be found dead. The remainder should be dosed with 5 g of sodium thiosulfate by mouth.

Brassica napus (rape)

This brassica is grown as a field crop worldwide. It can cause haemoglobinuria in SACs but the actual trigger factor is not fully understood except that normally it occurs soon after the animals have ingested large quantities. The animals will be anaemic, similar to Haemonchus contortus infestation. Normally they will survive if taken off the rape.

Brassica oleracea (marrowstem kale)

This is grown worldwide as a fodder plant for cattle. Toxicity in SACs is extremely rare. The toxicity signs are haemoglobinuria and resulting anaemia. Animals will survive if taken off the kale.

Brodiaea spp. (brodiaea, cluster lilies)

This erect flowering plant has purple flowers and is found on the west coast of the USA. It only causes poisoning if eaten by starving SACs. There is no antidote but symptomatic treatment for the diarrhoea is helpful.

Brunfelsia pauciflora floribunda (lady-of-the-night)

This is an evergreen shrub or small tree found in gardens worldwide. It is not palatable but contains a lethal cocktail of atropine, scopolamine and hyoscyamine, which causes ataxia and dilated pupils. The specific antidote is neostigmine at 0.01 mg/kg given subcutaneously.

Bryonia dioica (white bryony)

This plant, like black bryony, is a hedge-climbing plant; however, it comes from a totally different plant family. The toxin is a violent purgative. SACs rarely eat enough to cause real toxicity, unless the roots are dug up and fed. The roots, like the berries, are highly toxic as they contain large amounts of a glycoside called bryonin. Intravenous fluids are the only realistic treatment available.

Buxus sempervirens (box)

This cultivated ornamental evergreen shrub is common on chalky limestone soils. It is usually trimmed as a hedge but can grow to more than 6 m. It is used for topiary in the UK and Europe and also in Northern America. It originated in North Africa and western Asia. Like so many poisons, it was historically used in small amounts as a medicine to bring down fever. SACs will not touch the growing plant but may ingest hedge clippings. Box contains a toxic alkaloid, which causes intense bowel irritation. There is no specific antidote. Bowel protectants may be helpful.

Caesalpinia spp. (grey nicker bean)

This tree is found in the tropical areas of the south-west of the USA. It contains tannins, which cause acute diarrhoea. Treatment is symptomatic and normally successful.

Camassia quamash (camas)

This plant is found in the wild in western parts of the USA. It is rarely eaten by SACs. It will cause a transitory diarrhoea. No treatment is required.

Cannabis sativa (marijuana)

This plant, known as cannabis, which is grown illegally as a recreational drug for humans, may be eaten by SACs. They become depressed, ataxic and will vocalize. They should be given supportive care, with intravenous fluids. They are often cold, so this hypothermia should be addressed. The prognosis is good unless seizures are seen. These can be controlled with diazepam but the outcome then is rarely good.

Capsicum annuum (chili pepper)

This annual shrub is grown as a crop throughout the world. It is very irritant to the bowel and causes diarrhoea. It is not life threatening to SACs. Treatment should be symptomatic.

Cassia occidentalis (coffee weed)

This annual leguminous shrub is found in eastern areas of North America. It is also called wild coffee or septic weed. It causes recumbency as it contains an anthraquinone alkaloid. There is no specific antidote. Recovery is unlikely after the animal has gone down. There is a plant of the same genus, coffeepod (Cassia obtusifolia), which causes less severe symptoms. The animals are usually found to be ataxic. If treated symptomatically, they normally recover.

Cassia spp. (Senna)

These plants of the legume family are common in North America. The seeds are the most toxic but the green plant of many of the species contains enough anthraquinone to cause toxic signs. The plants often cause problems after the first frost when they are wilted, which seems to make them more palatable. Diarrhoea is followed by recumbency. The chance of recovery after recumbency is very unlikely. As there is no specific antidote, euthanasia is indicated. It should be noted that the use of vitamin E and selenium is contraindicated in treatment as they increase myodegeneration.

Cenchrus ciliaris (buffel grass)

This grass is found in tropical areas of Australia, the Far East, North and South America, and is a native of Africa. It is an extremely invasive plant. It is only eaten by SACs if there is no other forage or food available, e.g. in tethered llamas. It contains oxalates and causes 'milk fever'-like symptoms of hypocalcaemia. Treatment, which is normally successful, is with 20% calcium borogluconate given slowly intravenously. The dose is 80 ml for a SAC.

Cestrum parquet (green cestrum)

This is a cultivated garden shrub with yellow flowers. It is a native of Central and South America and has become wild in New South Wales, Australia. Diterpenoid glycosides are found in the black berries, which are consumed by inquisitive SACs. They cause acute liver damage and resulting encephalopathy. Once neurological signs have developed, death is inevitable and euthanasia is indicated. If the toxicity is caught early enough, vitamin B injections and a low-protein diet can be tried.

Cheilanthes sieberi (mulga fern)

This small fern is found in all subtropical and temperate areas of Australia. It is not readily eaten by SACs unless there is no other food available. It is cumulative and causes irreversible progressive retinal atrophy.

Chenopodium album (fat hen)

This weed grows on waste ground and in cultivated areas between fruit trees throughout Europe. It is not normally eaten in sufficient quantities by SACs to cause toxicity unless they are starving, e.g. a neglected animal. It contains high levels of oxalates and so causes hypocalcaemia. Treatment is 20% calcium borogluconate given slowly intravenously. The dose is 80 ml. Treatment is normally successful.

Cicuta virosa (water hemlock)

This is commonly called cowbane for obvious reasons as it is poisonous to all livestock. It is the roots, which look like parsnips, that are normally eaten after dredging of ditches. They are still toxic when dry. A piece the size of a walnut is sufficient to kill a cow (Stratton, 1919). The species Cicuta douglasii found in North America is also poisonous.

Claviceps purpurea (ergot)

This parasitic plant fungus produces a toxin that causes the well-known ergot poisoning. It grows on various grain crops worldwide. The main sign of toxicity is gangrene of the extremities. This is only seen in cold climates. Abortion will also be seen. There is no specific treatment. Normally if the condition is noticed early enough for the diet to be corrected, the animals will then recover from the gangrene but pregnant females will invariably abort.

Clematis vitalba (wild clematis)

This is often called old man's beard as the fruits resemble a white silky beard. It originated in the UK, but has spread and become a very invasive plant in New Zealand. It has an acid taste and is very irritant so is not attractive to SACs. However, if ingested it can cause violent diarrhoea and death.

Colchicum autumnale (autumn crocus)

This is also called meadow saffron when found outside of gardens. It is found in gardens throughout the world. The toxin is colchicine. The signs in SACs are gastroenteric. There is no specific antidote but demulcents are helpful and survival rates are very good.

Conium maculatum (hemlock)

This herbaceous plant, with white flowers, found in ditches, is rarely eaten by SACs except after ditch clearance. It can be distinguished from other members of the Umbelliferae family, which include carrots, parsnips, celery and parsley, by a smooth, spotted stem and the distinct smell of mice. It is a native of Europe, North Africa, West Africa and South Africa. It has spread to North America, Australia and New Zealand. It contains a very potent alkaloid. Ingestion causes severe nervous signs, staggering and dilated pupils. Death occurs from respiratory depression. There is no specific antidote. However, like all alkaloids, some authors report success with tannic acid or acetic acid (Copithorne, 1937).

Convallaria majalis (lily-of-the-valley)

This is a herbaceous perennial found in gardens worldwide. It has small bell-like flowers. It contains potent cardiac glycosides. As it is irritant, adult SACs do not normally touch the plant. Crias will show trembling and an atrial-ventricular block. They should be put on fluids intravenously and be given very small doses of atropine (e.g. 100 μg) very slowly intravenously while monitoring the heart.

Crotalaria spp. (rattlebox)

This perennial legume with yellow flowers is found throughout North America. It is called rattlepods in Australia. This should not be confused with Daubentonia punicea, which is also called 'rattlebox'. It causes a cumulative poisoning when fed dried in hay. SACs will not touch the growing plant. The toxic principle is a pyrrolizidine alkaloid, which causes jaundice, oedema and ataxia. There is no treatment.

Cycas spp. (cycad palm)

Poisoning has been reported in many subtropical and tropical areas throughout the world. These trees originated in the Far East. The signs reported are neurological and appear to be irreversible. Euthanasia is indicated.

Cynodon dactylon (Bermuda grass)

This fodder crop grown in semi-tropical areas can become toxic in the late summer and autumn. Animals will shake and become ataxic. The ataxia is made worse by movement. The animals should be coaxed very slowly off the pasture with the promise of hard feed. If they are driven they will stagger and become recumbent. The prognosis is then very poor. If the grass is cut for hay it will remain toxic for over 2 years. The specific antidote is sodium thiosulfate. This should be given intravenously at the rate of 20 mg/kg, well diluted in warm normal saline.

Cynodon nlemfuensis (African star grass)

This grass is grown as a forage crop in tropical and semi-tropical areas, particularly the south-eastern parts of the USA. It is really only toxic when the plant is young, particularly if it suffers physical damage from the frost when grown in higher areas. The toxin produced is cyanide. The animals will show ataxia and collapse. The specific antidote is sodium thiosulfate. This should be given intravenously at the rate of 20 mg/kg, well diluted in warm normal saline.

Cynoglossum officinale (hound's tongue)

This biennial plant is common on waste ground throughout North America. SACs will not eat the growing plant on account of its unpleasant smell; however, it becomes palatable when dry in hay. Luckily it is not found on hay fields. Poisoning only occurs when hay is made on waste ground. It contains two alkaloids, helio-supine and echinatine. These cause dysentery and necrotic liver damage. It is invariably fatal once jaundice is seen. There is no antidote. Euthanasia is indicated. All the other animals must be given hay not containing the plant and vitamin B injections together with antibiotics.

Dactyloctenium radulans (button grass)

This grass is not widespread in Australia, but restricted to New South Wales. It causes nitrate poisoning if large amounts are consumed rapidly. There is vasodilatation and shock. The antidote is intravenous 1% methylene blue at the rate of 5 mg/kg. Alpaca owners should avoid heavy nitrogen fertilization.

Datura stramonium (thorn-apple)

This weed is only found in southern England, not in the rest of the UK. It is called jimsonweed in the USA. It is rarely eaten in the fresh state but can be ingested in hay. All parts of this annual plant are toxic. The plant contains the alkaloids atropine, hyoscamine and hyoscine. It causes symptoms similar to deadly nightshade. The specific antidote is neostigmine, which should be given at the rate of 0.01 mg/kg subcutaneously.

Daubentonia punicea (purple sesbane)

This is a flowering shrub cultivated in gardens in North America and the UK. It is also found wild in northern America, where it is called rattlebox. It should not be confused with *Crotalaria* spp., which is also called 'rattlebox'. It has legume pods that are poisonous. These are not normally eaten but if ingested by curious llamas will cause circulatory signs and death if sufficient is ingested. There is no specific antidote. Treatment has to be supportive and is often successful if sufficient has not been eaten.

Delphinium nuttallii (larkspur)

This herbaceous plant has purple flowers. The first sign of poisoning will be generalized muscular weakness and trembling. Alpacas seem to be unable to defecate completely.

Delphinium spp. (delphinium)

This common blue garden flower in the UK is rarely a problem when growing. However, animals may eat the dried young plants on garden compost heaps. It is called larkspur in North America. The toxic alkaloids cause initial gastroenteric signs and then neurological signs. There is no specific treatment.

Dieffenbachia seguine (Dumbcane)

One author (Johnson, 1989) reported some mild toxicity signs were shown by a llama when this weed was fed dry. The llama recovered in 30 min.

Digitalis purpurea (foxglove)

This erect herb with purple flowers is a native of Europe but is now found throughout the world. The signs of poisoning are those of digitalis overdose as the Latin name of the plant would suggest, i.e. bradycardia, cyanosis and collapse. Animals will not eat the fresh plant but may ingest small amounts in hay. In the event of collapse a SAC should be given lidocaine intravenously at the rate of 3µg/min until the bradycardia improves. In the event of ingestion of a limited amount of foxglove causing bradycardia a SAC should be given 5 g of potassium chloride by mouth.

Drymaria pachyphyllia (inkweed)

This creeping annual plant is found in the south-west of North America. It is only consumed by SACs in drought conditions. The toxin is unknown but is thought to be a saponin. It causes depression, coma and death. There is no antidote. Animals should be fed quality roughage immediately.

Dryopteris filix-mas (male fern)

This is one of the most common ferns found in the northern hemisphere. It is doubtful if a SAC could ingest enough of this plant to cause toxicity.

However, if the roots are eaten then it will cause progressive retinal atrophy and irreversible blindness. There is no antidote.

Duboisia hopwoodii (pituri)

This large shrub is found in arid regions in Australia. It has black berries. It is not normally consumed if other food is available. It contains nicotine, which causes neurological signs. There is no antidote but if the animals are left alone and not stimulated they will often recover. This shrub is in the same genus as corkwoods, which contain an alkaloid, tropane, not unlike nicotine.

Duboisia leichhardtii (corkwood)

These small trees have small white flowers, which become green berries. They are found in tropical areas of the USA. They contain an alkaloid, tropane, which is not unlike nicotine. The signs shown by tropane and nicotine toxicity are similar. They both show marked dilation of the pupils and other neurological signs. There is a specific antidote, physostigmine. This should be given at the rate of 0.06 mg/kg by slow intravenous injection.

Duboisia myoporoides (corkwood)

These small trees are of the same genus as pituri. They have small white flowers and are mainly found in the east of Australia and New Caledonia. They contain an alkaloid, tropane, which is not unlike nicotine. The signs shown by tropane and nicotine toxicity are similar. They both show marked dilation of the pupils and other neurological signs. There is a specific antidote, physostigmine. This should be given at the rate of 0.06 mg/kg by slow intravenous injection.

Echium plantagineum (Patterson's curse)

This annual herb with blue flowers is found in the UK and Europe, particularly around the Mediterranean and Black Seas. It is also found in southern regions of Australia. The toxic principles are pyrrolizidine alkaloids. These cause chronic weight loss as they damage the liver over a length of time. There is no specific antidote. However, if the animals are removed from the weed their livers will regenerate on a low-protein diet. Vitamin B injections may be helpful.

Equisetum spp. (mare's tail)

This plant, which is seen on some pastures worldwide, is very toxic. However, it is not palatable and is only eaten by animals that are starving. It causes ataxia and convulsions. The specific antidote is thiamine (vitamin B1). Care should be taken on the administration of this vitamin intravenously as deaths have been reported. Normally it is given in a solution with other B vitamins. It should be given intramuscularly at the rate of 1 mg/kg daily.

Eremophila accuminatum (boobialla)

This small tree with white, bell-shaped flowers, grows in the central areas of Australia. It has red fruit and is also called the 'wild peach'. The author has eaten them cooked in a pie with no ill effects. Some plants but not all contain furanosequiterpenes. These cause acute or chronic liver toxicity. There is no antidote.

Eremophila deserti (turkey bush)

This small tree with white, bell-shaped flowers grows in the central areas of Australia. Some plants but not all contain furanosequiterpenes. These cause acute liver toxicity. There is no antidote.

Eremophila maculata (spotted emu bush)

This shrub has red tubular flowers and is found throughout the centre of Australia. The young leaves, which are attractive to SACs in drought conditions, contain cyanogenic glycosides. These cause rapid death if large amounts are ingested.

Treatment is with 30 mg/kg of sodium thiosulfate given as a warm solution intravenously twice daily for 3 days. All in-contact animals should be given 5 g sodium thiosulfate by mouth. This should be repeated 24 h later as relapses can occur.

Erythrophleum chlorostachys (camel poison)

This substantial tree has yellow-green flowers, which become dry brown flat seed pods. It is restricted to the north of Western Australia. It contains diterpenoid alkaloids, which cause sudden death. Luckily SACs rarely touch the plant. There is no effective antidote.

Eucalyptus cladocalyx (sugar gum)

This tall tree is found in the south-eastern states of Australia, in East Africa in areas over 1500 m above sea level and in gardens in the UK. It has white flowers and barrel-shaped fruit. It contains cyanogenic glycosides, which cause sudden death. The young leaves are the most toxic. Poisoning only occurs after a high wind early in the growing season. All in-contact SACs should be given 5 g sodium thiosulfate by mouth.

Euonymus europaeus (spindle tree)

This shrub, whose leaves are most toxic in the spring, is rarely eaten by SACs as it is bitter and gives off an unpleasant odour. It is a purgative. Treatment is symptomatic. It has small yellowish green flowers. It is found throughout Europe up to the Caucasus.

Eupatorium rugosum (white snakeroot)

This is a North American tall perennial herb. Poisoned llamas become ketotic with fatty degeneration of the liver with chronic poisoning. Although the heart is affected, the clinician has a dilemma as corticosteroids are normally helpful for the liver but risky with the cardiac signs.

Euphorbia pulcherrima (poinsettia)

This is a very common pot plant found worldwide. It causes acute diarrhoea in alpacas. It is not life threatening. Treatment is symptomatic.

Euphorbia spp. (spurges)

These plants occur worldwide. Poisoning has been reported in North America, Australia, New Zealand and Europe. The seeds look like small capers and indeed there is a species called the caper spurge in North America. The plant produces a very irritant juice, which burns the mouth of alpacas, giving an 'orf'-like appearance. The treatment is the application of topical oily creams. Fly control is also important.

Festuca arundinacea (fescue)

This is a common pasture grass in North America. Like ryegrass, it can harbour a fungus. The normal culprit is *Epichloe typhina*. The mycotoxicosis has been reported in llamas to cause ill-thrift and general malaise. This latter condition will resolve if the animals are removed from the pasture. An endophyte-free strain of fescue grass has been developed in the USA.

Galega officinalis (goat's rue)

As the name indicates this legume is toxic in large quantities to goats and also to SACs. It is a herb with purple flowers and is native to Europe, the Middle East and western Asia. It was used in the USA, South America and New Zealand as a forage crop. It has now become a weed in all these areas. It causes inappetence, so after the initial gorging the plant poisoning is self-limiting. Animals should be removed from the plant and fed good grass. Liver toxicity is extremely rare and recovery rates are good.

Gastrolobium spp. (poison bushes)

These bushes are found throughout Australia and there are over 30 different species. They contain fluoroacetate, which causes sudden death. They are not readily eaten by SACs. There is no antidote.

Gelsemium sempervirens (evening trumpet flower)

This trailing plant is found in open woods in the south-east of North America and in Latin America. It has yellow trumpet-like flowers. It contains alkaloids related to strychnine. The signs are dilated pupils, convulsions, coma and death. It is only eaten by tethered llamas. Immediate treatment with sedatives and relaxants is required to control the convulsions. There is no specific treatment.

Glyceria maxima (reed sweet grass)

This semi-aquatic grass is found in all the temperate areas of Australia. It causes sudden death as it contains cyanogenic glycosides. It is only eaten by very hungry animals. All in-contact animals should be given 5 g sodium thiosulfate by mouth.

Gutierrezia microcephala (snakeweed)

This perennial shrub is found throughout North America. The toxin is unknown. It causes abortion and haematuria. The animals can normally be saved if put on to good forage but the abortions cannot be prevented.

Halogeton glomeratus (halogeton)

This annual herb is found in desert areas in the western part of North America. It contains high levels of oxalic acid, which makes it unpalatable. However, if it is eaten by starving SACs it causes peracute hypocalcaemia. Unless given intravenous calcium borogluconate immediately the animals will die. A 20% calcium borogluconate solution should be given slowly. The dose is 80 ml.

Haplopappus heterophyllius (goldenrod)

This perennial bush found in gardens in the UK grows wild in North America, where it is called burroweed. It does not affect adults but only suckling crias, which will be weak and tremble. The nursing mother should immediately be taken away from the goldenrod and given other feed. If possible it should be milked out every 12 h. The young cria should be given warm electrolytes for 48 h before being returned to its mother.

Helenium hoopesii (western sneezeweed)

This perennial herb is found in North America and is often called orange sneezeweed after the colour of the flowers. It is a cumulative poison and so is rarely fatal. Owners will notice the stiff gait, weakness and emaciation. If the animals are removed from access to the plant they will recover.

Helenium microcephalum (smallheaded sneezeweed)

This annual herb is found in North America, as is its near relative orange sneezeweed, *H. hoopesii*. Both cause a cumulative poisoning and so are rarely fatal. Owners will notice the stiff gait, weakness and emaciation. If the animals are removed from access to the plant they will recover.

Heliotrope spp. (viper's bugloss)

This plant, which is found in Texas, contains a toxic alkaloid that will cause acute diarrhoea in SACs. It is not normally fatal but there is no specific treatment. Demulcents and NSAIDs are helpful. Not all species are toxic. *H. europaeum* was used in the Middle Ages to colour food and is still used in modern French cuisine.

Heliotropium amplexicaule (blue heliotrope)

This annual herb with blue flowers is found throughout the UK, Europe and southern areas of

Australia. It is not normally eaten by SACs unless they are starving. It contains pyrrolizidine alkaloids, which cause chronic liver damage. Animals should be removed from access to the plant and fed on a low-protein diet, e.g. cereals or sugarbeet pulp.

Heliotropium europaeum (common heliotrope)

This annual herb with white flowers is found throughout the UK, Europe and southern areas of Australia. It is not normally eaten by SACs unless they are starving. It contains pyrrolizidine alkaloids, which cause chronic liver damage. Animals should be removed from access to the plant and fed on a low-protein diet, e.g. cereals or sugarbeet pulp.

Helleborus niger (Christmas rose)

This garden flower is found throughout Europe. The toxic principle is a cardiac glycoside. The plant is very bitter so is not eaten by SACs when it is growing. However, it may be consumed when cut and dried on garden rubbish tips. It causes acute bloody diarrhoea. Treatment is symptomatic and is normally successful.

Heterodendron oleifolium (rosewood)

This small tree with flaky bark has linear leaves and is found in central areas of Australia. It contains cyanogenic glycosides and causes sudden death. All in-contact SACs should be given 5 g of sodium thiosulfate by mouth.

Homeria spp. (cape tulip)

This tulip is found in the UK, Europe, North America and Australia. It originated in South Africa. There are two species: the one-leaf cape tulip *H. flaccida*; and the two-leaf cape tulip *H. miniata*. They both contain cardiac glycosides. The growing plant is not touched by SACs. However, they may ingest it in hay. Even a small amount will cause rapid death.

Hoya australis (wax flower)

This is a vine with bunches of waxy white flowers and is found in subtropical areas of eastern Australia. It contains an unidentified neurotoxin, which causes convulsions. There is no effective treatment and so euthanasia is recommended.

Hymenoxys odorata (bitterweed)

This plant is found in North America, mainly in the south-west. It prefers wet areas. It has bright yellow flowers. It has an unpleasant smell and so is not normally a problem except if there is no other food available. It causes anorexia and depression. As it is a cumulative poison the symptoms regress when animals are moved on to good fresh pastures.

Hymenoxys richardsonii (Colorado rubberweed)

This North American perennial herb with yellow flowers is also called pinque. It is a cumulative poison causing depression and colic. Immediate removal from the plant will normally solve the problem.

Hyoscyamus niger (henbane)

This is an extremely poisonous herbaceous plant with pale yellow flowers. All parts are toxic. It has the same alkaloids as deadly nightshade and gives the same signs if eaten. It originated in Europe and Asia and is now global.

Hypericum perforatum (St John's wort)

This marshland plant rarely causes problems in temperate climates. It causes chronic liver damage. The first sign will be photosensitization. It is therefore much more serious in subtropical areas. Any affected animals should be brought in out of the sun. Vitamin B injections are helpful. The animals should be put on a low protein diet.

Ipomoea batatus (sweet potato)

These potatoes will cause poisoning worldwide if they are fed mouldy to animals. They contain pneumotoxic furanoterpenes, which cause respiratory signs. Animals will recover if the mouldy tubers are removed.

Ipomoea calobra (weir vine)

This vine has trumpet-shaped pink flowers and is found in localized areas of Queensland. It is a chronic poison. Animals develop a craving for the plant. If access is denied, less severely affected animals will recover. There is no known antidote.

Ipomoea muelleri (poison morning glory)

This is a vine with trumpet-shaped pink flowers, found in gardens in the UK and Europe. It is found wild in central and north-west areas of Australia. It contains an unknown neurotoxin. There is no known antidote. It is rare for SACs to eat the vines.

Isotropis spp. (lamb poisons)

These herbs have pea-type flowers of many colours and are found in gardens in the UK. Distinct species are found in south-western Australia and another in central Australia. They contain a heterocyclic alkaloid, which causes nephrosis in older crias. There is no known antidote.

Kallstroemia hirsutissima (carpetweed)

This weed is not readily eaten by livestock except under drought conditions. It is found in the south-west of North America. It causes paresis in single animals but does not affect the majority of the others. The toxin is unknown and hence any treatment is only supportive.

Kalmia angustifolia (lambkill)

This member of the Ericaceae family found in the south-east parts of the USA will kill SACs. It contains grayano-toxins and gives similar toxic signs as *Rhododendron* spp., i.e. projectile vomiting and abdominal pain. The only treatment is a mixture of morphine and atropine. The dose is 2 ml twice daily of a 5% w/v solution of morphine sulfate injected intramuscularly. Atropine will aid recovery by reducing the massive amount of saliva produced. A SAC should be given 2 ml of a 0.5% w/v solution of atropine sulfate intramuscularly.

Kalmia latifolia (mountain laurel)

This evergreen shrub of the Ericaceae family is found in the south-east of the USA. It is highly toxic but SACs tend to give it a wide berth. It contains grayano-toxins and gives similar toxic signs as *Rhododendron* spp., i.e. projectile vomiting and abdominal pain. The only treatment is a mixture of morphine and atropine. The dose is 2 ml twice daily of a 5% w/v solution of morphine sulfate injected intramuscularly. Atropine will aid recovery by reducing the massive amount of saliva produced. A SAC should be given 2 ml of a 0.5% w/v solution of atropine sulfate intramuscularly.

Kalmia spp. (kalmia)

This flowering plant found in gardens in the UK causes acute gastritis and abdominal pain. The pain should be controlled with morphine 2 ml twice daily of a 5% w/v solution of morphine sulfate injected intramuscularly. Atropine will aid recovery by reducing the massive amount of saliva produced. A dose of 2 ml of a 0.5% w/v solution of atropine sulfate should be given twice daily intramuscularly.

Karwinskia humboldtiana (coyotillo)

This woody shrub is common in the southern areas of North America. It has small black berries. It is the fruit that is toxic, causing generalized neurological signs. There is no specific antidote. If the animals are removed from the plant early enough recovery is possible. However, when the nervous signs are advanced euthanasia is indicated.

Kochia scoparia (Mexican fireweed)

This plant is found in many southern areas of North America and of course in Mexico. It causes neurological signs. Recovery rates are good if there is good nursing. NSAIDs are helpful.

Laburnum anagyroides (laburnum)

After yew this is the most poisonous tree in the UK. It is a native tree of Europe but is found in gardens throughout the world. The most poisonous parts of the tree are the seeds, which form from yellow flowers, but the whole tree is in fact poisonous. Alpacas will be poisoned by grazing under the tree and picking up the seeds. The main toxin is an alkaloid called cytosine, which gives similar signs as nicotine. These are incoordination, convulsions and death from asphyxia. There is no antidote.

Lamium amplexicaule (dead nettle)

This is a herb with pinkish tubular flowers. It is found as a weed after cultivation throughout Australia. It contains an unknown neurotoxin causing incoordination. There is no known treatment but removal from the toxic plants will normally result in a recovery.

Lantana camara (lantana)

This flowering shrub may be found in the wild as well as in gardens. It is a native of tropical Africa and America. It causes chronic liver damage with resulting jaundice and photosensitization. The treatment is vitamin B injections to help the liver and the animal should be kept out of direct sunlight.

Laurus spp. (laurel)

This plant is rarely eaten in sufficient quantities to cause toxicity. Quite large amounts need to be ingested. It is still toxic when dry so it can be eaten by animals on garden waste tips. It causes severe symptoms of cyanide poisoning.

Ledum glandulosum (Labrador tea)

This North American herb, which grows in wettish areas, contains andromedotoxin and has small white to cream flowers. It causes colic and paresis. There is no specific antidote but recovery can be expected with pain control and good nursing. The toxin is denatured by boiling, so the plant can be boiled to make a tea-like drink.

Leiocarpa brevicompta (flat billy buttons)

This shrub is also called plains plover daisy. It grows in the heavy clay soils of the floodplains of the Darling River system in Queensland and New South Wales. It has dense yellow flower heads. These develop into seed heads, which cause toxicity if eaten in quantity. They contain crepenynic acid and other fatty acids, which cause striated muscle degeneration. The main sign is recumbency. There is no specific antidote but with careful nursing most animals will recover.

Leucothoe davisiae (black laurel)

This is a shrub found in North America and Asia around lakes and along the banks of streams. It is not found in Africa except in Madagascar. It has white flowers. It causes colic and recumbency. There is no specific treatment. The colic signs should be controlled with NSAIDs. Provided only a little has been ingested, which is likely as it also causes anorexia, there is a good chance of survival.

Ligustrum spp. (privet)

This hedge plant is found worldwide. Large quantities have to be eaten by SACs to cause toxicity. The main sign is diarrhoea. Treatment is symptomatic.

Linum spp. (linseed)

This is often included as an oil in food. It causes diarrhoea and its use should be avoided. There is no specific antidote. One species *L. catharticum* is actually called purging flax.

Lolium spp. (ryegrass)

There are two main types of poisoning. The first poisoning is caused by an endophyte fungus, *Claviceps purpurea*, which causes gangrene of the extremities like ergot. The second is caused by another endophyte fungus, *Acremonium lolii*, which causes neurological signs, mainly stiffness. The condition seen in sheep and SACs is called 'ryegrass staggers'. It has been reported in the UK, New Zealand and in several states of Australia. Exercise will make the condition much worse. The SACs should be quietly walked off the offending pasture. Improvement will be quite rapid (i.e. 3 or 4 days) without any treatment. A third very rare condition of facial eczema has been reported in alpacas caused by the fungus *Pithomyces chartarum* in both New Zealand and Australia. It is a photosensitivity and the animals will recover if brought inside.

Lotus corniculatus (bird's-foot-trefoil)

The toxic substance found in this plant, which is common in cleared woodland in the UK, Europe and Australasia, is a cyanogenic glycoside. It will cause acute diarrhoea, which is followed by ataxia and collapse, when it is invariably fatal. However, if others are less affected they should be given the specific antidote, sodium thiosulfate, which should be given intravenously at a rate of 20 mg/kg well diluted in warm normal saline.

Lupinus spp. (lupines)

These plants are found in hedgerows and gardens. They also are grown commercially as nitrogen-fixing plants to improve the fertility of the soil in Europe, central Asia, Australasia and the USA. Alpacas can eat the green young plants without any problems. However, the seeds contain a poisonous alkaloid. The main sign is inappetence and so the poisoning is self-limiting. The animals should be moved quietly on to a grass pasture.

This will avoid the acute neurological symptoms that have been described. There is liver damage and jaundice has been reported (Brash, 1943). Animals will recover but it is slow.

Lythrum hyssopifolia (lesser loosestrife)

This herb has single pink or purple tubular flowers and is found in pastures in temperate areas of Australia. It contains an unidentified toxin that causes kidney and liver damage. Poisoning only occurs when this plant becomes very dominant in stubbles. There is no known treatment.

Malva parviflora (marsh mallow)

This is found on waste ground in the UK and in North America where it is known as cheeseweed. It is also found as a widespread weed throughout Australia. It seems to cause poisoning in suckling young with the mothers being unaffected. The crias will show convulsions, or be found dead. The post-mortem will reveal dark haemorrhages in many internal organs. There will be high nitrate/nitrite levels in the aqueous humor. There is a specific antidote, which is methylene blue at 10 mg/kg given slowly intravenously. The best approach is to set up an intravenous drip of warm isotonic saline and then slowly add the methylene blue.

Marsilea drummondii (common nardoo)

This aquatic fern is widespread in both eastern and western Australia. It looks like a four-leafed clover. It is eaten locally by man and does not appear to be toxic. However, it contains a thiaminase enzyme, which causes cerebro-cortico-necrosis (CCN). Prompt injections of thiamine hopefully given intravenously bring about a recovery.

Melia azedarach (chinaberry)

The yellow fruit of this tree found in the southeast of North America contains several alkaloids that cause gastroenteritis. It is a native of India and is also now found in southern China and Australia. Recovery is spontaneous provided not too large amounts are eaten. There is no specific antidote.

Melilotus officinalis (sweet clover)

This only causes poisoning when the plant has been spoilt or made into hay, haylage or silage. Fungal spores then convert the natural harmless coumarins into dicumarol. This interferes with the clotting mechanism. Haemorrhages are seen on the mucous membranes. Haematomas are rare but have been reported in alpacas. They should be removed from the pasture and given an injection of 3 mg/kg of vitamin K1 intramuscularly.

Menziesia pilosa (minniebush)

This member of the Ericaceae family found in the south-eastern parts of the USA is very toxic to SACs. It contains grayano-toxins and gives similar toxic signs as Rhododendron spp., i.e. projectile vomiting and abdominal pain. The only treatment is a mixture of morphine and atropine. The dose is 2 ml twice daily of a 5% w/v solution of morphine sulfate injected intramuscularly. Atropine will aid recovery by reducing the massive amount of saliva produced. A SAC should be given 2 ml of a 0.5% w/v solution of atropine sulfate intramuscularly.

Mercurialis perennis (dogs mercury)

This is said to be toxic. However, the only documented reported incident was in lambs that developed diarrhoea but the toxicity was not serious.

Mesembryanthemum spp. (ice plants)

These succulent prostrate herbs originated in South Africa and now grow wild in south-western Australia and are found cultivated in gardens throughout the world. They contain oxalates, which cause hypocalcaemia. Treatment, which is normally successful, is with 20% calcium borogluconate given slowly intravenously. The dose is 80 ml.

Nandina domestica (Chinese sacred bamboo)

This evergreen shrub has cyanogenic glycosides in its foliage. As the name suggests it is a native of China. It is also called heavenly bamboo. It is found wild in Japan and elsewhere in gardens and parks throughout the world. The treatment is specific: 30 mg/kg of sodium thiosulfate should be given intravenously. At the same time 3–5 g/h should be given by mouth to detoxify any remaining hydrogen cyanide (HCN; prussic acid) in C1. Affected animals show dyspnoea and tachycardia.

Narcissus spp. (daffodil)

The growing flowers are rarely eaten by SACs. Llamas have been reported to eat the bulbs, which caused mild diarrhoea.

Narthecium ossifragum (bog asphodel)

This plant is found growing in marshes in the UK and Scandinavia. It is not normally eaten fresh by SACs. However, it may be ingested in hay from rough pastures. It causes photosensitization on the white areas of llamas' faces. It is thought that the toxic effect is caused by microfungi that live on the plant. It may cause jaundice. Affected animals should be housed and treated with vitamin B injections.

Neobassia proceriflora (soda bush)

This small shrub grows in central Australia. It contains oxalates and so causes hypocalcaemia. Treatment, which is normally successful, is with 20% calcium borogluconate given slowly intravenously. The dose is 80 ml.

Nerium oleander (oleander)

This is a very toxic garden plant with pink flowers, which originated in Morocco. Animals will not eat it except in cut prunings. It causes sudden death. There is no treatment. As it is so toxic if any animal has eaten some, immediate gastrotomy should be carried out.

Nicotiana tabacum (tobacco)

Nicotine historically was used as a drench to control bowel worms in sheep. It had an extremely narrow safety margin. Deaths following convulsions were common. If SACs eat dried tobacco they will die. There is no antidote.

Nolina texana (sacahuista beargrass)

This perennial North American plant contains a heptatoxin in its flowers and fruit. The toxin causes photosensitization. SACs should be kept off the plant in the spring and early summer. If signs develop the animals should be kept out of the sunlight. Vitamin B injections may be helpful.

Notholaena sinuata cochisensis (jimmy fern)

This evergreen perennial fern is found in the south-west of North America. Its ingestion is rare. It causes nervous signs, which are more apparent when llamas are on the trek. Dehydration appears also to bring on the signs. With rest and fresh water the animals normally recover.

Oenanthe crocata (water dropwort)

The roots of this plant, which are called 'dead men's fingers', are eaten by livestock after dredging of ditches (Forsyth, 1954). They are still toxic when dry. The signs shown are convulsions, salivation, dilated pupils and death. Approximately 50% will recover from the convulsions and get diarrhoea for 48 h and then recover. There is no specific antidote. The plant occurs worldwide. The leaves are not toxic.

Osteospermum echionis (South African daisy)

This annual garden plant may be eaten by escaping SACs. It contains cyanogenic glycosides. Animals may be found dead. All in-contact animals should be given 5 g sodium thiosulfate by mouth.

Oxalis corniculata (wood sorrel)

As the Latin name implies this herb contains oxalates and so causes toxicity in SACs as it causes hypocalcaemia. It occurs in temperate areas of North America. It is most dangerous in the spring and autumn. Treatment, which is normally successful, is with 20% calcium borogluconate given slowly intravenously. The dose is 80 ml.

Oxalis pes-caprae (soursob)

As the Latin name implies this herb contains oxalates and so causes toxicity in SACs as it causes hypocalcaemia. It occurs in temperate areas of Australia. Treatment, which is normally successful, is with 20% calcium borogluconate given slowly intravenously. The dose is 80 ml.

Oxytenia acerosa (copperweed)

This herb is found wild in North America, mainly in the south-western states of the USA, where it is called 'sagebud'. It has been imported into gardens in the UK. The cause of the toxicity is unknown. It is not palatable so the only likely poisoning is curious SACs. It causes anorexia so poisoning is normally self-limited. Survival depends on changing the diet.

Panicum spp. (panicum grass)

These grasses are grown worldwide as fodder crops. They may contain steroidal saponins, which cause liver damage that results in photo-sensitization. Affected animals need to be brought in out of the sunlight and put on a low-protein diet. Vitamin B injections are helpful.

Peganum harmala (African rue)

This is a leafy perennial found in semi-desert areas, worldwide. It originated in the eastern Mediterranean area but is now also found in India, where it is used to make red dye for carpets. It is found in North America. It is unpalatable so is very rarely eaten unless there is absolutely no other food available. It causes anorexia and so is really self-limiting. Survival is likely if other food is provided.

Pennisetum clandestinum (kikuyu grass)

This forage grass originated in the highlands of Kenya but is grown in tropical and subtropical areas throughout the world. The leaves have very small spines, which cause alimentary irritation in certain animals. Normally the diarrhoea is short lived. However, in unvaccinated SACs pathogenic clostridial bacteria may multiply and release toxins causing death.

Perilla frutescens (perilla mint)

This herb originates in India, Pakistan and central Asia. It is also called purple mint. It has been imported into the UK, Europe and North America. It has an unpleasant smell. It may be eaten by tethered llamas but it needs a considerable amount to cause toxicity. The main signs are respiratory and result in mouth-breathing, which is very serious. Treatment with either steroids, diuretics or NSAIDs is rarely successful after the animal is recumbent.

Persea americana (avocado)

The toxic principle of this tree is persin, which is mainly found in the leaves and skin of the fruit. Individual animals may become addicted to this fruit and ingest toxic doses of the skin of the fruit. It will cause diarrhoea, which should be treated symptomatically.

Persicaria spp. (smart weeds)

These pink-flowered herbs are found near water in eastern areas of Australia. They contain an unknown toxin, which causes photosensitization. Animals need to be brought in. Vitamin B injections may be helpful.

Phalaris aquatica (Australian phalaris)

This grass grown in temperate areas throughout Australia is also called Toowoomba canary grass. It can contain indole alkaloids, which cause convulsions and recumbency, looking very like hypomagnesaemia; in fact the condition is called 'phalaris staggers'. There is no specific antidote.

Phoradendron flavescens (mistletoe)

This is a parasitic perennial evergreen plant with white berries. It is eaten by SACs on rubbish dumps after it has been discarded after Christmas. It contains acetylcholine, and causes acute diarrhoea and dilated pupils. Treatment is symptomatic. Physostigmine should not be injected as that is liable to make the symptoms worse.

Photinia fraseri (Chinese photinia)

This evergreen shrub is used as a hedge in North America and is also seen in gardens in Europe and the UK. It is a native of China. It contains a cyanogenic glycoside in its foliage. Affected animals show dyspnoea and tachycardia. There is a specific treatment available: 30 mg/kg of sodium thiosulfate should be given intravenously. At the same time, 3–5 g/h should be given by mouth to detoxify any remaining HCN in C1. Treatment may often be successful.

Phytolacca americana (poke weed)

This North American weed is found on waste ground in the eastern states, and has been introduced to gardens in the UK. The whole plant is toxic but poisoning seems to occur when the roots have been dug up and left on the ground. The main signs are violent colic and diarrhoea. There is no specific antidote but gastro-protectants are helpful plus intravenous fluids.

Pieris japonica variegated (pieris)

As the Latin name suggests, this flower grows wild in Japan and has been introduced into European gardens. It is extremely toxic to SACs. It is a member of the Ericaceae family and causes a similar toxicity to rhododendron. It contains a grayano-toxin, which acts on the autonomic nervous system via the vagal nerve stimulating the vomiting centre; only a very small dose is required. The only treatment is a mixture of morphine and atropine. The dose is 2 ml twice daily of a 5% w/v solution of morphine sulfate injected intramuscularly. Atropine will aid recovery by reducing the massive amount of saliva produced. The twice daily dose is 2 ml of a 0.5% w/v solution of atropine sulfate intramuscularly. The prognosis is good.

Pinus spp. (pine needles)

Several different species found in many countries will cause poisoning. The signs shown are depression, anorexia, C1 stasis, dyspnoea and even death. Pregnant animals will abort. There is no specific treatment.

Polypogon monspeliensis (annual beard grass)

This grass is found in seasonally flooded areas of subtropical and temperate regions of Australia. It is also found throughout North America, except it is absent from the mid-west. In northern America it is called 'rabbits foot grass'. There is a complex toxicological process, which results in convulsions and death, called 'Stewart range syndrome'. The toxic principle is a corynetoxin, which is produced by *Rathayibacter toxicus*, a bacterium in the seed-head nematode galls on the grass. There is a hope to develop cyclodextrin, a toxin binding agent, to be an antidote, but as yet trials have not been successful.

Portulaca oleracea (pigweed)

This weed is found throughout Australia, particularly in stockyards. It is often consumed when SACs are left penned in a stockyard with nothing else to eat. It contains oxalates, which cause hypocalcaemia. Treatment, which is normally successful, is with 20% calcium borogluconate given slowly intravenously. The dose is 80 ml.

Prosopis glandulosa (mesquite)

This small leguminous tree found in the southwest of North America has a long pod containing an unknown toxin, which causes partial paralysis of the tongue and atony of C1. The affected animals appear similar to animals that have been given oral antibiotics. They seem to have improper digestion. Probiotics and good grass seem to affect a cure.

Prunus caroliniana (cherry laurel)

This tree is found worldwide and is also called laurel cherry. It contains a cyanogenic glycoside, which causes convulsions and rapid death. Once the animal is convulsing euthanasia should be carried out as the prognosis is hopeless. However, if others are affected they should be given the specific antidote, sodium thiosulfate, which should be given intravenously at a rate of 30 mg/kg well diluted in warm normal saline.

Prunus serotina (black cherry)

This tree is found in Europe and North America. Like other *Prunus* spp. it contains a cyanogenic glycoside, which causes convulsions and rapid death. Once the animal is convulsing euthanasia should be carried out as the prognosis is hopeless. However, if others are affected they should be given the specific antidote, sodium thiosulfate, which should be given intravenously at a rate of 30 mg/kg well diluted in warm normal saline.

Prunus virginiana (choke cherry)

This tree is found in the south-east of the USA and in gardens in the UK. It contains a cyanogenic glycoside. SACs will show neurological signs. The specific antidote is sodium thiosulfate. This should be given intravenously at a rate of 20 mg/kg well diluted in warm normal saline. If animals are having convulsions they should be destroyed as the prognosis is hopeless.

Psilostrophe spp. (paperflowers)

This small erect, woody perennial is found on the range in the south-west of North America. Only poisoning in sheep has been reported. However, it is reasonable to suspect SACs will be affected by the sesquiterpene lactone, which the plant contains. The signs apart from general weakness are respiratory. Aspiration pneumonia is a possibility, so great care should be taken drenching animals. The animals should be kept away from the plant and stabilized. The toxic substance upsets the microflora in C1, so it is recommended that the diet is supplemented with sodium sulfate and large amounts of protein.

Pteridium aquilinum (bracken)

This common plant is not toxic in small quantities. However, if other food is not available SACs will ingest toxic doses. It causes a specific symptom of progressive retinal atrophy. This is called bright blindness and is irreversible. Bright blindness should not be confused with CCN. This also causes blindness in SACs. CCN can be brought on by eating bracken. This blindness caused by CCN is reversible with treatment with thiamine at 10 mg/kg, ideally given by intravenous injection for 3 days. Some clinicians consider it worthwhile to inject thiamine every 6 h for the first 24 h. If thiamine is not available on its own, a suitable multivitamin preparation may be given. The clinician must ensure that in so doing the same dose of thiamine is given. Cumulative bracken poisoning can also cause the development of cancerous changes in the wall of the bladder in SACs. This can be recognized by the clinician as haemoglobinuria. It is irreversible.

Quercus spp. (acorns)

Llamas and alpacas require quite large quantities of acorns to be poisoned. Poisoning can occur on a poor pasture in the early autumn in the UK after a high wind. Certain animals get a craving for green acorns. The toxin is tannin. The animals will be inappetent with lack of movement in C1. The faeces will be very dry. The animals will be dull. Animals may show colic pains. The colic should be controlled with NSAIDs. Liquid paraffin should be given by mouth, carefully to avoid inhalation. The animals should be given electrolytes in their drinking water. They should be moved off the contaminated area, ideally on to fresh grass. Ingestion can be prevented by rolling the area to push the acorns into the ground to make it hard for the animals to eat them. Areas around oak trees can be fenced off during the danger period.

Ranunculus spp. (buttercups)

These are very common but are not normally eaten by SACs and do not seem to be toxic in hay. They do contain a gastrointestinal irritant toxin and so in theory could cause diarrhoea in llamas and alpacas.

Raphanus raphanistrum (wild radish)

This herb is widespread throughout the temperate regions of the world. It is not palatable so SACs need to be starving to eat it. It contains S-methylcysteine sulfoxide (SMCO). This causes haemolysis. There is no effective treatment. Euthanasia should be carried out without delay.

Rapistrum rugosum (turnip weed)

This herb is widespread throughout the temperate regions of the world. It is not palatable so animals need to be starving to eat it. It contains S-methylcysteine sulfoxide (SMCO). This causes haemolysis. It may also cause polioencephalomalacia. There is no symptomatic effective treatment. Thiamine injections are not helpful. Euthanasia should be carried out without delay.

Rheum rhaponticum (rhubarb)

The stems of this plant have been cooked and eaten by humans for hundreds of years. It originated in Europe but is now worldwide. It is ingestion of the leaves by SACs that cause poisoning. They contain oxalates, which cause hypocalcaemia. The signs are anorexia, C1 stasis and recumbency. Treatment, which is normally successful, is with 20% calcium borogluconate given slowly intravenously. The dose is 80 ml.

Rhododendron occidentale (azalea)

This flower found in gardens and ornamental woods is very toxic but is not as attractive to alpacas and llamas as other *Rhododendron* spp. and other members of the Ericaceae family. All these plants contain a grayano-toxin, which acts on the autonomic nervous system via the vagal nerve and stimulates the vomiting centre. A very small dose is required. It will cause projectile vomiting, as it causes acute gastritis and excess salivation. The only treatment is a mixture of morphine and atropine. The dose is 2 ml twice daily of a 5% w/v solution of morphine sulfate injected intramuscularly. Atropine will aid recovery by reducing the massive amount of saliva produced. An adult alpaca should be given 2 ml of a 0.5% w/v solution of atropine sulfate intramuscularly. With an early diagnosis and treatment the prognosis is good.

Rhododendron ponticum (rhododendron)

This is the most common cause of plant poisoning in animals in the UK. It is found throughout the northern hemisphere, South-east Asia and northern Australia. Rhododendrons are very rare in Africa and South America. They may have originated in Nepal, where they are the national flower. It is one of the few causes of projectile vomiting in SACs. They have acute gastritis and excess salivation. It is a member of the Ericaceae family, which includes pieris and azaleas. These plants contain a grayano-toxin, acting on the autonomic nervous system via the vagal nerve stimulating the vomiting centre, and a very small dose is required. The only treatment is a mixture of morphine and atropine. The dose is 2 ml twice daily of a 5% w/v solution of morphine sulfate injected intramuscularly. Atropine will aid recovery by reducing the massive amount of saliva produced. A SAC should be given 2 ml of a 0.5% w/v solution of atropine sulfate intramuscularly. The prognosis is good.

Rhodomyrtus macrocarpa (finger cherry)

This small tree is also called native loquat or Wannakai. It is found in the rainforests of eastern Queensland. It has white flowers, which are followed by fleshy cylindrical red fruit. Both the leaves and the fruit are poisonous to SACs. They contain an unidentified toxin that causes permanent blindness. There is no effective treatment.

Ricinus communis (castor bean)

These may be included in animal feed and are not a problem in small quantities. However, it will cause diarrhoea and dysentery in alpacas if fed in large amounts.

Robinia pseudoacacia (black locust)

This large tree found in North America can cause diarrhoea and even collapse but it is rarely eaten by SACs unless they are tethered and there is no other food available. It has white flowers and is also found in southern Europe, central Asia and South Africa. There is no specific antidote so treatment should be symptomatic.

Rumex acetosa (sorrel)

This weed normally called common sorrel and its relative sheep's sorrel *Rumex acetosella* are common in pastures in Europe, Australia and New Zealand. Their relative curly dock *Rumex crispus* occurs in North America. All the sorrels are extremely acid and so are not readily eaten by livestock. In fact small quantities are not toxic but if animals eat small quantities over long periods of time they become hypocalcaemic. This will then give a picture after stress of a sudden onset. The main signs are recumbency, inappetence and gut stasis. The treatment, which is normally successful, is with 20% calcium borogluconate solution given slowly intravenously. The dose is 80 ml.

Salsola kali (soft roly-poly)

An annual herb that originated in Eurasia. It is now a very invasive weed found all over Australia and North America. It contains oxalates. If a large amount is consumed by a SAC over a short period of time they become hypocalcaemic. The main signs are recumbency, inappetence and gut stasis. The treatment, which is normally successful, is with 20% calcium borogluconate solution given slowly intravenously. The dose is 80 ml.

Salvia reflexa (mint weed)

This herb is widespread in inland areas of Queensland and New South Wales. It has pale blue tubular flowers. It will not be eaten by SACs fresh as it is not palatable. However, if it is cut and baled in hay then there are dangers. A large quantity consumed quickly would cause nitrate poisoning. The main sign is methaemoglobinaemia. There is a specific antidote, which is methylene blue at 10 mg/kg given slowly intravenously. The best approach is to set up an intravenous drip of warm isotonic saline and then slowly add the methylene blue.

Sambucus ebulus (ground elder)

This herb has white flowers, which become clusters of black berries. It is a native of Europe and south-west Asia. It is reported to be a purgative but no specific poisoning instances have been recorded.

Sambucus nigra (common elder)

This large shrub is a native of Europe. It is also found in north-west Africa and south-west Asia. It has been reported in western areas of northern Australia. It has pink flowers, which mature to dark red berries. This plant is said to be poisonous. However, there have never been any cases reported. Most animals do not seem to like the smell and therefore do not eat it.

Sapium sebiferum (Chinese tallow tree)

This tree found in the tropical parts of southeastern USA originated in China. Llamas will browse it with little toxic effects as it causes anorexia and therefore the danger is self-limiting. On recovery the llamas will have a brief period of diarrhoea.

Sarcobatus vermiculatus (grease-wood)

This large deciduous North American shrub is toxic in large quantities. It is also found in Mexico. It contains oxalates, which bind up blood calcium. It therefore causes hypocalcaemia. The signs are anorexia, lack of C1 movement and recumbency. Treatment is 20% calcium borogluconate given slowly intravenously. The dose is 80 ml. Treatment is normally successful.

Sarcostemma brevipedicellatum (caustic vine)

This vine has small bunches of waxy white flowers, which develop into long pods. It grows in tropical areas of Australia and in the nearby islands. It is not palatable so it really is only a problem with starving animals, e.g. tethered llamas. It contains an unidentified neurotoxin, which causes convulsions and death. There is no known antidote.

Sarothamnus scoparius (broom)

There is another species, Spanish broom *Sarothamnus junceum*. They are both very mildly poisonous.

It would be unlikely that any SAC could ingest enough to cause toxic signs.

Schoenus asperocarpus (poison sedge)

This grass grows in south-western Australia. It is avoided by grazing alpacas. However, it can cause problems when cut and baled in hay. It contains galegine, an alkaloid, which causes acute pulmonary oedema. There is no known antidote and euthanasia is advised.

Senecio jacobea (ragwort)

This plant is found throughout Europe. It was thought not to be toxic to SACs. Workers at Oregon maintain that llamas will not eat the plant and do not show signs of toxicity when they are given the plant as a slurry by stomach tube.

Senna obtusifolia (sicklepod)

This annual shrub is found in the wild in eastern USA. The plant is rarely eaten by SACs even on the trek. It contains anthraquinones, which cause neurological signs. If these are severe treatment is hopeless and euthanasia is advised.

Senna occidentalis (coffee senna)

This small shrub has yellow flowers. There is another plant of the same genus, *Senna obtusifolia*. They look alike and are both found in tropical parts of Australia and on the nearby islands. They are also found in the south-eastern states of the USA. The pods, which would only be eaten by starving animals, contain an unidentified toxin that causes striated muscle degeneration and necrosis. This results in myoglobinuria. There is no known antidote. Intravenous fluids may be successful.

Sesbania herbacea (dangle pod)

This used to be called *Sesbania exaltata*. It is also wrongly called coffee weed, which is really *Cassia*

occidentalis. SACs will eat this weed and get transitory diarrhoea. Treatment is unnecessary.

Sesbania vesicara (bladder pod)

This is a tall annual legume with yellow flowers. It is also called sesbane. It grows wild in the south-east of the USA. It can be consumed by SACs. The toxic principle is unknown but the signs are mainly gastroenteric. Treatment is with intravenous fluids, which is normally successful.

Setaria sphacelata (setaria grass)

This grass is found in pastures throughout the tropics. It very rarely causes poisoning. The animals need to be starving and then to be offered a large amount of this grass, which contains oxalates. These cause hypocalcaemia, which normally results in recumbency. The treatment, which is normally successful, is with 20% calcium borogluconate solution given slowly intravenously. The dose is 80 ml.

Silybum marianum (variegated thistle)

This herb originates in southern and eastern regions of Australia on land that has been cultivated. It has been imported in to the UK and Europe as a garden plant. Rapid intake by tethered animals can lead to nitrate poisoning, shown as methaemoglobinaemia. There is a specific antidote, which is methylene blue at 10 mg/kg given slowly intravenously. The best approach is to set up an intravenous drip of warm isotonic saline and then slowly add the methylene blue.

Sinapis arvensis (charlock)

This common weed is a brassica with bright yellow flowers. It is commonly seen in cornfields, particularly on organic farms. It is a native of Europe but is also now found throughout the northern states of the USA. It is only poisonous when the pods have formed. It causes acute gastroenteritis in SACs, with violent colic.

Survival is unlikely. Oil of camphor is the recommended antidote. NSAIDs are supportive.

Solanum dulcamara (woody nightshade)

Like the other nightshades it contains solanine, but like black nightshade it does not appear to be as toxic as deadly nightshade. It is a trailing type of plant and does not seem attractive to SACs.

Solanum esuriale (solly weed)

This plant causes neurological signs in alpacas in Australia. The animals show a characteristic hump-back appearance. Treatment is non-specific with B vitamins and NSAIDs.

Solanum nigrum (black nightshade)

This is a weed commonly found in gardens worldwide. It grows up to 30 cm high. It contains solanine and other allied alkaloids but does not seem as toxic as deadly nightshade. There have been few cases of toxicity reported. However, it will grow in maize and then can be cut and be made into silage. Maize silage is unlikely to be fed to SACs but clinicians should be aware that black nightshade will cause severe enteritis and maybe even death. There is no specific antidote. Fluids and NSAIDs will be helpful.

Solanum pseudocapsicum (Jerusalem cherry)

This shrub, which has bright red cherry-like fruit, is found in gardens worldwide. It contains solanocapsine and other alkaloids. It causes abdominal pain and anorexia, so that it is self-limiting. Treatment is symptomatic.

Solanum tuberosum (potatoes)

These can safely be fed to SACs but only in small quantities. If they are allowed to gorge on them they will get a toxic acidosis. They will have violent diarrhoea. Treatment should be symptomatic. Green potatoes should never be fed as they are very toxic. Also there is a bad reaction when potatoes and either pea straw or pea silage are fed together. Animals will die rapidly. Both feeds are acceptable in moderation separately but they should never be fed together.

Sophora secundiflora (mescal bean)

The beans from this tree found in Mexico, Texas and New Mexico contain a quinolizidine alkaloid. If large quantities are consumed quickly by SACs they will show nervous signs and fall over but remain alert. They will continue to eat. If they are prevented from eating more beans and given good-quality forage they will recover in a few minutes.

Sorghum halepense (Johnson grass)

This is very similar to Sudan grass. It causes the same toxicities of cyanide and nitrate poisoning.

Sorghum vulgare (Sudan grass)

This forage grass, which originated in Africa, is now grown throughout North America and is safe when cut as hay from a hydrocyanic acid poisoning perspective. However, when it is fed fresh in drought conditions or when it has been damaged by trampling or frost then it is toxic. The toxicity is that of cyanide poisoning. The pathognomic sign shown is the blood is bright red. Sudan grass can cause another problem if it has been heavily fertilized with nitrogen. It can cause nitrate poisoning. This can be avoided by not top-dressing with large quantities of nitrogen and accepting the lower yields. An alternative is to get the crop tested for nitrates and feed accordingly. The pathognomic sign for nitrate poisoning is when the blood is chocolate brown. Sudan grass toxicity is primarily a problem for cattle farmers. It is rarely grown to be the sole feed for SACs.

Stachys arvensis (stagger weed)

This herb with pink tubular flowers is a widespread weed of cultivation throughout Australia. The toxic principle is unknown but as the name suggests it causes incoordination. There is no specific treatment but animals normally get better on their own if they are not chased or stressed.

Stemodia kingii (woolly twintip)

This herb has blue tubular flowers and grows in the inland regions of Western Australia. A very similar species is found in more arid areas of North America. It contains cucurbitacins, which cause peracute irritation to the gastro-enteric tract. The resulting severe diarrhoea can cause death unless the animal is rehydrated immediately by intravenous normal saline. There is no specific antidote.

Stypandra glauca (blind grass)

This is not really a grass but a perennial herb with blue flowers. It is found in the temperate areas of Australia. It is also found in gardens, where it is called the 'nodding blue lily'. It contains stypandrol. This causes irreversible blindness by retinal and optic nerve degeneration. There is no effective treatment. Toxicity is rare as SACs rarely eat the growing plant. Ingestion can occur in hay.

Swainsona spp. (Darling or Swainson peas)

These herbs can have a variety of colours of flower. They originate in subtropical regions of Australia. However, they now can be found in gardens throughout the world. They contain an indolizidine alkaloid, which primarily causes incoordination but may also cause abortion. SACs need over 4 weeks of exposure before there are signs of toxicity. Poisoning is therefore only likely in subtropical areas of Australia. There is no antidote. However, if the animals are denied access to the plant they will recover except abortions cannot be prevented. It is reputed that certain animals develop a craving for the plant.

Tamus communis (black bryony)

This common hedge-climbing plant, with greenish white flowers, is found in England but not in Scotland. SACs can eat the leaves without ill effects. The author has eaten it as a boiled vegetable served with butter in Algeria. It is found throughout Africa north of the Sahara, where it originated. However, the bright red berries contain a glycoside, which is irritant but more importantly is a strong narcotic. It causes colic, paralysis and rapid death. Treatment is unlikely to be successful. Demulcents (e.g. egg whites) have been recommended.

Taxus baccata (yew)

Established veterinary opinion is that this is an extremely poisonous plant. In theory SACs need very little of the foliage or the berries to die. However, they do not eat the live tree. The danger is clippings from yew hedges. The toxicity is normally peracute and the animal is found either dead or totally collapsed. There is no realistic treatment. However, one author (Angus, 2010) reported after heavy snow in early January 2009 that three adult roe deer (*Capreolus capreolus*) ate large quantities of yew branches. A second author (Scott, 2010) confirms seeing muntjac deer (*Muntiacus reevesi*) and Soay sheep browsing yew branches on trees during snowy periods with no ill effects. The tolerance to yew is confirmed by a third author (Stevenson, 2010), having seen his own Lleyn sheep eating the branches. A fourth author (Swarbrick, 2010) confirms resistance to yew by roe deer and muntjac deer. This author considers that the profession should be prepared to review its views on the toxicity of yew in at least sheep. There is no doubt that the berries are more toxic. It is still prudent to deny access to yew to SACs as yew is definitely extremely toxic to cattle in the author's own experience. It is reasonable to expect it to be toxic to SACs. Other yew species (e.g. Japanese yew *Taxus cuspidate*) appear to be more toxic to SACs in the author's experience.

Terminalia oblongata (yellow wood)

This deciduous tree has small white flowers. It is only found in the McKenzie River basin of north-eastern Queensland, Australia. SACs are poisoned by large intakes of fallen branches. The tannins cause convulsions. There is no antidote. Euthanasia is indicated.

Tetradymia spp. (horsebrush)

This is a shrub found in arid areas of western North America. It causes photosensitization of the non-woolly white areas of llamas' faces. Affected animals should be brought in and treated with vitamin B injections.

Trachyandra divaricata (branched onion weed)

This herb originated in south-west Australia and is found throughout the world. It has white flowers and a rhizome, which contains an unknown toxin, which causes ataxia and recumbency. There is no known antidote. If the llamas or alpacas are recumbent but still eating they will normally recover. If they have stopped eating euthanasia is indicated.

Trema tomentosa (poison peach)

This small tree has small white flowers, which develop into small black fruit. The trees are found in northern and north-eastern areas of Australia and on tropical islands nearby. Llamas are not normally poisoned unless the branches are broken or cut for browse. The unidentified toxin affects the liver and can cause death from hepatoencephalopathy. There is no known treatment.

Trianthema spp. (red spinach)

This succulent prostrate herb is found in the arid and semi-arid areas of northern Australia. It requires rapid intake by SACs so poisoning is only likely when the animals are starving. Toxicity therefore is extremely rare. The plant contains oxalates, which cause hypocalcaemia and result in recumbency. Treatment, which is normally successful, is 80 ml of 20% calcium borogluconate given slowly intravenously.

Tribulus terrestris (caltrop)

This prostrate creeping herb originated in southern Europe and is found throughout the world. It has small yellow flowers. The plant contains steroidal saponins, which are enhanced by wilting. Toxicity is only seen if this plant is the main part of the diet of llamas for several weeks. The main sign is photosensitization. The affected animals should be brought in. Vitamin B injections and a low-protein diet will help the affected liver to regenerate. Like so many poisonous plants, this herb may have medicinal effects. It may stimulate sexual behaviour in male SACs.

Triglochin maritima (arrowgrass)

This plant contains a cyanogenic glycoside, which causes not only neurotoxic signs but also dyspnoea with bright red blood. The plant is found worldwide. The specific antidote is sodium thiosulfate, which should be given intravenously at a rate of 30 mg/kg, well diluted in warm normal saline twice daily for 3 days.

Urochloa panicoides (liverseed grass)

This grass grows throughout the tropics and originated in southern Africa. If consumed lush and in large quantities it can cause nitrate poisoning in SACs. The specific antidote is methylene blue, which should be given at 10 mg/kg slowly intravenously. The best approach is to set up an intravenous drip of warm isotonic saline and then slowly add the methylene blue.

Veratrum californicum (false hellebore)

This plant is also called the 'corn lily'. It is an erect herb with white flowers. It is found throughout North America. The signs of poisoning are vomiting, convulsions and a fast irregular heartbeat. There is no specific antidote and symptomatic treatment is unlikely to be successful. It is not normally eaten by SACs.

Verbesina encelioides (crownbeard)

This herb has daisy-like yellow flowers. It causes problems in sandy soils in eastern Australia. It is also found in gardens in the UK and wild in parts of southern Europe, the Middle East and central Asia. The toxic principle galegine causes acute pulmonary oedema. There is no treatment and euthanasia is indicated. However, large intakes are required to cause toxicity. These are unlikely except with starved or tethered animals.

Viburnum spp. (viburnum)

There are over 150 species of this garden shrub, bush or small tree. They are all toxic to SACs to varying extents. The symptoms are the same as poisoning with rhododendron, i.e. gastritis making the animal vomit. The treatment is the same as for rhododendron poisoning, i.e. morphine and atropine.

Wedelia asperrima (yellow daisy)

This herb is a native of northern Australia. It is also called the sunflower daisy. Toxicity is rare as large intakes are required. It contains kaurene, which causes acute liver toxicity with a resulting encephalopathy. There is no effective treatment known.

Wikstroemia indica (tie bush)

This shrub is a native of the coastal areas of eastern Australia. It is liable to cause acute diarrhoea in SACs that have been tethered. There is no specific treatment. However, warm intravenous fluids and other supportive treatments are worthwhile.

Xanthium occidentale (Noogoora burr)

This upright annual herb is found in eastern Australia. As the name implies it has burrs, which contain the active toxin, kaurene. It is an acute liver toxin, which leads to an encephalopathy. There is no effective treatment and euthanasia is

indicated. Trekking llamas are at risk but otherwise toxicity is extremely rare.

Xanthium spp. (cocklebur)

This plant found in the south-east of the USA causes liver damage. It is a cumulative poison and so is unlikely to cause problems in alpacas or llamas. In theory it might cause photosensitization of the white areas of the faces of individual llamas.

Zamia pumila (coontie)

This cycad palm is found in gardens in many subtropical and tropical areas throughout the world. These trees originated in the Far East. SACs are unlikely to eat it unless it is on rubbish dumps. It causes neurological signs, which appear to be irreversible. Euthanasia is indicated.

Zantedeschia aethiopica (arum lily)

These striking large white lilies are found throughout the world as well as in gardens. They are also called calla lilies. They contain actual oxalate crystals, which irritate the buccal mucosa. The animals will froth at the mouth and even get laryngeal oedema with dyspnoea. There is little need for any anti-inflammatory treatment as the condition soon resolves. It normally occurs when animals escape into gardens.

Zea mays (maize)

This cultivated crop grown for maize or for silage is highly palatable. On non-organic farms it is normally top-dressed with large amounts of nitrogen fertilizer. This is what causes the problem for alpacas if they are allowed to gorge on the young green growing plants. They develop nitrate poisoning. The specific antidote is methylene blue, which should be given at 10 mg/kg slowly intravenously. The best approach is to set up an intravenous drip of warm isotonic saline and then slowly add the methylene blue.

Zephyranthes atamasco (rain lily)

This woodland plant is also called the Easter lily. It is at springtime that it is most toxic to llamas on the trek. It contains alkaloids with anticholinergic properties, mainly vomiting and excessive salivation. It is self-limiting and the effects although violent only last for an hour or so. Treatment is symptomatic but hardly required.

Zigadenus venenosus (death camas)

This poisonous plant is found in North America and has star-shaped white flowers. It is often called 'snakeroot'. It is also found in Asia. It will not normally be eaten by llamas except when they are tethered on a trek with little else to eat. The alkaloid will cause ataxia. There is no specific antidote. Recovery is likely unless large quantities have been eaten.

A Guide to Plants Found in the UK That Cause Poisoning Classified by the Signs Shown by the Affected Camelids

Plants that contain cardiac glycosides and therefore cause vasodilation with signs of acute shock

1. Cape tulip, *Homeria* spp.: Both the one-leaf and two-leaf varieties are toxic.
2. Christmas rose, *Helleborous niger*: A common garden flower. Very bitter so only a danger when cut.
3. Foxglove, *Digitalis purpurea*: An erect herbaceous summer flowering plant with purple flowers.
4. Purple sesbane, *Daubentonia punicea*: The orange flowering type are seen in gardens.

Plants that cause neurological signs

1. Aconite monkshood, *Aconite napellus*: A small purple flower found in gardens.
2. Blind grass, *Stypandra glauca*: Not a grass but a small purple flowering perennial.
3. Bracken, *Pteridium aquilinum*: Only toxic in large amounts.
4. Branched onion weed, *Trachyandra divaricatea*: Originally from Australia. A perennial plant with a white flower and a rhizome,

5. Fool's parsley, *Aethusa cynapium*: A herbaceous plant with white flowers found as a weed in gardens.
6. Golden rod, *Haplopappu heterophyllius*: This garden flower will cause neurological signs in suckling crias.
7. Hemlock, *Conium maculatum*: A plant with a white flower found in ditches. A danger after ditch dredging.
8. Laburnum, *Laburnham anagyroides*: A very toxic tree with yellow hanging flowers.
9. Lupines, *Lupinus* spp.: Found in gardens and grown as a nitrogen storing plant. The seed pods are toxic.
10. Male fern, *Dryopteris filix-mas*: Unlikely to be consumed in sufficient quantities. The roots are very toxic.
11. Mare's tail, *Equisetum* spp.: A very common pasture plant. Only consumed if the camelid is starving.
12. Marijuana, *Cannabis sativa*: A problem in illegally grown plants.
13. Marsh mallow, *Malva parviflora*: A common wasteland plant that only causes problems in suckling crias.
14. Poison morning glory, *Ipomoes muelleri*: A vine grown in gardens with pink trumpet flowers.
15. Rushes, *Juncus* spp.: A marshland plant only eaten when starving.
16. Rye grass, *Lolium* spp.: The poisoning is caused by two species of saprophytic fungi living on the grass.
17. Tobacco, *Nicotiana tabacum*: **Normally** eaten as a plant but poisoning seen in a camelid that had eaten cigarettes.
18. Water dropwort, *Oenanthe crocata*: The roots are very toxic and are eaten after ditch dredging.
19. Water hemlock, *Cicuta virosa*: The roots are very toxic and are eaten after ditch dredging.

Plants that cause blood clotting deficiency

1. Sweet clover, *Melilotus officinalis*: Only cause poisoning when crushed or made into hay. The specific treatment is vitamin K injections.

Plants that cause colic

1. Black bryony, *Tamus communis*: A common hedge climbing plant with white-green flowers. Only the berries are toxic.

2. Poke weed, *Phytolacca americana*: Originally from the USA but now common in gardens in the UK.
3. White bryony, *Bryonia dioica*: A hedge growing plant that is very toxic.

Plants that cause bloat

1. Clover, *Trifolium* spp.: An excess in pastures can cause problems.
2. Onions, *Allium* spp.: Large quantities need to be ingested.

Plants that contain taxine

1. Yew, *Taxus baccata*: A very common evergreen tree found in church yards and as hedges in gardens.

Plants that cause irritation of the oral mucous membranes

1. Spurges, *Euphorbia* spp.: Found as hedges or on wasteland.

Plants that cause gastroenteric signs with constipation

1. Acorns, *Quercus* spp.: Acorns are much more toxic than oak leaves, which are often browsed by camelids. Problems occur in dry autumns when there are high winds bringing down green acorns. Certain animals have a craving for them. They are best to be rolled into the soil to prevent ingestion.
2. Chickweed, *Stella media*: A small white flowering plant, traditionally grown to be fed to hens.
3. Pine needles, *Pinus* spp.: Various pine trees throughout the UK.

Plants that cause gastroenteric signs with diarrhoea

1. Autumn crocus, *Colchicum autumnale* (also called meadow saffron): It causes problems in crias which are suckling.

2. Avocado, *Persea americana*: The skins, which are toxic, are often consumed from compost heaps. The toxin, persin, affects the udder and causes mastitis.
3. Box, *Buxus sempervirens*: It is a common hedge plant in gardens. It is not touched when growing but toxicity occurs when animals are fed trimmings.
4. Castor bean, *Ricinus communis*: They are often included in animal feeds and are only toxic when consumed in large quantities.
5. Charlock, *Sinapis arvensis*: A common brassica weed with yellow flowers found in cornfields.
6. Cuckoo-pint, *Arum maculatum* (also called 'lords and ladies'): It is very bitter but animals are attracted by the very toxic red berries.
7. Daffodil, *Narcissus* spp.: The bulbs are mildly toxic.
8. Delphinium, *Delphinium* spp.: It is not eaten except when it is cut and dried.
9. Dog's mercury, *Mercurialis perennis*: It is only mildly toxic.
10. Ground elder, *Sambucus ebulus*: It is a common garden weed and is only mildly toxic.
11. Linseed, *Linum* spp.: It is often included in animal feed. It is purgative in large quantities.
12. Potatoes, *Solanum tuberosum*: The green leaves are toxic, and if the potato is green then they are toxic.
13. Privet, *Ligustrum* spp.: It is a common hedge plant. Large quantities of cuttings are cathartic.
14. Wild clematis, *Clematis vitalba* (also called 'Oldman's beard'): It is very irritant to the gastric mucosa but is rarely eaten.

Plants that cause haematuria

1. Marrowstem kale, *Brassica oleracea*: A fodder crop often eaten to excess.
2. Rape, *Brassica napus*: A fodder crop often eaten to excess.
3. Turnip weed, *Rapstrum rugosum*: This herb is not very palatable but requires only small amounts to cause toxicity. It contains S-methylcysteine sulphoxide (SMCO).
4. Wild radish, *Raphanus raphanistrum*: This herb also contains SMCO.

Plants that cause acute respiratory signs

1. Algae, *Microcystis* spp., *Anabena* spp. and *Aphanizomenon* spp.: These are all found in inland lakes and ponds.
2. Arum lily, *Zantedeschia aethiopica*: This is a garden plant that causes laryngeal oedema resulting in frothing at the mouth. The condition soon subsides.
3. Golden crown beard, *Verbesina encelioides*: This is a common herb with yellow daisy-like flowers.
4. Perilla mint, *Perilla frutescents* (also called curly perilla): It is found in gardens but is rarely eaten on account of its unpleasant smell.
5. Sweet potatoes, *Ipomoea batatas*: Large quantities are required to cause toxic signs. Usually fed by mistake.

Plants that contain a cyanogenic glycoside

These require a specific treatment of 20 mg/kg sodium thiosulphate intravenously together with 1 g/20 kg *per os* to detoxicate the remaining HCN in C1. This can be repeated in an hour.

1. Arrow grass, *Triglochin maritima*: Found in gardens but imported from the USA.
2. Bird's foot trefoil, *Lotus corniculatus*: Commonly found in cleared woodland.
3. Chinese photinia, *Photinia fraseri*: Found in gardens but imported from China.
4. Chinese sacred bamboo, *Nandina domestica*: Found in gardens but imported from China.
5. Laurel, *Laurus* spp. Large amounts need to be ingested so toxicity is rare except in animals given access to garden rubbish.
6. Wild cherry, *Prunus* spp. Found in gardens and woodland.

Plants that contain oxalic acid

These require a specific treatment of vitamin B preparations and 60 ml of 20% calcium borogluconate given intravenously.

1. Fat hen, *Chenopodium album*: Commonly found on waste ground and in cultivated areas between fruit trees. Large amounts are required so poisoning is rare except in animals tethered on a trek.
2. Ice plants, *Mesembryanthemum* spp. Only found in gardens having been imported from South Africa.
3. Rhubarb, *Rheum rhaponticum*: Found in vegetable gardens or on rubbish dumps.
4. Soft roly-poly, *Salsola kali*: A weed found in open woodland.
5. Sorrel, *Rumex acetosa*: A weed found in certain pastures, a relative of sheep sorrel *R. acelosella*. Poisoning is very rare.
6. Sugar beet, *Beta vulgaris*: Only causes problems if animals are suddenly fed large quantities.

Plants that contain hyoscamine and/or atropine and solanine

These require a specific treatment of neostigmine. This should be given at 0.01 mg/kg subcutaneously. Flunexin is useful to control the ileus.

1. Black nightshade, *Solanum nigrum*: It is not as toxic as deadly nightshade.
2. Deadly nightshade, *Atropa belladonna*: It is found in hedgerows. Normally animals will not touch this very toxic plant, except when it is in hay.
3. Henbane, *Hyoscyamus niger*: It is a very toxic ubiquitous garden plant.
4. Pheasant's eye, *Adonis macrocarpa*: It is originally from Australia but now it is commonly found in gardens.
5. Thorn apple, *Datura stramonium*: It is a very toxic woodland plant.
6. Woody nightshade, *Solanum dulcamara*: It is a trailing woodland plant not normally eaten.

Plants that contain nitrate/nitrite

These require a specific treatment of methylene blue. This should be given very slowly intravenously at 10 mg/kg.

1. Maize, *Zea mays*: A cultivated crop that is highly palatable and can easily be fed to excess.
2. Variegated thistle, *Silybum marianum*: Originated in Australia but is now a garden plant, which has purple flower-heads with spiny bracts, in the second year.

Plants that cause acute gastritis

These require a specific treatment of 2 ml twice daily of a 5% w/v solution of morphine sulphate and 2 l twice daily of a 0.5% w/v solution of atropine sulphate intramuscularly.

1. Azalea, *Rhododendron occidentale*: Found in gardens and ornamental woods. Animals show marked salivation and projectile vomiting. Flowers are seen in early summer.
2. Kalima, *Kalima* spp.: A common garden plant. Flowers are seen late spring.
3. Oleander, *Nerium oleander*: A flowering garden plant from Morocco. Eaten when cut.
4. Peris/white rim peris, *Pieris japonicum variegate*: A common garden plant from Japan. Urn-shaped flowers borne in panicles in spring.
5. Rhododendron, *Rhododendron ponticum*: This shrub originated in Nepal. It is very common in gardens and woodlands. It is particularly dangerous as it is very palatable to camelids.
6. Viburnum, *Viburn* spp.: There are many different species in this genus, which can be shrubs, bushes or small trees. They are readily eaten.

Plants that cause liver toxicity

These require a specific treatment of doses of vitamin B and a low-protein diet.

1. Algae, *Microcystis* spp., *Anabena spp.* and *Aphanizomenon* spp.: These are found in inland lakes, e.g. the Norfolk Broads.
2. Blue heliotrope, *Heliotropium amplexicaule*: An annual flower found commonly in gardens.
3. Bog asphodel, *Narthecium ossifagum*: Found in marshy ground. The main danger is when it is cut in hay.
4. Caltrop, *Tribulus terrestris*: A creeping herb with yellow flowers.
5. Common heliotrope, *Heliotropium europaeum*: An annual herb with white flowers.
6. Goats rue, *Galega officinalis*: A large herb with purple flowers. Large amounts are required to produce toxic signs.
7. Lantana, *Lantana camara*: Found in the wild as well as in gardens. Flowers throughout spring, summer and autumn.
8. Panicum, *Panicum* spp.: Grown as a fodder crop. Large quantities are required for toxicity.

9. Paterson's curse, *Echium plantagineum*: An annual garden herb with blue flowers.
10. Ragwort, *Senecio jacobea*: An annual plant with yellow flowers, Found in large quantities on wayside verges and horse pastures.
11. St John's wort, *Hypericum perforatum*: A common marshland plant that flowers in the summer.

Fungus Poisoning

Psilocybe cyanesciens (wavy caps)

This fungus found in the UK normally grows on dry bark, e.g. under swings in children's playgrounds. It will grow in paddocks normally in the autumn. The fungi are attractive to alpacas. The toxic signs shown are swollen lips, dyspnoea and slight tremors. Consumption of large amounts will cause ataxia and death. There is no antidote so treatment must be supportive.

Amanita spp.

These fungi found in the UK are very toxic to humans and to other mammals but have not been implicated in toxicity in SACs. They are *A. muscaria*, the fly agaric, *A. pantherina*, the panther cap, *A. phalloides*, the death cap, and *A. verna*, the destroying angel. The most toxic is the death cap. There is no antidote. Clinicians faced with a possible poisoning should set up a fluid line and carry out an emergency emptying of C1. Dexamethasone and glucose should be given intravenously. Morphine may help as the animals will suffer severe cramping pain. The prognosis is very poor and euthanasia must always be considered.

Chemical Poisons

Alphachloralose

Alphachloralose is the active ingredient of mouse bait. It causes death in mice by coma and hypothermia. SACs are unlikely to consume enough to cause problems. It is possible that crias might be affected. They should be warmed in a hot box to raise their core temperature. There are no references in the literature of incidents of toxicity.

Aluminium

Although this metal is potentially toxic because it binds up phosphorus, it does not appear to be toxic to SACs.

Amitraz

This acaricide used for dipping and spraying cattle is toxic to SACs. Alpacas may absorb a toxic dose from massive fleece contamination. It normally causes C1 atony and constipation, with resulting colic. Treatment is NSAIDs and oral liquid paraffin. Obviously the animal should be bathed to remove further chemical.

Antimony

This metal is not found free in nature but may cause toxicity from wastes associated with mining or indeed by discarded alloys containing antimony. Acute poisoning causes diarrhoea. Treatment is with oral magnesium oxide to precipitate the antimony and other demulcents to protect the mucous membranes. Chronic poisoning causes liver damage. The animals should be removed from further ingestion and treated with B vitamins by injection.

Arsenic

Poisoning from arsenic can be in two ways, as an inorganic source, or as an organic source. The source for inorganic poisoning is from rat bait, or acaricides. The principle sign is severe dysentery. The diagnosis can be confirmed by analysis of the ingesta, liver or kidney. Low doses of arsenic were included in tonics for horses to improve their coats. These should not be given to SACs. The specific treatment for toxicity is sodium thiosulfate at the rate of 30 mg/kg twice daily. Ideally this should be given by very slow intravenous injection. If a very dilute solution is used it can be given subcutaneously. It may cause a severe reaction and damage the fleece in alpacas. Oral administration is not effective. Historically, arsenic used to be included in pig food to prevent swine dysentery and as a growth promoter. This is the source of organic arsenic. Organic poisoning has a slower onset compared with the acute inorganic poisoning and shows neurological signs. There may also be diarrhoea. This should be controlled symptomatically as there is no specific treatment.

Battery acid

If animals lick the acid from batteries they will get ulcers on their tongues reminiscent of foot-and-mouth disease lesions. The condition is not life threatening.

Cadmium

Direct toxicity in SACs has not been recorded.

Caesium

Radioactive caesium was recorded in sheep in the UK after the Chernobyl disaster in 1986. However, no toxic effects were observed.

Cantharidin

Blister beetles of *Epicauta* spp. swarm on to lucerne during harvesting. The beetles contain cantharidin, which is very toxic to all animals. Cantharidin causes acute abdominal pain with diarrhoea. Shreds of mucosa will be seen in the faeces. It also causes haematuria. Animals will die unless stabilized by an isotonic saline drip. The toxicity of cantharidin does not diminish in stored hay.

Carbamate

These substances, which are herbicides and insecticides, will cause poisoning in all animals.

The signs and treatment are the same as for organophosphorous poisoning.

Chlorinated hydrocarbons

These insecticides and acaricides are very potent poisons in all animals. They cause nervous signs from overstimulation of the central nervous system. There are no specific antidotes and supportive treatment is rarely effective.

Closantel

Closantel is a salicylanilide drug used for the treatment and control of fasciolosis in sheep. It is also active against *Haemonchus contortus* and the nasal bot, *Oestrus ovis* (Barlow *et al.*, 2002). When it was given at four times the recommended dose rate it caused blindness 2 weeks later on account of retinal degeneration. This drug should not be used in SACs if possible as it has a very narrow safety margin.

Copper

There is a very fine margin of safety with copper in SACs. They all require some copper supplementation, particularly on copper-deficient land. Although this is rare, what is more likely is land that is high in molybdenum or sulfur. These two elements bind up the copper so it is not available for the animal. However, copper is very toxic to SACs and so supplementation has to be carried out with care. Copper ingestion can be cumulative. Historically, pigs used to be fed diets high in copper to act as a growth promoter. If such pig food is fed to SACs it will cause copper toxicity. The main sign is jaundice. This will be mirrored in the increase in liver enzymes, e.g. GLDH, AST and GGT. The SAC will be ataxic. If this is evident then the outcome is death. For a definitive diagnosis at post-mortem liver copper levels need to be above 8000 µmols/kg dry matter (DM) or kidney levels higher than 650 µmols/kg DM. Kidney samples are more reliable as there is not the same interference by iron as in the liver. There is no reliable antidote when the disease

has developed that far. However, a subcutaneous injection of 3.4 mg/kg ammonium tetrathiomolbdate on 3 alternate days has been successfully used for treatment of copper poisoning in sheep (Sargison, 2001). This author suggests treating the entire in-contact group. Young animals of all species are more susceptible to toxicity and deficiency. Soil ingestion may account for up to 30% of DM intake of copper.

The availability of dietary copper varies between different feeds. Feeds with high concentrations of available copper, which are liable to cause toxicity, include:

- Pasture, silage and root crops grown on ground to which large quantities of pig or poultry manure has been applied.
- Distillery by-product feeds such as dark grains produced from copper stills.
- Concentrate feeds containing palm oil or molassed sugarbeet pulp (wholegrain cereals are relatively poor sources of copper).
- Milk provides a highly available source of copper, and copper absorption is very efficient in young animals, hence crias suckling dams fed on copper-rich diets are at risk of copper poisoning.

Other potential sources of copper include access to cattle minerals, copper sulfate foot baths and fungicide-treated timber or vines.

The concentrations of copper antagonists are often low in preserved rations fed to housed animals.

Cyanide

Although this poison could potentially be ingested by SACs when used in the inorganic form as a rodenticide, this is not the normal type of poisoning seen. Many plants such as linseed, flax, wild black cherry, sorghum and Sudan grass contain cyanogenetic glycosides. These glycosides can be released by damage to the plants by herbicides or wilting. SACs are very susceptible. The main sign is bright red mucous membranes and severe asphyxia convulsions followed by death. The blood will appear bright red on post-mortem. Tests for hydrocyanic acid can be performed on the stomach contents to confirm the diagnosis, although the smell of 'bitter almonds' is strongly indicative of poisoning.

Treatment is specific: 30 mg/kg of sodium thiosulfate should be given intravenously. At the same time 3–5 g/h should be given by mouth to detoxify any remaining HCN in C1.

Fluoride

This element will cause chronic poisoning from factory contamination. There is marked excessive wearing of the teeth, together with some enlargement of the long bones, including the mandible. There are increased levels of fluorine in the urine and plasma. Obviously the animals should be removed from the contaminated pasture. Feeding of calcium carbonate will reduce the fluoride in the gut contents. If pastures may contain toxic levels of fluorine, animals should be fed rock phosphate to lower the danger of toxicity. The provision of salt licks will help prevent animals licking the soil. Provision of uncontaminated water is important. Any ponds or other sources of water should be fenced off. Acute fluorosis is extremely rare. It will only occur if there are several millimetres of ash on a pasture. The initial signs are gastroenteric, quickly leading on to collapse and death.

Formaldyde

This is used in a diluted form in foot baths. It is normally stored in a concentrated form and would not be attractive to animals. It is therefore unlikely to cause severe toxicity with nervous signs but is more likely to cause mild signs of abdominal discomfort and salivation if animals eat contaminated straw. Symptomatic treatment would be indicated.

Lead

Lead poisoning is possible if animals are kept in an enclosure constructed of very old farm gates with flaking lead paint. This cause of poisoning is relatively rare nowadays as lead paint has been banned in the UK for over 50 years. However, other causes have arisen, e.g. lead-acid batteries, burned building materials and contaminated soil from mining or even clay pigeon shooting (Payne and Liversey, 2010). Most cases are going to be seen when animals are out on pasture or on waste ground.

Animals may be found dead. However, more often they will be showing advanced neurological signs. Death is caused by convulsions leading to respiratory failure. There is a raised temperature, which may confuse the practitioner into thinking an infection is involved. Pregnant animals will abort. Colic is seen. There is blindness like in cases of cerebral-corticonecrosis, which is the main differential, but the high temperature is absent in CCN. Diagnosis can be made from whole blood in a lithium heparin tube (normally a green top). There is marked anaemia but no jaundice, unlike in copper poisoning. Haemonchosis must be ruled out. Chelation therapy with sodium calcium edetate will give rapid improvement. The dose is 75 mg/kg dissolved in normal saline given intravenously. This dose can be repeated several times. A daily injection of thiamine is helpful to reduce the deposition of lead in the tissues. The dose is 20 mg/kg. The use of thiamine will also reassure the practitioner that CCN is being treated in case the diagnosis is in doubt.

For prevention, owners are urged to dispose of all waste carefully, particularly batteries and building materials. Owners are strongly advised to check all over any waste ground before turn out, especially old bonfire sites. If land is going to be used that is likely to have high levels of geochemical lead, owners are advised to make sure the grass is not grazed too short. A minimum depth of 3 cm has been suggested for sheep by two authors (Payne and Liversey, 2010). It is vital that good water is supplied in troughs and that animals are not allowed to drink from run-off water.

Levamisole

SACs have a very small safety margin with this useful anthelmintic. Mild signs of diarrhoea will be seen when dosages are doubled as recommended by some authorities (see Chapter 6). Greater overdosing will cause neurological signs and even death. There is no specific antidote. Treatment is supportive.

Mercury

Organic mercury compounds used to be used as a dressing for seed. SACs might have access to a bag of old maize. They will show neurological signs, which may have a delayed onset. There are two recommended treatments. Sodium thiosulfate can be given intravenously at the rate of 30 mg/kg well diluted in normal saline or the easy option is to give British Anti Lewisite by mouth at the rate of 6.5 mg/kg. Both these treatments are a one off.

Metaldehyde

This lethal poison is found in slug and snail bait, which is normally blue/green. It can be spread on the ground surrounding crops. Animals are liable to be poisoned by spillage. It is very palatable and animals will actively seek it out. It is very toxic, causing neurological signs. There is no specific antidote but 2 ml of diazepam given intravenously for an adult will help to control the convulsions. To help to control the animal for the intravenous injection, 1 ml of acetyl promazine (ACP) 10 mg/ml should be given intramuscularly first, which is not easy in an animal convulsing. B vitamins will aid the liver in detoxicating the poison and will help to prevent liver damage, which has been reported. Sadly, in the author's experience death has resulted if convulsions have occurred, even if they are controlled with medication.

Monensin

This poisoning only occurs if cattle feed containing monensin (used as a growth promoter) is fed to SACs in high doses. It is extremely toxic and will cause total collapse and death from cardiac failure. Treatment is unrealistic but oral vitamin E has been recommended. Monensin is used in some parts of the world as a coccidiostat. It is not licensed in the UK.

Mycotoxins

Poisoning results from the ingestion of food contaminated with toxins produced by moulds, which occur throughout the environment. They may be found in a variety of feedstuffs. Mycotoxins affect animals in a wide variety of ways and as there are also many different types, diagnosis and identification are inherently difficult. In fact animals are rarely poisoned. There are three common moulds and mycotoxins that affect SACs. They are *Fusarium*, *Penicillium* and *Aspergillus*. *Aspergillus* is typically associated with warm climates whereas the other two are common in the UK. There are toxins that are found in specific plants, e.g. ergot, perennial ryegrass, sweet clover and fescue grass. However, the majority are found when there is poor harvesting and storage of feed, e.g. slow clamp filling and poor clamp consolidation leading to poor fermentation. There may also be a problem when feeding out with poor face management.

Nitrate

This is a fertilizer. It rarely causes poisoning. However, it is advisable not to put alpacas on to a treated pasture until after a shower of rain. It is bitter and alpacas will not willingly eat it. The signs are those of vasodilatation, similar to shock, i.e. a weak rapid pulse and low rectal temperature. There may be haemoglobinuria and petichial haemorrhages. The blood is said to be chocolate brown. The treatment is specific. It is a slow intravenous injection of 1% methylene blue at the rate of 5 mg/kg.

Organochlorine pesticides

These are very potent poisons. They cause peracute neurological signs, quickly followed by collapse and death. There is no antidote.

Organophosphate insecticides

These insecticides are very potent poisons. Their acute toxicity is due to cholinergic overstimulation. Poisoned animals will show neurological signs. Initially they will be ataxic with continuous attempts to urinate. This will lead on to convulsions and death. In theory an adult should be given 5 mg of atropine sulfate intravenously and a further 20 mg subcutaneously. However, the prognosis is extremely grave. There is also a danger of a delayed neurotoxicity.

Paraquat

This common weedkiller is very toxic to animals. There is no antidote. Death is relatively rapid in 6–8 h and is the result of massive pulmonary oedema. It is likely to contaminate water as recorded in Australia (Philbey and Morton, 2001).

Propylene glycol

This oily chemical is used as antifreeze in cars as well as being given to cattle with ketoacidosis. It is toxic if given to SACs in too large a dose. Practitioners should avoid its use.

Prostaglandin

Great care with these medicines should be taken in SACs. Acute pulmonary oedema has been reported in all species. There is no antidote. Oxygen may be helpful but normally they are found dead, 12 h after the injection.

Salt

Some animals can be remarkably stupid when offered large quantities of salt. Obviously they become very thirsty, then have diarrhoea and then start to stagger. Severe nervous signs will follow. Water should be given little and often as large amounts sccm to make the symptoms worse. Dexamethasone by intravenous injection is helpful. However, fluid therapy must be the treatment of choice.

Selenium

Selenium normally causes a chronic poisoning in grazing alpacas that ingest herbage containing very high levels of selenium. The first signs are loss of hair with cracking of the feet. Animals will recover totally when removed from the selenium-high diet. However if the animals are left on these pastures they will be found dead. Liver and kidney should be sent to the laboratory to confirm the diagnosis.

Sodium chlorate

This is an old-fashioned weedkiller. Its modern equivalent is sodium monochloroacetate. Sodium chlorate is palatable to SACs and causes convulsions and death. There is no specific treatment but diazepam should be used to control the convulsions. Fluid therapy will be helpful.

Urea

This can cause poisoning when animals manage to break up molasses blocks containing urea. If they eat chunks of these blocks rather than licking them they will suffer with urea poisoning. This will be manifest as neurological signs, mainly of hyper-excitement. Treatment with tranquillizers (e.g. acetylpromazine or diazepam) is recommended, followed by intravenous fluids.

Warfarin

This is found in rat bait. It is an anticoagulant. SACs appear to detoxicate them in C1. There are no problems with poisoning in the literature. If SACs are found to have consumed some quantity, their mucous membranes should be checked regularly for pallor. If that occurs, injections of vitamin K should be administered.

Wood preservatives

These are phenol-containing substances. They are very corrosive and unlikely to be drunk. The author understands that creosote has been banned in the UK. However, the modern compounds are still toxic. The only likely problem would be an alpaca knocking over a large container and getting its wool soaked. The phenol can be absorbed through the skin. The animal will show depression, diarrhoea and a very subnormal rectal temperature. Shearing may be the best course of action so that the substance can be washed off with warm soapy water. The animal should be kept warm.

Zinc

Zinc is much less toxic than copper and so it has replaced copper in sheep foot baths. However, it is toxic and will cause diarrhoea and weight loss in SACs if it is fed to excess to try to control skin disease.

Other Toxic Products

Cloth

This is mainly a problem in alpacas kept as pets in gardens and around houses. They may ingest anything from string to washing off the line. The problem arises if the cloth or string balls up in C1. The animal will become inappetent. Diagnosis is difficult. Removal by opening C1 surgically is the only treatment as liquid paraffin will be ineffective.

Stale concentrate feed

This is likely to be attractive to SACs and can cause many problems. First of all excessive hard feed will cause acute acidosis. Treatment will consist of fluids by mouth and intravenous fluids spiked with bicarbonate. Vitamin B injections will be useful. Stale food also is liable to contain aflatoxins. This will result in ataxia, convulsions and hyperammonaemia leading to hepatic encephalopathy. There is no helpful treatment and therefore euthanasia must be advised.

Stored fruit

This is normally a problem in animals that break into food stores. If they ingest large quantities of fruit, particularly if is fermenting, they will get alcoholic poisoning and diarrhoea. Treatment is with large doses of vitamin B by injection.

17

Zoonotic Diseases

General

Zoonotic diseases have always been important. However, they are even more important now as the number of emerging diseases with zoonotic implications is increasing rapidly. Veterinarians have a large role to play in controlling these diseases and in advising their medical colleagues on the real risks that animal diseases pose to humans. Zoonotic diseases can be viral, bacterial, fungal, protozoal and parasitic in origin. Veterinarians are uniquely qualified to advise on prevention and reduce the chances of transmission to humans by proper education and management techniques. Veterinarians have a duty of care to the general populace, the owners and carers of the animals concerned, their own staff and of course to themselves. Washable protective clothing should be worn if possible.

There are some very simple measures that can be taken to protect yourself, your family and your staff from zoonotic diseases. You can also advise your clients how to protect themselves and their families as well as visitors to their farms:

- Never cuddle SACs or give newly born crias mouth-to-mouth resuscitation.
- Always wash your hands thoroughly after handling SACs.
- Always wash your hands before handling food.

- Remove dirty clothes before entering the kitchen.
- Pay particular attention to the hygiene of children.

As farmers, if you have an open farm, you have an obligation to:

- keep the farm clean;
- keep animals, their feed and water clean;
- handle dung, manure, slurry and sewage safely;
- protect water supplies and water courses;
- reduce transport stress of animals; and
- keep transport vehicles clean.

Viral Zoonotic Diseases of SACs Categorized by Their Human Medical Name

Contagious pustular dermatitis

This viral sheep disease is extremely common. It is also seen in SACs. Animals do build up immunity. There are vaccines available for sheep but they should not be used in SACs. However, the virus is very hard to eradicate and survives for a considerable length of time in organic matter, whether inside or out on the pasture (Gallina and Scagliarini, 2010). It is very contagious to

© Graham R. Duncanson 2023. *Veterinary Treatment of Llamas and Alpacas,* 2nd Edition (G.R. Duncanson)
DOI: 10.1079/9781800623576.0017

humans and only requires a small abrasion to infect the skin, normally on the hands or forearm. The lesions tend to develop into what used to be called a 'cold abscess'. These should not be lanced as the open wound will take weeks to heal.

Foot-and-mouth disease

This is obviously a very important livestock disease. It infects SACs. Humans are very resistant to the disease. It is therefore a very rare zoonotic disease. Transmission of the virus either between humans or from humans back to animals has never been confirmed. The disease in humans is primarily in people in close contact with infected animals. The incubation period is 2–4 days. Normally there is a skin wound or wound on the oral mucosa where the primary vesicle appears. Other vesicles may appear in the mouth or on the hands and feet. Normally after brief pyrexia the person is fully recovered in 1 week.

Louping-ill

This disease of sheep is caused by a flavivirus and is spread by the sheep tick *Ixodes ricinus*. It will infect SACs. It is primarily a neurological disease. Some pregnant animals will abort or produce live crias that show neurological signs. The disease in humans is extremely rare and requires the bite of the tick. In humans there is an incubation period of 2–8 days. The disease is biphasic with the first few days of fever. Then there are 5 days where there are no symptoms and then in the odd case there will be neurological signs resembling poliomyelitis. These cases may need a long convalescence but all cases will recover.

Middle East respiratory syndrome coronavirus

This severe respiratory disease (MERS-CoV) has a high case fatality in humans. Dromedary camels are considered the major reservoir host. Camelids are certainly susceptible. They demonstrate a mild to moderate upper respiratory infection. There is no specific treatment. Hopefully a vaccine will be developed (Te *et al.*, 2022).

Rabies

This dreaded disease is caused by a lyssavirus. SACs are the end host and do not exhibit the furious form and so they are not a real danger to humans. However, it is possible in certain cases for there to be virus particles in the saliva and so clinicians should take care when carrying out examinations on any suspect cases. The signs of disease shown by SACs are at first nondescript. They move away from the others and appear to be depressed with dilated pupils. They normally contract the disease from the bite of an infected carnivore or an infected bat. Often the clinician will be drawn to the place of the bite wound as the animal will show a hypersensitivity reaction at that site. They will normally develop progressive neurological signs starting with muscle tremors and slight incoordination progressing to collapse, convulsions and death. The disease is invariably fatal in these animals as it is in humans once there are severe neurological signs. There is no treatment but there are very good vaccines available for humans and SACs.

Vesicular stomatitis

This disease called 'sore mouth' mainly affects horses and cattle. However, it has been seen in SACs in South America. The disease is of little importance except that it resembles foot-and-mouth disease (FMD) and causes problems with diagnosis. Small papules and vesicles appear on the mouth, teats and interdigital areas. They very quickly regress. In humans the disease resembles a mild infection of influenza with a few vesicles in the mouth.

West Nile fever

This disease has risen to prominence as although it is a flavivirus and spread by mosquitoes it is very prevalent in veterinary surgeons, particularly those dealing with horses. The main reservoir for the virus is wild birds. The horse is just an incidental host. It could infect SACs. The human also is an incidental host, but the virus can cause fatal encephalitis. The disease can also be severe in horses. A vaccine is still in the experimental stage. Controlling the vector is difficult as the mosquitoes are ornithophilic, but are not always anthropophilic.

Bacterial Zoonotic Diseases of SACs Categorized by Their Human Medical Name

Actinomycosis

Although it is just possible that this is a zoonosis, in reality it is extremely unlikely. Actinomycosis in humans is normally caused by *Actinomyces israelii*. These bacteria are found in the normal flora of the human buccal cavity. They invade the soft tissue and bones when teeth are extracted. They also invade the genital tract of women using intrauterine contraceptive devices. The organism has never been isolated from animals. However, *Actinomyces bovis* is a common pathogen in cattle, causing the condition of 'lumpy jaw'. *Actinobacillus ligniersii* causes the condition called 'wooden tongue', and has been isolated in SACs. It causes granulomatous lesions in the soft tissues of the oral cavity and in the mandible. *Actinomyces bovis* has been found in oral lesions in humans, but it is extremely rare. Treatments in animals rely on high doses of streptomycin given over long periods if the organism has invaded the bone, but for shorter periods if just soft tissue is involved. Both organisms are found worldwide.

Animal erysipelas (human erysipeloid)

There is considerable confusion concerning this condition as a zoonosis. The zoonosis is caused by the bacteria *Erysipelas rhusiopathiae*. This organism is found in the soil all over the world. It commonly causes disease in pigs. SACs kept in close contact with pigs will develop an endocarditis when infected with this organism. The disease in humans caused by *E. rhusiopathiae* is a skin disease found in persons working in close proximity to pigs. The organism needs an abrasion to cause the infection. The organism is readily cured by penicillin in both humans and animals except when there is long-term vegetative endocarditis in SACs.

The confusion arises as there is a condition in humans termed erysipelas or 'fish sorters disease', which is not caused by *E. rhusiopathiae* but by a streptococcus. This organism is found in fish and in marine mammals. It is a systemic disease as well as a skin disease and so is a more serious condition in humans. However, it also is sensitive to penicillin.

Anthrax

This disease is perhaps the most notorious zoonosis. The organism *Bacillus anthracis* occurs in all mammals. It has three manifestations in man. 'Wool-sorters disease' is the invariably fatal pneumonic form caught from the skins of sheep and goats. There is an enteric form from eating carcasses contaminated with *B. anthracis*. This has been recorded in the Andes from eating SACs that have died from the disease. Although this is an acute form, liaison between veterinary surgeons and doctors can prevent deaths by prompt treatment with penicillin. The third form, which is the most common, is the skin form. This occurs in slaughterhouse workers, knackermen and even veterinary surgeons who handle diseased carcasses. Although it has a slower onset, it is still a very serious disease. The disease starts as a malignant pustule. The bacteria then rapidly move up the lymphatics. Once again prompt penicillin treatment will prevent deaths.

Anthrax is renowned for causing sudden death in cattle. It can do this in SACs if they eat large numbers of spores in contaminated feed. This has normally occurred by feed being transported in containers that have previously contained contaminated hides and skins. The very resistant spores are only formed when carcasses are opened and the bacteria are in an oxygen-rich environment. This should be avoided as the soil, or even worse a watercourse, will become contaminated. SACs may get an acute form. They will have a high fever with bloody diarrhoea and even haematuria. The organisms in their chains with their distinctive staining capsules can be found on a blood smear. These smears after heat fixing need to be stained for 30 s in old methylene blue stain (called McFadyeans stain). This is then washed off with tap water and the slide is examined under oil emersion. Treatment in these cases can be successful with intravenous crystalline penicillin in high doses. This does not lead to contamination of the environment.

Botulism

This disease is caused by the toxin produced by the anaerobic spore-forming bacterium, *Clostridium botulinum*. All warm-blooded animals are affected. There is a high mortality both in animals and in humans. The picture is confusing as there are four groups of organism, which produce seven antigenic types of toxin. Most human deaths are caused by eating contaminated food. There is an infant form where the organism colonizes the intestine and produces toxin. There is a third form where the organism can enter the skin through an abrasion and then produce toxin in an anaerobic environment.

Botulism is normally not an actual zoonosis as humans are poisoned by eating food in which the bacteria has produced toxin, e.g. in contaminated fish. Cases have been recorded worldwide. Camelids have been shown to die from the disease, so in theory it could kill SACs but it has never been reported.

Brucellosis

Brucella melitensis is not found in the UK but is common in the Mediterranean basin, the Middle East and central Asia. *B. melitensis* is a very serious disease in humans. It causes high fever, which may undulate over 24 h and also undulate in attacks separated by several days. It causes severe headaches and depression. It causes splenomegaly and therefore may be confused with malaria. Attacks may keep recurring for several years. It principally occurs in SACs when they are run together with sheep and goats. In this way it can be spread to SACs and has been reported in Peru, Argentina and Chile. *B. ovis* and *B. abortus* have not been isolated in SACs.

Campylobacteriosis

This is caused by *Campylobacter jejuni*. It is the main cause of acute bacterial enteritis in the UK. The most common animal host to be a danger to

humans is the chicken. In humans the organism causes acute diarrhoea, which is self-limiting. Care should be taken to protect a child if they are vomiting as severe dehydration has very serious consequences. It is extremely rare in SACs.

Clostridial food poisoning

Although these many species of bacteria are very important and prevalent in SACs, it is not an important zoonosis. The organism is found in soil and dust and so animals are not the main cause of infection. The *Clostridium* spp. that occur in SACs cause very mild enteritis in humans, which rarely lasts more than 24 h. It is self-limiting. The important pathogen in humans is *C. difficile*, which is not pathogenic, or found in SACs.

Clostridial wound infections

The most important bacteria in this group is *Clostridium tetani*, which receives a large amount of media hype. Tetanus is a very serious disease in humans, causing neurological signs. However, an animal is not required for the infection, which normally comes from a contaminated deep puncture wound. *C. tetani* is a ubiquitous organism in the soil throughout the world. It requires anaerobic conditions to multiply and release its sometimes fatal toxin. Tetanus is a very serious disease in SACs; however, they are not contagious to humans. Other *Clostridium* spp. will infect the wounds in humans or in SACs. They cause serious gangrene and death but humans cannot become infected from animals. The main organisms are *C. novyi*, *C. septicum* and *C. sordellii*. These organisms may infect humans and SACs by injections with contaminated needles.

Colibacillosis

This is a very important life-threatening zoonotic disease. It is particularly serious in the old and in children. The most important highly pathogenic *Escherichia coli* is the verocytotoxigenic strain *E. coli* O157. In other countries there are other verocytotoxigenic strains, e.g.

O26. Verocytotoxigenic strains of *E. coli* do occur in SACs but they are not pathogenic to them. A survey in the UK (Featherstone *et al.*, 2011) indicated that approximately 2% of SACs were carrying VTEC O157 although they were not indicated in an outbreak on an open farm in Surrey, UK (Griffin, 2010). VTEC O157 is carried asymptomatically by animals, and owners of SACs should be aware of the potential for zoonotic transmission of VTEC O157 even from healthy animals. Avoiding contact with animal faeces and adopting principles of good hygiene following animal contact is crucial in reducing the risk of zoonotic infections. The tendency of SACs to spit occasionally is another potential risk factor to consider, given that VTEC O157 has been isolated from the saliva of other animals (Keen and Elder, 2002).

However, hygiene for humans when handling animals is very important, particularly in children who are really at risk on open recreational farms. The greatest danger to man is from cattle. However, SACs are well recognized as animals harbouring the organism and therefore are a risk to humans. Avoiding contact with animal faeces and adopting principles of good hygiene following animal contact is crucial in reducing the risk of zoonotic infections. O157 infection is acquired from animals either directly or indirectly. The organism colonizes the rectal-anal junction of certain individual animals and these become supershedders. The routes of infection in humans are: contaminated food or water, direct animal contact, indirect animal contact through the environment and person-to-person spread.

Corynebacteriosis

Corynebacterium diphtheria is a very serious condition in humans but it does not occur in animals. *Corynebacterium pseudotuberculosis* is a very important pathogen in SACs. It is called caseous lymphadenitis. It has a long incubation period of one to two months and can be shown in sera by an ELISA test. Although the organism is susceptible to most antibiotics, treatment is rarely successful (Sting *et al.*, 2022a). However, although there are cases of *C. pseudotuberculosis* reported in humans they are extremely rare. The

disease causes caseous lymphadenitis in animals and this is seen in man but only in immune-suppressed individuals.

Dermatophilosis

This is a skin condition in SACs. It causes extensive mycotic dermatitis called lumpy wool in alpacas. However, the cases recorded in humans can be counted on one hand and so it is not an important zoonosis.

Leptospirosis

There is considerable confusion with this zoonotic disease. *Leptospira icterohaemorrhagiae* is a very serious often fatal disease in humans, called Weil's disease. It manifests as jaundice, fever and vomiting. However, sometimes jaundice is not a feature but it is just as serious. This disease is passed to humans from rodents, which are normally symptomless carriers. Pigs can get the disease and infect humans. This serovar is not a known pathogen of SACs in the Antipodes. Leptospira species have been found in SACs in Austria (Steinparzer *et al.*,2022). However, SACs will become infected with *Leptospira harjo*. This infection is rare unlike in cattle where it is a very common pathogen. If SACs do show symptoms it is usually a widespread short-term malaise but sometimes abortions will occur. *Leptospira harjo* is not a serious disease in humans. It is caught from drinking contaminated fresh milk or more commonly in farmers from infected urine. SACs are rarely a zoonotic focus as they are rarely affected. In humans the disease is similar to a short influenza attack, often over in 48 h.

Listeriosis

This disease is caused by *Listeria monocytogenes*. It is a very serious infection in very young babies and will cause abortion in humans. It can also cause fatalities in elderly patients. It is found throughout the world. Humans become infected by eating contaminated food, e.g. cheese made from contaminated milk. Neonates can become infected in late pregnancy. Although SACs can be infected with the disease, which causes encephalitis, neonatal mortality and septicaemia, giving mortalities as high as 30%, they are unlikely to transmit the disease to humans. It is seen in animals eating poor quality silage and so infections are rare in SACs.

Pasteurellosis

There is confusion in the nomenclature of the two agents causing this disease. They used to be called *Pasteurella multocida* and *Pasteurella haemolytica*. They are now called *Mannheimia*. They do occur in SACs, where they cause severe pneumonia. The disease in humans is extremely rare and even more rarely related to SACs. It normally occurs in humans from bites or scratches from dogs and cats. The organism lives asymptomatically in their mouths. It is not found in the mouths of SACs.

Rhodococcus

Rhodococcus equi is a pathogen primarily known for infections in equine foals, but it is also present in SACs as reported by Sting *et al.*, 2022b. The authors suggest that it should be considered as a zoonotic infection in the One Health approach.

Salmonellosis

Salmonella typhimurium

This organism has been recorded in SACs but has never been recorded as a zoonosis from them. However, it is a common cause of enteritis in humans. *Salmonella enteritidis* is a very common cause of enteritis in humans but is caught from chickens and does not occur in SACs. There are other causes of salmonellosis that are ever-present on farms, namely *Salmonella enterica* ssp. *Salmonella diarizonae*, *Salmonella montevideo* and *Salmonella dublin*. These organisms are not renowned for being present in SACs and are more commonly found in other farm animals.

Most human salmonella infections are acquired as a result of eating contaminated food.

Infection acquired on farms, however, is more commonly acquired by mouth from hands contaminated by infected animals, their bedding and surroundings. People who are ill with salmonellosis often have diarrhoea, vomiting or a flu-like illness. Children, pregnant women, the elderly and occasionally healthy adults may become seriously ill and require hospital treatment.

These simple precautions will go a long way to prevent people associated with livestock from becoming infected with salmonellosis:

- Do observe high standards of personal hygiene; wear rubber boots and protective overgarments when working with animals.
- Do change and launder overalls frequently and disinfect boots to avoid spreading the infection to other animals and people.
- Do wash your hands using hot water and soap immediately after working with infected animals.
- Do wash hands before eating, drinking or smoking.
- Do ensure that anyone with diarrhoea, vomiting or flu-like illness consults a doctor, and informs the doctor if salmonellas have been isolated from livestock.
- Do not take or wear dirty clothing and boots into the home.
- Do not allow vulnerable people, including children, the elderly and pregnant women to come into contact with infected animals.
- Do not bring infected animals into any room where food is prepared or eaten.
- Do not allow pets to come in contact with infected animals.

Zoonotic tuberculosis

Tuberculosis in humans is normally caused by the human pathogen *Mycobacterium tuberculosis*. However, humans can become infected by *Mycobacterium bovis*. This is primarily a disease affecting cattle and badgers. It is a chronic condition eventually leading to severe caseous pneumonia and death in both cattle and badgers. Humans become infected by drinking unpasteurized contaminated milk. *M. bovis* is now quite commonly seen in SACs. They will quite readily become infected either from badgers, cattle or other SACs. It is thought that the main mode of transmission between SACs is respiratory as many SACs have active lesions in the lungs. However, a case of *M. bovis* has been reported in the mammary gland of an alpaca (Richey *et al.*, 2011). This animal had a chronic discharging sinus in the mammary gland, which was flushed continuously by the owner and the practitioner creating bacterial aerosols with obvious serious zoonotic implications. It is a real zoonotic problem as humans can readily become infected by close contact (Twomey *et al.*, 2010c). The intradermal skin test is not very reliable in cattle and it is even worse in SACs. At the time of writing the blood test is little better. In SACs the disease can be of a very chronic nature and therefore very difficult to recognize clinically. There is no suitable treatment.

Chlamydioses and Rickettsioses of SACs Categorized by Their Human Medical Name

Chlamydiosis

This is caused by *Chlamydophila abortus*, which is found in SACs. The medical profession is very aware of the disease and its zoonotic implications. The general public is also alarmed. A large amount of investigation into the condition in humans has been carried out. It is now thought that the organism is not nearly as dangerous as had been suggested. The organism is a very common specific ovine pathogen causing abortion, and it is rare that it infects humans. Only three cases had been recorded in the last 20 years in the UK. However, it is advisable for pregnant ladies not to have close contact with SACs that are aborting. The infection has been found in Austria (Steinparzer *et al.*, 2022).

Q fever

Coxiella burnetti causes 'Q' fever. It can be spread from animals to humans through close contact and through the drinking water. It can also be spread by ticks. There has been a recent 'Q' fever epidemic in the Netherlands, which is the largest ever epidemic reported globally. The source of

infection was aerosol transmission from a very high concentration of large, infected dairy goat units located close to the human population (Harwood *et al.*, 2010). It has also been found in Austria (Steinparzer *et al.*, 2022). The disease is an influenza-type condition in humans. It does respond to oxytetracyclines in high doses. It causes abortion in SACs and the results of abortion are contagious to humans. The best test would appear to be an immunofluorescence assay (Tellis *et al.*, 2022). *Coxiella burnetti* is shed in large numbers from the reproductive tracts in a spore-like form, which is very resistant in the environment.

Fungal Zoonotic Diseases of SACs Categorized by Their Human Medical Name

Dermatophytosis

Compared to cattle, ringworm in SACs is extremely rare. However, SACs will contract *Trichophyton verrucosum* from cattle. The lesions are normally around the face in alpacas but will occur elsewhere in llamas. The organism is very contagious to humans. Prevention by thorough washing with soap and water must be recommended. Violent scrubbing and very strong disinfectants should be avoided as these will damage the skin. *Microsporum canis* has been recorded in SACs following bite wounds from dogs on the hindlegs and rump. *Microsporum gypseum* has been recorded in llamas. However, neither of the *Microsporum* species is very contagious to man.

Protozoal Zoonotic Diseases of SACs Categorized by Their Human Medical Name

Babesiosis

Although this protozoan has a worldwide incidence, it is not an important zoonosis. It is spread by ticks. However, humans seem resistant to the disease so infections are extremely rare. It is also rare in SACs, being primarily a cattle parasite.

The disease in humans is characterized by a severe illness with jaundice and haemoglobinuria.

Cryptosporidiosis

This protozoan has a worldwide distribution. It can cause a very serious disease in humans, either meningitis or pneumonia. However, such manifestations are extremely rare. The normal manifestation is acute diarrhoea, which is unpleasant but normally self-limiting. SACs will become infected by the organism, particularly in young animals. They may show quite severe diarrhoea or they may be symptomless carriers. Bottle-fed animals are particularly often symptomless carriers. The main human danger is from children visiting open, educational farms. The disease can be well contained by strict hygiene, involving/including hand washing and not allowing eating and drinking near the animals.

Toxoplasmosis

The causal organism is *Toxoplasma gondii*. There is no doubt that this organism is pathogenic to humans. Equally there is no doubt that it causes abortion in SACs. It has been recorded in Austria (Steinparzer *et al.*, 2022). However, the level of infection in aborted fetuses and their membranes is extremely low. On the other hand the level of infection in the faeces of certain cats is extremely high. It is the cats and rodents that need to be controlled to prevent the danger of this disease.

Parasitic Zoonotic Diseases of SACs Categorized by Their Human Medical Name

Coenurosis

This disease is caused by the larval stage of the tapeworm *Taenia multiceps*, which is called *Coenurus cerebralis*. The normal life cycle occurs in the dog or wild canid, e.g. the fox, the jackal or the coyote. They harbour the tapeworm in their intestine as the definitive host. The life cycle starts with the expulsion of gravid proglottids or eggs within the faeces of the definitive host. Intermediate hosts are affected by ingesting the eggs with grass or water. The normal intermediate host is the sheep or rarely the SAC. The oncospheres penetrate the wall of the small intestine and, via the blood vessels, are distributed to different tissues and organs. The cycle is completed when a dog or wild canid ingests tissue or an organ containing the coenuri. In the case of *C. cerebralis* the organ is the brain. In SACs the cystic *C. cerebralis* will reach a size of 5 cm in 6 months and cause neurological signs. The disease is caused 'gid'. Humans are not the normal intermediate host; however, rare cases have been recorded. The tapeworm is found worldwide in temperate areas.

Dicroceliasis

Dicrocoelium dendriticum is a lancet-shaped trematode that lives in the bile ducts of SACs as well as other domestic and wild herbivores. It requires two intermediate hosts for its development, the first being a land snail and the second an ant. The adult trematodes deposit their eggs in the bile ducts of the definitive host; the eggs move with the bile and are eventually carried by the faecal matter to the exterior. The eggs contain a miracidium and can survive for many months. This is released when the egg is ingested by the mollusc. In the snail's tissues, the miracidium gives rise to two generations of sporocysts, the second of which produces large numbers of cercariae. These are eaten by the ant, which in turn is eaten by the herbivore. The parasite is found in North and South America, Europe, Asia and North Africa. The disease is rare in humans as it relies on a human ingesting an infected ant. The disease in humans is not serious, causing dyspepsia and flatulence or it may be asymptomatic. In SACs the disease is not nearly as serious as fascioliasis but anaemia and diarrhoea have been reported. It can be treated with flukicides.

Fascioliasis

This is a very serious disease in SACs (see Chapter 9). It is caused by *Fasciola hepatica* throughout the world and by *Fasciola gigantica* in Africa and Asia. The herbivore is the main host. The flukes live in the liver and lay eggs. The amphibious snail *Lymnaea truncatula* is the main intermediate host and sheds metacercaria on to the vegetation. In some areas other *Lymnaea* spp. are also involved. Humans are a rare host but normally become infected by consuming contaminated watercress. The severity of the disease in humans is related to the number of metacercaria ingested. Normally there is some liver disease, which is transitory. Some cases may cause anaemia and serious liver disease. It can be treated with flukicides.

Hydatidosis

The normal life cycle for this tapeworm is between the sheep and the dog, however humans can become infected. The adult tapeworm *Echinococcus granulosus* infects dogs and wild canids. It lives in the small intestine and sheds gravid proglottids, which contain several hundred eggs. These are then ingested by the intermediate host, which is commonly the sheep but can also be the SAC. There are other herbivores or omnivores that can be the intermediate host. The human is in this last group. In humans the egg, which is ingested, may take years to become a cyst. The symptoms caused by the cyst vary with its location. It may be asymptomatic but normally the large amount of fluid will cause some mild malaise. The normal site is the abdomen. It can attach to the liver or any other organ, and abdominal swelling will be observed. If it occurs in the lungs it will be walled off by fibrous tissue. The main danger to the patient is rupture of the cyst. This will cause an anaphylactic reaction in many cases, which may be fatal. It may also cause seeding of eggs to multiple other sites.

In the SAC often the disease is only diagnosed on post-mortem, although it could be diagnosed on abdominal ultrasonography or thoracosonography. If the cyst or cysts are in the lung, respiratory symptoms may be observed. These will be chronic and in SACs may be confused with tuberculosis. The life cycle is complete if the SAC is eaten by a dog. Treatment of dogs is very effective. In untreated dogs the tapeworm

develops in the intestine. Obviously, unlike the SAC, the human is an end host. The disease is worldwide but is relatively common in the Andes in South America.

Linguatuliasis

This disease is caused by *Linguatula serrata*. The female of this linguiform parasite measures 10 cm and the male 2 cm. It is found in the nasal passages and frontal sinuses of dogs and cats. Eggs are laid and pass to the environment by sneezing or spitting. They need to be eaten by a secondary host, the SAC. These develop into larvae, which penetrate the wall of the intestine. After 6 months the larvae, after a series of moults in the abdominal cavity, penetrate into various tissues. These are consumed by the carnivore. The nymph travels up the oesophagus to the nasopharynx and the life cycle is complete.

This pentastomid worm is found in Europe, the Middle East and North Africa. It is also found throughout the New World. The larvae are asymptomatic in SACs. Humans can become infected in two ways. First, by ingesting eggs from vegetables or water. The larvae then may cause gastroenteric signs or the nymphs may cause ocular infection by invading the anterior chamber of the eye. However, the second type of infection in humans is more common, when humans ingest contaminated offal from herbivores. The infection is immediate as the nymphs invade the nasopharynx and cause pain in the throat and a runny nose.

Myiasis caused by larvae of *Oestrus ovis*

The adult of *Oestrus ovis*, a grey fly 12 mm in length, is larviparous, depositing larvae in the nostrils of sheep, goats, SACs and, occasionally, humans. It is found throughout the world. First the larvae enter the nasal fossae and feed on mucus. They then penetrate the sinuses where they mature. After a period of months the mature larva migrates again to the nasal fossae where it is expelled by sneezing, falls to the ground, and pupates for a month. The fly that emerges can live for another month. The condition is easily controlled by ivermectins in SACs.

Trichostrongyliasis

These short slender nematodes inhabit the small intestine and third compartment of the stomach (C3) of SACs. They cause severe problems and have become resistant to several anthelmintics. Humans are only very rarely infected by chance ingestion of the eggs. On the whole the disease is asymptomatic. It should not be confused with the specific human parasite *Trichostrongylus orientalis*, which is passed indirectly from human to human via the faeces. This pathogen has been seen very rarely and in small numbers in sheep. It does not cause disease in this species. In humans the signs are variable with low-grade gut pain being a feature. Control with anthelmintics is easy as this species is not resistant. The nematode is found in central Asia and the Far East. It is particularly prevalent in central Iran.

Zoonotic scabies

Whether this is a zoonotic disease found in SACs is contentious. *Sarcoptes scabiei* is definitely a mite that can cause severe skin disease in humans. Some authorities suggest that this mite can infest animals. Most authorities think that the *Sarcoptes* spp. mites, which infect SACs, are a different species. There was only one definitive animal to human infestation and that involved pigs. There has been no proven link with SACs. *Sarcoptes scabiei* does cause severe disease in SACs.

References

Angus, K.W. (2010) Apparent low toxicity of yew for roe deer (*Capreolus capreolus*). *Veterinary Record* 166, 216.

Arroyo, E., Patino, C., Ciccarelli, M., Raudsepp, T., Conley, A. and Tibary, A. (2022) Clinical and histological features of ovarian hypoplasia/dysgenesis in alpacas. *Frontiers in Veterinary Science* 9, 837684.

Baird, G. (2003) Current perspectives on caseous lymphadenitis. *In Practice* 25, 62–68.

Barlow, A.M., Sharpe, J.A.E. and Kincaid, E.A. (2002) Blindness in lambs due to inadvertent closantel overdose. *Veterinary Record* 151, 25–26.

Bedenice D., Bright, A., Pedersen, D.D. and Dibb, J.. (2009) Humoral response to an equine encephalitis vaccine in healthy alpacas. *Journal of Veterinary Internal Medicine* 234, 530–534.

Bennett, S.J., Adkins, P.R.F., Schultz, L.G. and Walker, K.E. (2022) Assessment of cerebrospinal fluid analysis and short-term survival outcomes in SACs: A retrospective study of 54 cases (2005-2021). *Journal of Veterinary Internal Medicine* 36, 2263–2269.

Bradbury, L. (2008) Field anaesthesia in camelids. *In Practice* 30, 460–463.

Brash, A.G. (1943) Lupinosis. *New Zealand Journal of Agriculture* 67, 83–84.

Bravo, P.W., Bazan, P.J., Troedsson, M.H.T., Vallata, R.P. and Garnica, J.P. (1996) Induction of parturition in alpacas and subsequent survival of neonates. *Journal of American Veterinary Medical Association* 209, 1760–1762.

Buxton, D. (1989) Toxoplasmosis in sheep and other farm animals. *In Practice* 11, 9–12.

Carmichael, I.H., Ponzoni, R.W., Judson, G.J., Hubbard, D.J., Howse, A. and McGegor, B.A. (1998) Studies on parasitism in alpacas in southern Australia. *Proceedings: 'Crossing Boundaries'*, pp. 75–82.

Copithorne, B. (1937) Hemlock poisoning. *Veterinary Record* 49, 1018–1019.

Cubero, M.J., Gonzalez, M. and Leon, L. (2002) *Enfermedades infecciosas de las poblaciones de cabra montes*. In: Perez, J.M. (ed.) Distribucion, genetica y estatus sanitaria de las poblaciones andaluzas de cabra montes. Universidad de Jaen/Junta de Andulucia, Consejeria de Medio Ambiente, Jaen, Spain, pp. 199–253.

D'Alterio, G. (2005) Prevalence of *Chorioptes* sp. mite infestation in alpaca (*Lama pacos*) in the south-west of England: implications for skin health. *Small Ruminant Research* 57, 221–228.

D'Alterio, G.L. (2006) Introduction to the alpaca and its veterinary care in the UK. *In Practice* 28, 404–410.

Eichenberger, R.M., Karvountzis, S., Ziadinov, I. and Deplazes, P. (2011) Severe *Taenia ovis* outbreak in a sheep flock in south-west England. *Veterinary Record* 168, 619.

Featherstone, C.A., Foster, A.P., Chappell, S.A., Carson, T. and Pritchard, G.C. (2011) Verocytotoxigenic *Escherichia coli* O157 in camelids. *Veterinary Record* 168, 194–195.

Firshman, A.M., Wünschmann, A., Cebra, C.K., Bildfell, R., McClanahan, S.L. *et al.* (2008) Thrombotic endocarditis in alpacas. *Journal of the American Veterinary Medical Association* 22, 456–461.

Flanagan, A.M., Edgar, H.W.J., Foster, F., Gordon, A., Hanna, R.E.B. *et al.* (2011) Standardising a coproantigen reduction test for the diagnosis of triclabendazole resistance. *Veterinary Parasitology* 176, 34–42.

Forsyth, A.A. (1954) *British Poisonous Plants*. Bulletin No 161 of MAFF, published by Her Majesty's Stationery Office, London, pp. 42–43.

Foster, A. (2008) Skin diseases of South American camelids. *British Veterinary Zoological Society Proceedings of the Spring Meeting*. Woburn, 17 May to 18 May, 2008, pp. 30–32.

Gallina, L. and Scagliarini, A. (2010) Virucidal efficacy of common disinfectants against orf virus. *Veterinary Record* 166, 725.

Garcia Pereira, F.L., Greene, S.A., McEwen, M.M. and Keegan, R. (2006) Analgesia and anaesthesia in camelids. *Small Ruminant Research* 61, 227–233.

Garmendia, A.E. (1987) Failure of passive immunoglobulin transfer. *American Journal of Veterinary Research* 48, 1472–1475.

Gommez-Quispe, O.E., Rodriguez, E.L., Benites, R.M., Valenzuela, S., Moscoso-Munoz, J. *et al.* (2022) Analysis of alpaca (*Vicugna pacos*) cria survival under extensive management conditions in the high elevations of the Andes Mountains in Peru. *Small Ruminant Research* 217, 106839.

Goodchild, L.M., Dart, A.J., Collins, M.B., Dart, C.M., Hodgson, J.L. and Hodgson, D.R. (1996) Cryptococcal meningitis in an alpaca. *Australian Veterinary Journal* 74, 428–430.

Gordon, E., Cebra, C.K., Stang, B.V., Christensen, J.M., Alshahrani, S.M. *et al.* (2022) Plasma pharmacokinetics, pulmonary disposition, and safety of subcutaneous gamithromycin in alpacas. *Journal of Veterinary Pharmocology and Therapeutics* 45, 283–290.

Griffin, G. (2010) Review of the major outbreak of *E coli* O157 in Surrey 2009. Report of the Independent Investigation Committee, June 2010.

Harwood, D.G., McPherson, G.C. and Woodger, N.G.A. (2010) Possible horse chestnut poisoning in a Cashmere goat. *Veterinary Record* 167, 461–462.

Hay, L. (1990) Prevention and treatment of urolithiasis in sheep. *In Practice* 12, 87–91.

Hayes, C.J., O'Brien, P.J., Wolfe, A., Hoey, S., Chandler, C. *et al.* (2021) Acute fasciolosis in an alpaca: a case report. *BMC Veterinary Research* 17, 215.

Hubbs, J.C. (1947) Deadly nightshade poisoning. *Veterinary Medicine* 42, 428–429.

Jackson, P. (1986) Skin diseases of goats. *In Practice* 8, 5–10.

Johnson, L.W. (1989) Llama medicine update. *Veterinary Clinics of North America Food Animal Section* 5, 101–133.

Johnson, L.W. (2009) Camelid congenital/genetic defects. *Proceedings International Camelid Health Conference*, Oregon, pp. 151–154.

Kawaji, S., Begg, D.J., Plain, K.M. and Whittington, R.J. (2011) Use of faecal quantitative PCR testing to detect Johne's disease in sheep. *Journal of Veterinary Microbiology* 148, 35–44.

Keen, J.E. and Elder, R.O. (2002) Isolation of Shigatoxigenic *Escherichia coli* O157 from hide surfaces and the oral cavity of finished beef feedlot cattle. *Journal of American Veterinary Medical Association* 220, 756–763.

Kutzler, M.A., Baker, R.J. and Mattson, D.E. (2004) Humoral response to West Nile virus vaccination in alpacas and llamas. *Journal of the American Veterinary Medical Association* 225, 414–416 (2004).

Kutzler, M., Foreyt, W., Kaplan, R., Heidel, J., Jones, P. *et al.* (2009) Fascioliasis in Llamas: Treatment, mortality and difficulties in antemortem diagnosis. *Proceedings International Camelid Health Conference*, Oregon, USA 12–15 March 2009, p. 143.

Kwiatek, O., Ali, Y.H., Saeed, I.K., Khalafalla, A.I., Mohamed, O.I. *et al.* (2011) Isolation of Asian lineage of peste des petits ruminants virus in Africa. *Emerging Infectious Diseases* 17, 1223–1231.

Lopez, B. (2021) Approach to veterinary management of adult camelids. *In Practice* 43, 329–337.

MacDougall, D.F. (1991) Diagnosis, monitoring and prognosis of renal disease. *In Practice* 13, 250–256.

Malik, H., Fazili, M.R.U., Bhattacharyya, H.K., Buchoo, B.A., Moulvi, D.M. and Makhdoomi, D.M. (2010) Minimally invasive surgical tube cystotomy for treating obstructive urolithiasis in small ruminants with an intact urinary bladder. *Veterinary Record* 166, 528–531.

Michaely, L.M., Hoeltig, D., Ganter, M., Renteria-Solis, Z., Bauer, C. *et al.* (2022) First report about a cerebrospinal nematode infection in an alpaca (*Vicugna pacos*). *Tierarztl Prax Ausg G Grosstiere Nuttztiere* 50, 280–285.

Mitchell, S., Mearns, R., Richards, I., Donnan, A.A. and Bartley, D.J. (2011) Benzimidazole resistance in *Nematodirus battus*. *Veterinary Record* 168 (23), 623.

Neubert, S., Puff, C., Kleinschmidt, S., Kammeyer, P., von Altrok, A. *et al.* (2022) Gastric ulcers in alpacas – clinical, laboratory, and pathological findings. *Frontiers in Veterinary Science* 9, 877257.

Paul-Murphy J.R., Morgan J.P., Snyder J.R. and Fowler, M.E. (1991) Radiographic findings in young llamas with forelimb valgus deformities 28 cases (1980–1988). *Journal of the American Veterinary Medical Association* 198, 2107–2111.

Payne, J. and Liversey, C. (2010) Lead poisoning in cattle and sheep. *In Practice* 32, 64–69.

Philbey, A.W. and Morton, A.G. (2001) Paraquat poisoning in sheep from contaminated water. *Australian Veterinary Journal* 79, 842–843.

Po, E., Allen, M.J., Whitelock, R.G. and Elsayed, S.H. (2022) Use of antimicrobial impregnated calcium sulphate beads in the surgical management of mandidular osteomyelitis in an 8-year-old huacaya alpaca. *Veterinary Record Case Reports* 10, e301.

Proost, K., Pardon, B. and Vlaminck, L. (2022) Mandibular thickness measurements as predictive tool for specific dental disorders in alpacas (*Vicugna pacos*). *Frontiers in Veterinary Science* 9, 817050.

Rebhun, W.C., Jenkins, D.H., Riis, R.C., Dill, S.G., Dubovi, E.J. and Torres, A. (1988) An epizootic of blindness and encephalitis associated with a herpesvirus indistinguishable from equine herpesvirus 1 in a herd of alpacas and llamas. *Journal of the American Veterinary Medical Association* 192, 953–956.

Richardson, C., Taylor, W.P., Terlecki, S. and Gibbs, E.P.J. (1985) Observations on transplacental infection with bluetongue virus in sheep. *American Journal of Veterinary Research* 46, 1912–1922.

Richey, M.J., Foster, A.P., Crawshaw, T.R. and Schock, A. (2011) *Mycobacterium bovis* mastitis in an alpaca and its implications. *Veterinary Record* 168, 214.

Rodgerson, D.H., Baird, A.N., Lin, H.C. and Pugh, D.G. (1998) Ventral abdominal approach for laparoscopic ovariectomy in llamas. *Veterinary Surgery* 27, 331–336.

Rousseau, M., Anderson, D.E., Miesner, K.L., Schulz, C.E. and Whitehead, C.E. (2010) Scapulo-humeral joint luxation in alpacas. *Journal of the American Veterinary Medical Association* 237, 1186–1192.

Sargison, N. (2001) Copper poisoning in sheep and cattle. *UK VET* 6, 54–58.

Sargison, N.D. and Scott, P.R. (2011) Diagnosis and economic consequences of triclabendazole resistance in *Fasciola hepatica* in a sheep flock in south-east Scotland. *Veterinary Record* 168, 159.

Scott, W.A. (2010) Apparent low toxicity of yew in muntjac deer and Soay sheep. *Veterinary Record* 166, 246.

Song, Y., Wang, Z., Li,, R., Hao, D., Wang, Z. *et al.* (2022) Left displacement of the third gastric compartment in an alpaca: the first report in China. *BMC Veterinary Research* 18, 85.

Sponenberg, D.P. (2010) Suri and huacaya breeding results in North America. *Small Ruminant Research* 93 (2–3), 210–212.

Steinparzer, R, Knjzek, M., Zimpernik, I. and Schmoll, F. (2022) Serological detection of antibodies to *Coxiella burnetii, Chlamydia abortus, Toxoplasma gondii* and *Leptospira* spp. in New World camelids from Austria. *Wiener Tierärztlichen Monatsschrift Veterinary Medicine Austria* 109: 6.

Stevenson, M.J. and Swarbrick, O. (2010) Apparent low toxicity of yew in grazing animals. *Veterinary Record* 166, 307.

Sting, R., Geiger, C., Rietschel, W., Blazey, B., Schwabe, I. *et al.* (2022a) *Corynebacterium pseudotuberculosis* infections in alpacas (*Vicugna pacos*). *Animals* 12, 1612.

Sting, R., Schwabe I., Kieferle, M., Münch, M. and Rau, J. (2022b) Fatal infection in an alpaca (*Vicugna pacos*) caused by pathogenic *Rhodococcus equi*. *Animals* 19, 1303.

Stratton, M.R. (1919) Water hemlock poisoning. *Colorado Medicine* 16, 104–111.

Swarbrick, O. (2010) Apparent low toxicity of yew in grazing animals. *Veterinary Record* 166, 307.

Taylor, S.D., Baird, A.N., Well, A.B. and Ruple, A. (2017) Evaluation of three intravenous injectable anaesthesia protocols in healthy adult male alpacas. *The Veterinary Record* 181, 322.

Te, N, Ciurkiewicz, M., van den Brand, J.M.A., Rodon, J., Haverkamp, A.-K. *et al.* (2022) Middle East respiratory syndrome coronavirus infection in camelids. *Veterinary Pathology* 59, 546–555.

Tellis, A.N., Rowe, S.M. and Coilparampil, R. (2022) Evaluation of three immunological assays to mitigate the risk of transboundary spread of Coxiella burnetii by alpacas. *Transboundary and Emerging Diseases* 69, 793–804.

Tornquist, S.J., Boeder, L.J., Lubbers, S. and Cebra, C.K. (2011) Investigation of *Mycoplasma haemolamae* infection in crias born to infected dams. *Veterinary Record* 168, 380.

Twomey, D.F., Allen, K., Bell, S., Evans, C. and Thomas, S. (2010a) *Eimeria ivitaensis* in British alpacas. *Veterinary Record* 167, 797–798.

Twomey, D.F., Cooley, W.A. and Wood, R. (2010b) Conformation of the chewing louse, *Bovicola breviceps*, in a British llama *(Llama glama)*. *Veterinary Record* 166, 790.

Twomey, D.F., Higgins, R.J., Worth, D.R., Okker, M., Gover, K. *et al.* (2010c) Cutaneous TB caused by *Mycobacterium bovis* in a veterinary surgeon following exposure to a tuberculus alpaca (*Vicuna pacos*). *Veterinary Record* 166, 175–177.

Whitehead, C.E. (2017) Pregnancy diagnosis in camelids. *Livestock* 22, 330–334.

Woods, L.W., Puschner, B., Filigenzi, M.S., Woods, D.M. and George, L.W. (2011) Evaluation of the toxicity of *Adonis aestivalis* in sheep. *Veterinary Record* 168, 49.

Index

CABI – who we are and what we do

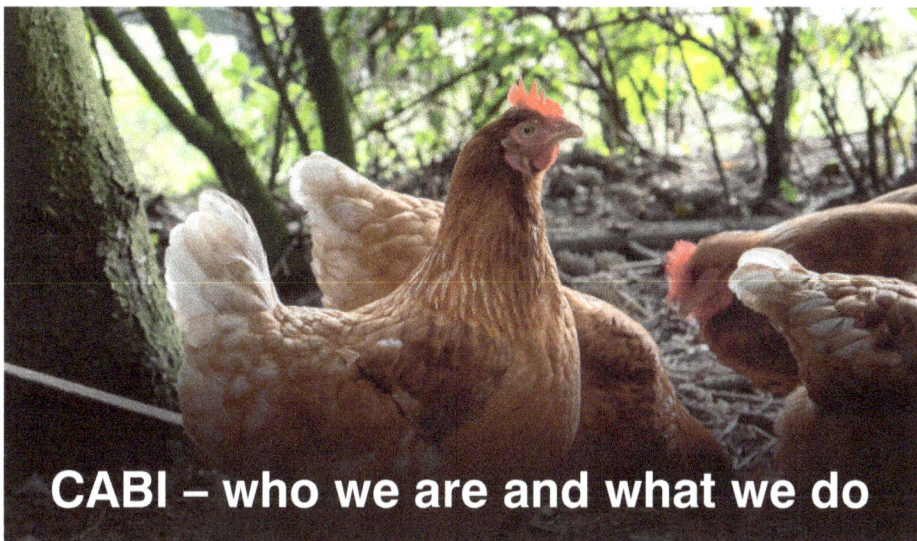

This book is published by **CABI**, an international not-for-profit organisation that improves people's lives worldwide by providing information and applying scientific expertise to solve problems in agriculture and the environment.

CABI is also a global publisher producing key scientific publications, including world renowned databases, as well as compendia, books, ebooks and full text electronic resources. We publish content in a wide range of subject areas including: agriculture and crop science / animal and veterinary sciences / ecology and conservation / environmental science / horticulture and plant sciences / human health, food science and nutrition / international development / leisure and tourism.

The profits from CABI's publishing activities enable us to work with farming communities around the world, supporting them as they battle with poor soil, invasive species and pests and diseases, to improve their livelihoods and help provide food for an ever growing population.

CABI is an international intergovernmental organisation, and we gratefully acknowledge the core financial support from our member countries (and lead agencies) including:

Discover more

To read more about CABI's work, please visit: **www.cabi.org**

Browse our books at: **www.cabi.org/bookshop**,
or explore our online products at: **www.cabi.org/publishing-products**

Interested in writing for CABI? Find our author guidelines here:
www.cabi.org/publishing-products/information-for-authors/

www.ingramcontent.com/pod-product-compliance
Lightning Source LLC
Chambersburg PA
CBHW040137200326
41458CB00025B/6295